ROUTLEDGE LIBRARY EDITIONS: PSYCHIATRY

Volume 1

PSYCHIATRY IN THE BRITISH ARMY IN THE SECOND WORLD WAR

PSYCHIATRY IN THE BRITISH ARMY IN THE SECOND WORLD WAR

ROBERT H. AHRENFELDT

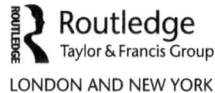

LONDON AND NEW YORK

First published in 1958 by Routledge & Kegan Paul Ltd
This edition first published in 2019
by Routledge
2 Park Square, Milton Park, Abingdon, Oxon OX14 4RN
and by Routledge
711 Third Avenue, New York, NY 10017

Routledge is an imprint of the Taylor & Francis Group, an informa business

© 1958 Robert H. Ahrenfeldt

All rights reserved. No part of this book may be reprinted or reproduced or utilised in any form or by any electronic, mechanical, or other means, now known or hereafter invented, including photocopying and recording, or in any information storage or retrieval system, without permission in writing from the publishers.

Trademark notice: Product or corporate names may be trademarks or registered trademarks, and are used only for identification and explanation without intent to infringe.

British Library Cataloguing in Publication Data
A catalogue record for this book is available from the British Library

ISBN: 978-1-138-60492-6 (Set)
ISBN: 978-0-429-43807-3 (Set) (ebk)
ISBN: 978-1-138-33366-6 (Volume 1) (hbk)
ISBN: 978-1-138-33375-8 (Volume 1) (pbk)
ISBN: 978-0-429-44581-1 (Volume 1) (ebk)

Publisher's Note
The publisher has gone to great lengths to ensure the quality of this reprint but points out that some imperfections in the original copies may be apparent.

Disclaimer
The publisher has made every effort to trace copyright holders and would welcome correspondence from those they have been unable to trace.

PSYCHIATRY
IN THE BRITISH ARMY
IN THE SECOND WORLD WAR

by

ROBERT H. AHRENFELDT

Late Major, R.A.M.C.
and Deputy Assistant Director of Army Psychiatry

Foreword by
J. R. REES

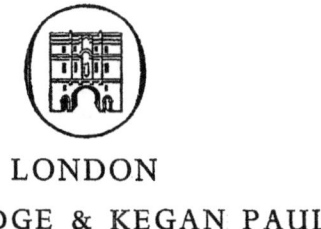

LONDON
ROUTLEDGE & KEGAN PAUL

*First published in 1958
by Routledge & Kegan Paul Ltd
Broadway House
68–74 Carter Lane
London, E.C.4
Printed in Great Britain
by Butler & Tanner Ltd
Frome & London*
© *Robert H. Ahrenfeldt 1958*

"All persons, however, who follow any particular pursuit, are often exposed to very mortifying questions respecting the use of their enquiries. . . .

Questions of this nature coming from the generality of mankind, may be easily answered, by telling them some striking fact, in which their health, safety, or profit is concerned. . . .

Critics . . . frequently molest the patient traveller in the path of science, as well as the honest investigator of moral truth, with questions tending only to perplex, and with remarks less calculated to assist than to confound. Unprofitable indeed may that pursuit be esteemed, the prosecution of which is not preferable to a controversy with such men! He whose good-nature should induce him to try to enlighten them, would probably find them as incapable of improvement as of candour; as unskilful perhaps in what they ought to know, as illiberal in their censures of what they do not even profess to understand.

But nothing affords a more humiliating view of human wisdom, than when we see men of real learning and skill in particular branches, treating the scientific pursuits of others with contempt. How much soever such men may excel in their own science, and how lofty and important soever that science may be, they can neither be esteemed true philosophers, nor friends of mankind."

JAMES EDWARD SMITH, M.D., F.R.S.
(*Tracts relating to Natural History*, 1785)

"I do not blame you for your exasperation at being ignored, but . . . you and your millions of charges deserve better champions and more articulate spokesmen than have risen from your ranks. . . . Must you forever rely on outsiders to tell the laity your overwhelming truths?"

ALAN GREGG, M.D.
(*A Critique of Psychiatry*, 1944)

FOREWORD

THE HISTORY of the medical and social services of an army at war for six years is necessarily a lengthy document. It is not surprising that in the official history of the British Army in the Second World War the section concerned with the therapeutic and prophylactic activities of psychiatrists and psychologists has rather a small space. There are many traditional factors which explain this.

Many of us are extremely grateful to Dr. Ahrenfeldt that he has devoted so much research and thought and time to the writing of this particular fragment of history. It needed to be written, and there is a great deal to be learned from it—not merely about the handling of similar catastrophic occurrences like fighting a war, but also about the management of the problems of human relationships in large industrial groups and the prophylaxis of psychiatric disturbances.

As Dr. Ahrenfeldt records in his Preface, he had originally written a much larger and more comprehensive document, which I read through several years ago. Unfortunately it seemed impossible, because of its length, to find a publisher. I marvel at the way in which he has now re-designed and reduced it to a fraction of its original length. That many useful things are missed out is inevitable; but from the angle of research and further enquiry, I am encouraged by Dr. Ahrenfeldt's statement in his Preface that he will welcome direct specific enquiries on particular points from those who need further information.

The operations carried through between 1939 and the end of the war by the psychiatrists who were brought into the British Army, and slightly later their psychological colleagues, were essentially a team activity. I would ask readers, when they notice the rather too frequent references to the Consulting Psychiatrist, who read this or said that, to bear in mind that as in all such team activities, the things that were committed to paper in memoranda or letters, or were said to committees, were in fact the recording of conclusions reached by the team as a whole, or by many individual members other than the Consulting Psychiatrist.

In the British Army we started the war with very little psychiatric help for the first consultant overseas, and with only one psychiatrist in the Army at home. Fortunately, however, a quite considerable team of competent men and women psychiatrists were expecting to come into the Army to help when they were called in, and this group by no means wasted their time. A great deal of reading of past documentation and history, much exploration of the Army's general organization and its training schemes, was being carried on by people who were still nominally in hospital or private practice, and their accumulated wisdom was available from the beginning. The consequences of their previous work became obvious almost immediately they were brought into the Army and found themselves in uniform. This group really provided 'the voice of psychiatry' in the Army. In reading through this historical record, I realize afresh how all my life I have been plagiarizing, and never more so than in the years 1939 to 1945.

The psychiatric team in the Army, which grew to over three hundred by the end of the war, was drawn from every branch of our profession—from the mental hospital service, from child guidance and psycho-analytic work, from research and from amongst the psychotherapeutic practitioners. Almost without exception, the change of role was easily accepted, and indeed welcomed. Prophylaxis and help in the creation of a really fit and competent Army was the urgent need, and in a realistic way (though treatment was by no means neglected) most of the skills which were needed and were used were those of applied or social psychiatry and psychology and, as this record will show, they were not altogether unsuccessful. Except for those who had the good fortune to be regimental medical officers, the psychiatrists in the Army perhaps got inside the skin of the Army better than any other group of temporary medical officers. The principle that an industrial medical officer must, to be competent, know a good deal about the jobs that the workers in all grades in his industry are faced with, holds true for an army, and it is necessary for Army medical officers, and particularly psychiatrists, to be good soldiers as well as good doctors with a public health outlook.

Those who actually served in Army psychiatry will of course be excited by this book. In reading through the manuscript, I have experienced nostalgia and, as all my colleagues will, I found myself

FOREWORD

ready to say, 'But do you remember this, or that?' I think that this is inevitable when a considerable group of men and women, working very often through group discussions either at the War Office or in the Commands at home and abroad, are excited about work which they feel to be a realistic contribution to winning a war, and also to the care and social betterment of very large numbers of the general population of their country.

This record will interest not only psychiatrists and psychologists who worked in or worked with the Army. Many of our colleagues who were combatants, administrators, or in other branches of the medical service, will find it a thought-provoking history. There certainly are lessons in it, not fully digested yet, for peace-time industry, for public health, for penology and for social psychiatry, as well as for the future management of an army at war.

J. R. REES

London, W.1
December, 1957

PREFACE

THE AUTHOR is, in the first place, very greatly indebted to Dr. J. R. Rees—as it were, the 'father of British Army psychiatry' in the recent war—for his encouragement and advice, and for the loan of a number of important documents. He is also most sincerely grateful to Professor Eli Ginzberg of Columbia University, whose continued interest in this work, and considerable and untiring efforts, eventually led to the possibility of its publication in the present form.

The present work is a revised and much abridged version of a most detailed 'departmental' history which was compiled by the author, in large part in 1948, originally at the request of the then Director of Army Psychiatry, Brigadier A. Torrie. The author is indebted to Dr. Torrie, and also to Dr. J. C. Penton (then Assistant Director) and Dr. E. H. Larkin (then Reader in Psychiatry, Royal Army Medical College), for their assistance, advice and encouragement. The original work was based on the study of all available relevant documents, including all those (unpublished) on file, at that time, at the Directorate of Army Psychiatry, and others in the sole possession of individual psychiatrists who had made important contributions to military psychiatry during the war. In particular, the author wishes to express his gratitude for assistance and advice in various respects, to Professor T. F. Rodger, and to Drs. E. A. Bennet, G. W. B. James, S. A. MacKeith, T. F. Main, A. A. White, and A. T. M. Wilson.

This is, however, not an 'official' history—with consequent advantages, and possibly some disadvantages. Indeed, the significance of the contribution of Army psychiatry in the Second World War has been acknowledged, in the official war history of the Medical Services of the United Kingdom, by the allotment to this subject of twenty-five pages (of which ten are devoted to the Middle East Force in 1940–3). It is perhaps true, on the other hand, that a somewhat inordinate amount of the author's time and that of others was

PREFACE

required to overcome appreciable resistances and not a little casuistry, with regard to the original manuscript, in official quarters; but, if the latter showed themselves at times a little over-zealous in their role of guardians of official secrets and of the nation's vital defences, it should be realized that their actions must inevitably be conditioned by the necessarily authoritarian structure of the organization of which they are a part.

It must be clearly understood that, while the War Office has agreed to the publication of this work, the author is to be held solely responsible for the presentation of the material, the accuracy of his statements, and, needless to say, for his opinions and conclusions. He has nevertheless made a sincere attempt to present, so far as possible, and on the basis of an obsessionally careful examination of every source of evidence available to him, a factual account and objective evaluation of the matters discussed in the present work. It has been necessary to omit a considerable amount of detail, and especially so with respect to the psychiatric services in theatres of operations overseas. The author would welcome any specific enquiries, where he might be in a position to assist professional workers and those engaged in research.

The author gratefully acknowledges his indebtedness for permission to quote from copyright material, as follows:

For the quotation, in Chapter III, from Robert Graves' translation of Suetonius, *The Twelve Caesars* (in The Penguin Classics), to Messrs. Penguin Books.

For the quotation, in Chapter II, from Alan Hackney's *Private's Progress*, to Messrs. Victor Gollancz, Ltd.

For the quotations, in Chapters I and VIII, from Rudyard Kipling's poem, 'Tommy', in *Barrack-Room Ballads*, to his executrix, Mrs. George Bambridge, and to Messrs. Methuen & Co., Ltd., the Macmillan Company of Canada, Ltd., and to Doubleday & Co., Inc. (the publishers in the United States of *Departmental Ditties and Ballads* and *Barrack-Room Ballads*).

For the quotations, in Chapter VII, from C. Day Lewis' poems, 'Word Over All' and 'Ode to Fear', in *Word Over All*, to Professor C. Day Lewis, and to Messrs. Jonathan Cape, Ltd.

For the quotation, in Chapter VII, from T. F. Main's contribution to the discussion on 'Forward Psychiatry in the Army', to Dr. T. F. Main, and to the Honorary Editors of the *Proceedings of the Royal Society of Medicine*.

PREFACE

And, finally, for the quotations, in Chapters I and IX, from Professor Gilbert Murray's admirable translation of Aeschylus, *The Agamemnon*, to Messrs. George Allen & Unwin, Ltd.

Finally, the author is sincerely and deeply grateful to his friend and colleague, Peter M. Robinson, without whose unfailing support, and invaluable editorial assistance, the revision of this work would never have been possible.

R. H. A.

Bransgore, Hampshire
September, 1957

CONTENTS

FOREWORD by Dr. J. R. Rees	*page*	vii
PREFACE		xi
I INTRODUCTION		1
II PERSONNEL SELECTION		29
III OFFICER SELECTION		51
IV MENTAL DEFECT AND DULLNESS		77
V DISCIPLINARY PROBLEMS		97
VI TREATMENT AND DISPOSAL OF PSYCHIATRIC CASES		141
VII FORWARD PSYCHIATRY		163
VIII PROBLEMS OF TRAINING AND MORALE		196
IX REHABILITATION AND CIVIL RESETTLEMENT OF REPATRIATED PRISONERS OF WAR		226
X CONCLUSION		251

APPENDICES

A Practical Considerations on the Disposal of Delinquents in the Army by R. H. Ahrenfeldt and P. R. A. May	260
B The Incidence of Desertion in the British Army in the First and Second World Wars, in relation to the death penalty and its abolition	271
C Statistics Relating to British Army Psychiatry in the Second World War	276
LIST OF ABBREVIATIONS	283
GENERAL BIBLIOGRAPHY	286
SUPPLEMENTARY (TECHNICAL) BIBLIOGRAPHY (published works on British Army psychiatry and related subjects)	293
INDEX	303

I
INTRODUCTION

THERE WILL NO DOUBT be not a few who will be quick to judge superfluous indeed the writing of yet another 'History', specialized in subject and localized in application, relating to the period of the Second World War—the addition of one more stone, albeit a small one, to this already vast edifice of historical records and pseudo-historical literature.

Thus, it may be that the present work will be regarded as redundant, by some because they have decided (as it were, without further appeal) that psychiatry and all its works are vanity; by others because of a failure, or inability, on their part to see more than a momentary (and now, therefore, debased or infinitesimal) value in psychiatric practice and activities developed to meet the immediate needs of a world-engulfing conflict which is receding rapidly in history, and still more so in the minds of many: these would say, with the herald returning from the wars, in the *Agamemnon* of Aeschylus:

> Why think of it? They are past and in the grave,
> All those long troubles. . . .
> Surely for us, who live, good doth prevail
> Unchallenged, with no wavering of the scale.

There will, assuredly, be others still, ready to emphasize the futility of compiling a work such as this, on the grounds that it is as misleading, in planning for the present and the future, to rely on the data provided by historical experience, as it is useless to attempt to draw from the latter any valid conclusions upon which to base subsequent investigations and practical developments and policies. It was, however, Leonardo da Vinci who observed:

INTRODUCTION

"Experience never errs; it is only your judgements that err by promising themselves effects such as are not caused by your experiments. . . . Men wrongly complain of experience; with great abuse they accuse her of leading them astray: but let experience alone, and turn your complaints against your own ignorance."

In appraising the psychological effects of grave social crises, such as revolutions and war, in the light of historical experience, it should be remembered that, in some instances, they may be temporarily more or less obscured by the severity and urgency, the dominant impact, of the physical forces of disruption and those threatening survival.

In the course of time, and with the emergence and gradual evolution of psychiatry and the social sciences, came an increasing awareness of the fact that, while such major upheavals need not invariably be immediately obvious either in the degree or in the extent of their influences on the individual and social organism alike, they can eventually have serious and protracted repercussions.*

There are, in the writer's opinion, three pertinent reasons for undertaking the present historical survey of the vicissitudes and achievements of psychiatry in the British Army during the Second World War. To those who are accustomed to visualize the field of medicine in general, or one of its several specialized branches, in relation to all cognate and interdependent disciplines, and as a dynamic entity, it will be apparent that these three 'reasons' constitute, in fact, a logical sequence, and not only reflect three aspects of the evolutionary course of Psychiatry, but, indeed, represent the three consecutive stages of development which have punctuated the entire history of Medicine.

The first purpose of this History is to place on record the work accomplished by Army psychiatrists, as the traditional duty and responsibility of the medical profession, in the alleviation of suffering, and the care and treatment of patients with psychiatric disorders.

---

* Thus, it has been said that "'if the [French] Revolution was a direct cause of insanity in but a limited number of cases, subsequently its ravages continued under the Empire and even under the Restoration. Esquirol believed 'that almost all of those who had escaped the revolutionary scythe have been stricken with mental derangement' " (M. Laignel-Lavastine & J. Vinchon, *Les Malades de l'Esprit et leurs Médecins du XVIe au XIXe Siècle*, Paris, 1930, p. 341). There were, it is true, a number of local instances of severe *mass* aberrations, particularly during *la Terreur*, but it must not be forgotten that all such periods provide full scope and a fertile medium for many unstable, psychopathic, and even psychotic, individuals. (Cf. A. Cabanès and L. Nass, *La Névrose Révolutionnaire*, 2 vols., Paris, 2nd ed., 1924; and Y. Dhotel, *Joseph Le Bon ou Arras sous la Terreur: Essai sur la Psychose Révolutionnaire*, Paris, 1934.)

INTRODUCTION

The second purpose is to show how, apart from these immediate tasks, psychiatrists were called upon to assist in solving, and dealing with, a number of urgent and vital social and psychological problems arising from conditions of total war and mobilization, and the consequent disruption and reorganization of the life of the individual and of the community. It is certainly no exaggeration to say that, in this field, the work of psychiatrists, with the professional and expert collaboration of others, was of the very greatest importance to the efficiency of the war effort, and indeed for the ultimate communal survival and welfare. Thus, for example, in their contribution to the selection of personnel, the social and vocational rehabilitation of the physically disabled and of psychiatric cases, and, later, to the successful readjustment and employment of ex-servicemen and repatriated prisoners of war, psychiatrists were largely instrumental in ensuring the fullest possible utilization of all available man-power, and preventing wastage through invalidism, disability, social or vocational maladjustment, of our very limited human resources.

The third purpose of this book is to emphasize, at least implicitly, that it is as a result of the above-mentioned developments during the war, and the urgency of the man-power problem, that there gradually emerged a clearer appreciation of the importance, in physical as in psychological medicine, of preventive measures. It was with this end in view that experienced psychiatrists devoted a large part of their time to studying the social and environmental factors which contributed to mental breakdown in the Army. As J. R. Rees has recently remarked, in this connection, "Perhaps we need the urgency of war to turn the thoughts of professional men and women to the practical problems of the application of their experience in the field of prophylaxis." [101] It may, in fact, be said that the principles of epidemiology were actually being used effectively in the British and American Armies, during the recent war, for the prevention of mental illness and inefficiency.* [12, 13, 100]

It should not be thought, therefore, that the history of experience and developments in military psychiatry and allied fields during the Second World War is of possible value only in relation to the Armed

---

* Cf. the view expressed by the World Health Organization's Expert Committee on Mental Health, "that it is only by the preventive application of psychiatric knowledge that mental health problems can ultimately be solved. In this field, the well-developed countries have set a bad example, since it is common to find in such countries highly developed therapeutic facilities for psychological disorders along with an absence of any planned application for preventive measures." [44]

INTRODUCTION

Forces. An objective appraisal of the facts outlined above should provide clear insight into the vast potentialities of their future application and further evolution, with a view to planning and establishing efficient mental health services, promoting the widespread use of preventive psychiatric methods and ensuring the conservation of human resources and the fullest utilization of man-power, in *civilian* life.*

These preliminary observations are intended to place in true perspective the matters discussed in the present History, in order that their significance may be correctly evaluated: it is with a view to orientation towards the future, not the embalming of the past, that this work has been undertaken.

BRITISH ARMY PSYCHIATRY BEFORE THE SECOND WORLD WAR

Military psychiatric planning, in so far as it existed at all in the period immediately preceding the outbreak of the Second World War, was principally based on experience gained in this field between 1914 and 1918. It is, therefore, relevant briefly to review some aspects of British Army psychiatry during and following the First World War.

The occurrence of cases of psychoneurosis in the armies of other nations during 1915 had compelled their authorities to take steps to deal with the problem. At an early date, the French sent medical experts to investigate these cases and to report on the conditions under which they arose. It was thus possible for French neurologists and psychiatrists, quite early in the war, to study the clinical material which soon became available in the special hospitals provided for these cases, and they were among the first to give a detailed and accurate description of the 'war neuroses'.

Dr. C. S. Myers has given an interesting and revealing account of the difficulties encountered, and the obstructions which had at that time to be overcome before it was possible even to initiate a rational and effective approach to the treatment and disposal of psychiatric casualties in the British Expeditionary Force.[84]

---

* Valuable and extensive research on the factors responsible for the wastage of man-power, including a reappraisal of the experience of the Second World War, is at present being undertaken in the United States by the Conservation of Human Resources Project: this was established at Columbia University in 1949, on the initiative of General Eisenhower, and is under the direction of Dr. Eli Ginzberg, Professor of Economics, Columbia University.[51]

INTRODUCTION

By August, 1916, there had been appointed a 'Consulting Psychologist' and a 'Consulting Neurologist' to the B.E.F. There was, however, considerable confusion as to which cases should be considered 'mental' and which should be considered 'neurological', and each of the two consultants had to advise on psychiatric as well as neurological cases, although each specialist was, in fact, only competent to deal with one of these two distinct groups of patients.[84]

The problem in the British Expeditionary Force did not become acute until July, 1916, when, during the first battle of the Somme, several thousand soldiers were, in the first few weeks, rapidly withdrawn from the battle zone on account of 'nervous disorders', and many of them were evacuated to England. This experience rendered obvious the very considerable wastage of fighting man-power which could result from this single cause, in the absence of any specific medical organization to deal with the problem. Yet the military authorities in the fighting zone still adopted the attitude that it was not possible to differentiate psychoneurosis from 'malingering', and that the establishment of special treatment centres would merely provide a means of evasion and invalidism, and would inevitably result in an unending and uncontrollable wastage of man-power. It was, indeed, largely because of such prevalent fears that this whole subject was constantly regarded with some degree of hostility and suspicion by the authorities.* The latter were, however, eventually compelled by the urgency of the problem to take some action. Towards the end of 1916, Lt.-Col. C. S. Myers was able to recommend the institution

---

* This attitude was still encountered in the Second World War, in the British and American Forces. It has been well expressed by the late General G. S. Patton, who also had his own psychotherapeutic theories: "Any man who says he has battle fatigue is avoiding danger and forcing on those who have more hardihood than himself the obligation of meeting it. If soldiers would make fun of those who begin to show battle fatigue, they would prevent its spread, and also save the man who allows himself to malinger by this means from an after-life of humiliation and regret."[89]

The psychiatric evaluation of the concept of 'malingering' has been clearly stated by two American psychiatrists, Lt.-Col. R. R. Grinker and Capt. J. P. Spiegel, of the Medical Corps, U.S. Army Air Forces, on the basis of extensive experience in the Second World War: "Malingering is extremely uncommon in this war to date [1943]. ... War neuroses cannot be malingered, even superficially. ... At the basis of malingering there is usually a highly neurotic background. The greatest problem associated with malingering is the ready conclusion by many medical officers that mild neurotic symptoms and [hysterical] conversion phenomena are simulated. Some physicians place great emphasis on the apparent secondary gain obtainable in release from combat duty. Education of medical officers is necessary to offset this viewpoint, often sadistically originated as a reaction or projection of the physician's own unconscious wishes. No secondary gain can offset the suffering of the war neurotic. Even as an obstacle to the final step of recovery, it is not an adequate explanation. Rather it is the apprehension of return to duty that re-stimulates the old anxieties and keeps the neurosis boiling."[54]

INTRODUCTION

of a special centre for diagnosis and treatment of such cases in each army area ('N.Y.D.N. Centres').[60] A number of 'neurologists', many of whom were, in fact, psychiatrists, were brought into the Army in response to the critical situation[97] and, by the end of 1916, specialists had been appointed to the various bases provided with 'Mental Wards'.[84]

How slight was the understanding of the psychiatric problems of the First World War was clearly shown by the use of the term 'shell-shock' which was so prevalent at the time. Medical and combatant officers alike indiscriminately grouped under this popular heading cases of psychosis, psychoneurosis, and instability occurring in high-grade mental defectives. The psychological determinants of these cases were largely disregarded and, indeed, seldom recognized.[9] The necessity for asserting the allegedly accidental, traumatic and physical nature of these conditions was due to a variety of causes. Among the latter were, no doubt, the organically biased trends of modern medical science; and strong, unconsciously determined psychological resistances based on the idea that the *British* soldier or 'hero' could not possibly show 'mental' symptoms*—(we might perhaps today refer this attitude to a 'master-race' ideology)—and on the guilt arising from a deeply rooted, Anglo-Saxon, puritanical tendency to regard all illness, but particularly psychoneurotic disorders, as evasion of duty and shameful evidence of 'moral weakness'. The condition of 'war neurosis' was thus stated to be *not an illness*, but attributable to an organic injury sustained as a result of blast, etc., in the course of actual fighting, and was, therefore, morally justified.† In

---

* —A view which was not shared by the British soldier! Cf. Rudyard Kipling (*Barrack-Room Ballads*):
> "Then it's Tommy this, an' Tommy that,
> an' 'Tommy, 'ow's yer soul?'
> But it's 'Thin red line of 'eroes' when the
> drums begin to roll. . . .
>
> We aren't no thin red 'eroes, nor we aren't no blackguards too,
> But single men in barracks, most remarkable like you;
> An' if sometimes our conduck isn't all your fancy paints,
> Why, single men in barricks don't grow into plaster saints. . . ."

† As Dr. Edward Glover has stated, "Naturally most observers find it convenient to explain mental manifestations in terms of . . . 'immediate' or 'exciting' causes, usually regarded as environmental in nature. Should this attempt miscarry their next step is to attribute the manifestations in question to 'constitutional' (innate) factors. Only when all other means have failed do they display a reluctant interest in 'developmental' factors 'predisposing' to normal or abnormal states. As a rule, therefore, it is easy to establish a direct ratio between the stress laid on constitutional and precipitating factors on the one hand and ignorance of developmental (individual) factors on the other." [52]

INTRODUCTION

this connection, it is interesting to note that, even in the Second World War, in the United States these cases have been referred to in the press as the 'mentally wounded', although there is, perhaps, more justification for this term—which had already been used by some British and American authors in the First War—than for that of 'shell-shock'.

It appears to have been largely a matter of chance, and of individual outlook, whether a soldier suffering from a psychoneurotic breakdown was considered to be ill from 'shell-shock', or to be a 'malingerer' or deserter. Dr. T. W. Salmon stated, in 1917, that "especially before the clinical characters and remarkable prevalence of war neuroses among soldiers had become familiar facts, not a few soldiers suffering from these disorders have been executed by firing squads as malingerers";[124] and, with reference to desertion in the First World War, it has been noted that "official figures . . . show that only 11% of the men on whom the death sentence was passed actually suffered the penalty. . . . The remainder were almost entirely cases of chronic and acute nerve exhaustion with a history of war sickness and wounds, who had suffered from a complete breakdown at the time of their action. A few were genuine 'fugues' who had wandered away in a dazed condition." [60]

In the light of these statements, one may be permitted to entertain some doubt as to the mental health and stability of the 'mere' 11% who were executed. As Dr. J. R. Rees has observed, there would appear to be a connection between the abolition of the death penalty for desertion, and the relatively small number of self-inflicted wounds in the Second World War: "Those of us who had to have first-hand experience of the men who were shot at dawn in the last war feel that we can perhaps understand that: . . . these men were in many cases quite obviously suffering from an acute neurosis." [97]

After studying the methods adopted in the French Army, and as a result of his own practical experience, Lt.-Col. Myers came to realize the great importance of organizing, in addition to the special centres at the bases and in the rear of army areas, advanced psychiatric centres. He recommended that a forward 'sorting centre' for psychiatric cases should be established in each army area not farther from the front than Army Headquarters, each accommodating some 250 cases received direct from field ambulances, and that a specialist, assisted by another medical officer, should be in charge of each centre. "In these 'sorting centres', the strictest attention should be paid to

INTRODUCTION

military discipline, to which the patients should be returned as soon as possible. No cases should be retained except those which, in the opinion of the specialist in charge, were likely to be cured within two or three days and to be fit for the front line after a further few days' 're-education', the severer and more obstinate cases being sent down at once to one of the special army 'centres' in the rear." [84]

The results of this recommendation have been described by Dr. Myers as follows: "Early in 1917, with the approval of the Director of Medical Services of one of the British armies in France, such an Advanced Sorting Centre had been experimentally established at my request, from which a large number of cases were returned to duty after a few days' stay. This trial lasted long enough to convince me that a still larger proportion of the 'shell-shock' cases at that time being evacuated from the front areas could be cured by more immediate attention and by the maintenance of the strictest discipline, which was inevitably lost by transfer farther away from the front line. But this Sorting Centre was soon abolished by instructions from General Headquarters." [84]

Nevertheless, by June, 1917, the situation had greatly improved, and Dr. Myers commented: "Thus, after more than twelve months of unremitting effort, despite persistent opposition and even misrepresentation of my views, I saw my main recommendations put into effect—the (virtual) abolition of the term 'shell-shock'; the provision of special receiving 'centres' both in the army areas and at the bases, and of an expert medical officer at each of these 'centres' and in each Mental Ward for the appropriate treatment and disposal of all 'nervous' and 'mental' patients . . ." [84]

Although the British at first profited little, even in knowledge, from their experience, this was not the case in the United States. Dr. T. W. Salmon visited this country in June, 1917, for the purpose of studying the psychiatric problems of the British Army, and his report to the U.S. Surgeon-General showed a penetrating insight into the nature and origin of 'shell-shock', and enabled the U.S. Army in its mobilization of 1917 to profit from our experience in the previous three years.*

---

* In the Second World War, however, despite their inadequacies, the British authorities at first showed more foresight in planning for military psychiatry than did those of the United States. Thus, Brigadier-General William C. Menninger, who was Chief Consultant in Neuropsychiatry to the Surgeon-General of the U.S. Army (1943–6), has stated: "The most severe indictment that can be made must be laid at the feet of the psychiatric profession as a whole—we permitted the military to forget almost all the lessons that we learned in the last war. As a consequence, we began this war

INTRODUCTION

"The high rate of mental disorders in the British Army (one-seventh of all discharges for disability had been due to mental conditions), the difficulties in which the Allies found themselves as a result of failure to prepare adequately for the management of mental and nervous cases developing in combat, and the great problem created by the acceptance of large numbers of recruits who had been in institutions for the insane or were of demonstrably psychopathic make-up—these and other significant observations were among the most important factors determining the course of American medico-military preparations. . . . Not only medical officers, but the line officers interviewed in England, had emphasized over and over again the importance of not accepting mentally unstable recruits for service at the front." [124]

The annual rate of admissions of psychiatric cases to British military hospitals was estimated (in 1917) at about 2 per 1,000 among the non-expeditionary troops and about 4 per 1,000 among expeditionary troops as compared with a rate of 1 per 1,000 among the adult civil population of Great Britain. In 1917, Dr. Salmon stated:

"Sorely pressed to meet the tremendous medical problems of war, England first used her existing civil facilities for caring for mental diseases among soldiers. Public disapproval, based chiefly upon a mistaken attitude towards the insane and towards the local institutions for their care, forced a different method of management. The military hospitals for the insane, created without exception by converting civil institutions for mental diseases, failed to do much more than provide places for receiving mental cases and giving temporary care, the clearing hospital is woefully inadequate in size and personnel to determine the important issues which should be determined there, and a solution to the problem presented by mental diseases among soldiers in England does not seem to be in sight. For the United States, this experience carries important lessons. More important than all others is the result of careless recruiting. . . . The

with hospital treatment forbidden, with no plan of treatment for combat troops, no unit to provide such, no plans for training, no psychiatrist in combat divisions, and not even a psychiatrist in the headquarters when war was declared." [78] Paradoxically, we, in Britain, "had at our disposal before the war the Report of the 1922 War Office Committee on Shell-Shock, and even more valuable Vol. X of the *U.S. Army Medical History* of the last war. . . . The American Vol. X on Neuropsychiatry provided us with a complete textbook on both the clinical and administrative sides of Army work, and much of the history of our allies contained in that volume has repeated itself in the British Army in this war. There was therefore a considerable amount of material to aid us in making plans before the outbreak of war. . . ." [96]

INTRODUCTION

next most important lesson is that of preparing in advance of an urgent need, a comprehensive plan for using existing civil facilities for treating mental disease in a manner which will serve the army effectively and at the same time safeguard the interests of the soldiers, of the Government, and of the community." [124]

Some idea may be given of the burden on the State of psychiatric disability in the First World War, in terms of the number of pensions granted. In March, 1939, there were about 120,000 pensioners who were still in receipt of pensions or had received final awards for primary psychiatric disability (including 'neurasthenia', 'shell-shock', effort syndrome, epilepsy and insanity). 'Neurasthenia' itself accounted for some 100,000 men, costing ten million pounds a year, and representing about 2% of total serving troops. These 120,000 cases represented about 15% of all pensioned disabilities.[91, 97]

Perhaps the most important effect of the psychiatric experience of the First War was that mentioned by Dr. Salmon in 1917: "It is freely predicted in England that the wide prevalence of neuroses among soldiers will direct attention to the fact that this kind of illness has been almost wholly ignored while great advances have been made in the treatment of all others. In civil life one still hears of detecting hysteria, as if it were a crime. . . . Today the enormous number of these cases among some of Europe's best fighting men is leading to a revision of the medical and popular attitude toward functional nervous diseases." [124]

Valuable experience in the U.S. Army in the First World War was also derived from area work and psychiatric examinations carried out in camps. The psychiatrists came across some cases of gross organic disease of the nervous system, and well-developed psychiatric disorders.

"Between these two extremes, there was a host of intermediary conditions, such as mild neuroses . . . neurasthenias, anxiety states, hysterias and hysteroid episodes, epileptoid conditions, psychopathic personalities, inferiors, military misfits, and otherwise near-normal individuals. . . . They constituted a greater menace to the military organization, by lowering the efficiency and impairing the general morale, than did the obviously diseased types which were readily recognized and without great difficulty eliminated. They were constant sources of annoyance and trouble to the officers, forming the larger number of the absentees, the discontented, the inefficients, the

INTRODUCTION

inmates of the guardhouse, and the frequenters of the regimental infirmary." [124]

The American military psychiatrists engaged on this area work also made some revealing comments on the attitudes towards psychiatry which they encountered in the Army:

"One hardly expected to be received with enthusiasm when one arrived at a camp to do neuropsychiatric work. There appeared to be, on the contrary, with very few exceptions a lack of interest or an indifference or a manifest scepticism; not infrequently there was a passive, or even an active, antagonism to any examination of this sort. Strangely enough, the medical officers were the chief passive obstacles and, in the very beginning, very little assistance or co-operation could be obtained from them. So the first effort at a cantonment had to be directed to the officers, especially the medical officers, with the view of demonstrating to them the practical value of such examination in order to enlist their sympathy and co-operation. They had to be made to appreciate the importance of neuropsychiatric examinations. In order to accomplish this, one frequently had to resort to tact, persuasion, or even strategy. . . . The greatest help to the neuropsychiatrist came, however, from the line officer, and particularly the company commander. It may seem strange, but it is nevertheless true, that the line officers appreciated the value of neuropsychiatric examinations much more readily than did the medical officers. The explanation for this was found in the fact that the line officer rated his men in terms of conduct, behaviour, and efficiency, which, after all, was equivalent to the standard of the neuropsychiatrist, who estimated conduct from the mental qualities and make-up of the individual. If a company of soldiers be carefully examined from the neuropsychiatric standpoint and the results compared with the reports furnished by the company commander of men in his organization who have been inapt, inefficient, slow, awkward, easily fatigued, delinquent, insubordinate, and difficult to get along with, a striking parallelism will be found between the two sets of observations. Experiences of this character naturally brought the line officer very close to the neuropsychiatrists. The officer eagerly sought counsel and aid, as he at once recognized that he and the examiner were dealing with similar problems." [124]

In an excellent review of the position of Army psychiatry in 1920,

INTRODUCTION

Dr. Stanford Read—formerly Officer-in-Charge, 'D' Block, Royal Victoria Hospital, Netley—wrote:

"It is certain that as psychiatric medicine is having its importance more recognized in civilian life, the military authorities will have to develop this branch in the Royal Army Medical Corps, and by its scientific application do much to improve the mental status of the soldier. The sooner officers become *thoroughly* trained in this speciality the better.* The late war has given an enormous impetus to the necessity for active interest in psychopathic disorders, and the lessons learnt should immediately instigate a line of organization by means of which the soldier's mentality can be judged accurately, so that his fitness for any particular form of service may be gauged. This would not only mean increased efficiency through elimination of the unfit, but increased efficiency by seeing that the soldier is psychologically suited for his particular work. Thorough psychiatric knowledge, too, would bring an added justice in its train, as the delinquent is then seen in the right perspective. All frequent offenders, and certainly a large proportion of court-martial cases, should be mentally examined in order to get at the basic root of their antisocial acts, and so treat the offender and not the offence. This certainly has been a lack in the Service organization during the war, when organic neurologists with no psychiatric training have been called on to determine the question of responsibility of such men." [95]

In April, 1920, a debate was initiated in the House of Lords by Lord Southborough, who wished "to call attention to the different types of hysteria and traumatic neurosis, commonly called 'shell-shock', from which many soldiers suffered during the war; to refer to the death penalty inflicted upon men by courts-martial on the charge of 'cowardice' (without inviting any re-opening of the evidence in such painful cases); and to move His Majesty's Government to make enquiry, either by a Select Committee of this House or by Departmental Committee, into the expert knowledge derived by the Army medical authorities and the medical profession with the object

---

* It is interesting, and not a little surprising in view of later developments, to find that, but a few years after the formation, in 1898, of a united Royal Army Medical Corps, specialist appointments were introduced, under the new Director-General, Sir William Taylor, with specialist pay, and the opportunity for professional study at the expense of the Crown: every officer in his qualifying examination for promotion to major was required to offer a special subject, and among these was psychological medicine. (Cf. J. B. Neal, 'Two Reformers in the Army Medical Services', *Proc. R. Soc. Med.*, 1953, **46**: 601–4.)

INTRODUCTION

of recording for use in time to come the experiences of the war, and to advise whether, by military education or otherwise, some scientific method of dealing with such cases cannot be devised. . . ." Lord Southborough further stated that "the history of the war cannot be complete unless we record for the benefit of those who come after us all our knowledge and experience of this fell disorder with its terrible effect upon the lives and health of so many of our soldiers".* The motion was accepted by the Government, and the Southborough Committee were accordingly appointed, in August, 1920, and issued their report in 1922.† [128]

The Committee, having considered the evidence of combatant officers and medical witnesses, made a series of recommendations, the majority of which still have the full approval of informed psychiatric opinion. The report stressed, in particular, the importance of careful selection and the promotion of good morale through adequate training and skilled leadership, in preventing psychiatric breakdown in the Armed Forces. It was emphasized that both executive and medical officers should co-operate in preventing and detecting mental instability, and that for this purpose they should receive special instruction in the management of men and in the nature of psychiatric illness.[128]

THE GENERAL DEVELOPMENT AND ADMINISTRATION OF BRITISH ARMY PSYCHIATRY DURING THE SECOND WORLD WAR

Before giving an outline of the development and administration of British Army psychiatry during the Second World War, mention may be made of some of the conclusions which had been reached by British psychiatrists as a result of experience gained during 1914–18, as summarized in two books which appeared in 1940.[80, 84]

Dr. C. S. Myers stated that the account of his experiences might "perhaps raise a doubt in some minds as to how far the present senior administrative officers of the Army Medical Service and the

---

* *Parliamentary Debates*, 5th ser., Lords, 39: 1094–1109; 28 April, 1920.
† The terms of reference submitted to the Committee by the Army Council differed in part from Lord Southborough's motion, and were as follows: "To consider the different types of hysteria and traumatic neurosis, commonly called 'shell-shock'; to collate the expert knowledge derived by the service medical authorities and the medical profession from the experience of the war, with a view to recording for future use the ascertained facts as to its origin, nature, and remedial treatment, and to advise whether by military training or education, some scientific method of guarding against its occurrence can be devised." [128]

INTRODUCTION

Adjutant-General's Department will be prevented from repeating the same mistakes—errors of commission, omission, and especially of wasteful procrastination—as arose during the last war". He expressed the hope that a book on so-called 'shell-shock' might "serve to re-enlighten members of the general public as to its nature, and to convince them how dependent it is on a previous psychoneurotic history and inherited predisposition, on inadequate examination and selection of soldiers fitted for the front line, and on the lack of proper discipline and esprit de corps".[84]

In another work on *The Neuroses in War*, Dr. Emanuel Miller observed that, from the experiences of the previous war, there was reason to expect a high incidence of neuroses in civil and military life in the Second World War. The contributors to this volume had studied and treated large numbers of so-called 'shell-shock' cases fresh from the line, or in hospitals abroad and at home: their clinical experiences and considered opinions should be placed at the service of the present military medical officers. Dr. Miller stressed the fact that, whereas in civil life medical practitioners could pass on their psychiatric cases to specialists in clinics, "those who are in the services will be obliged to recognize these conditions in the line if they are battalion M.O.s. They will be obliged to distinguish between minor and major disorders, from sudden panic which required firm and sympathetic handling, to major hysteria and psychosis. Indeed, they may be from time to time puzzled by disorders of character and discipline which call for considered judgement and rapid decision; a man's fate before a court-martial may depend upon such judgements. In training-camps, M.O.s will see raw recruits, passed as physically fit, with a mental equipment and disposition which make them quite unsuited for service. The so-called normal man is a dark horse where emotional control in times of stress is concerned; it is difficult to legislate psychologically for him. But nevertheless psychological foreknowledge may prove helpful in weeding out the doubtful characters and freeing the Army and other fighting forces of men who are potential neurotics, a misery to themselves and grit in the military machine from the point of view of morale." [80]

Finally, the following comments by Dr. Miller certainly deserved the careful consideration of those who might be inclined to adopt an attitude of moral superiority towards the neurotic soldier: "But let us not dismiss the man who breaks down with neurosis in wartime. As a group, the psychological patients of the last war served

INTRODUCTION

as long and at least as well as the average soldier. . . . There is official evidence to show that in a very large proportion of cases, before the breakdown, the man has done credit to himself and his unit. Against overwhelming mental forces calling him to abandon his struggle to fight on, he has frequently carried on. In fact the proportion of men with neuroses who received decorations for valour showed little difference from the proportion of other soldiers who received decorations." [80]

In the light of these statements, the development of British Army psychiatry during the recent war may now briefly be surveyed.*

Shortly before the outbreak of the Second World War, a conference called by the Ministry of Pensions expressed the intention of providing treatment but not giving pensions, except in special circumstances, in cases of neurosis developing during active service in the Forces. By this policy it was hoped to combat any possible 'epidemic' of 'war neurosis'.[96] These principles were also included in the recommendations of a conference of representatives of the Service Departments, Ministry of Health and Ministry of Pensions, in November, 1939.

It was clear enough, however, long before the commencement of the war, that the prophylactic approach to the problem of 'war neurosis' was by far the more important, and that scientific selection and placing of men would do more than anything else to avoid the development of widespread psychiatric disabilities. Unfortunately, it was not until much later that adequate measures were instituted to that end. Despite the unequivocal conclusions and recommendations of the Southborough Committee, a pre-war attempt, in April, 1939, to initiate the introduction into the Army of selection testing met with failure.[96]

Some half-dozen Regular Army medical officers with varying degrees of psychiatric training (including one or two very competent psychiatrists), who had acquired experience at 'D' Block, Netley, represented the total specialist personnel of the R.A.M.C. in this field of medicine prior to the outbreak of the Second World War. "As always happens, however, regular soldiers who have specialized are, after a certain point is reached in their careers, liable to be taken

---

* The official medical histories of the Second World War, published on behalf of the British and Dominion Governments, have appeared since the completion of the original manuscript of the present work: they contain chapters on psychiatric disorders in the Services, respectively, of the United Kingdom,[61] Australia,[15] Canada[86] and New Zealand.[87]

INTRODUCTION

off to fill other more senior posts, and at the outbreak of war the Army at home was stripped of its psychiatric help, and from the beginning had to rely on psychiatrists who came in with emergency commissions." [98]

This much provision had been made before the war, that two civilian psychiatrists were invited, in March, 1939, to act as Consultants in case of war, one for the B.E.F. (Dr. Henry Yellowlees), and the other for the Army at home (Dr. J. R. Rees). Both Consultants were called up and commissioned, with the rank of colonel, in the first week of September, 1939, and commenced their duties forthwith. Originally, it had been suggested that they should be called 'Consulting Psychologists', in accordance with the terminological precedent of the 1914–18 war, but it was fortunately possible to avoid the adoption of this misleading designation. It was not until some considerable time after the beginning of the war that Brigadier Rees was made Consulting Psychiatrist to the Army as a whole.

The Consultant in this country, working alone in the first few months of the war, could do little more than interview certain patients, lecture to the staffs of hospitals which were mobilizing and to groups of medical officers in training, establish contact with the medical administrative services throughout the United Kingdom, begin planning, and attempt to arouse in others the conviction and support necessary to enable these plans to be carried out. The Consultant to the B.E.F. was followed abroad by a small staff who were attached for duty to general hospitals. At home, no other Army psychiatrists were appointed until April, 1940.

However, illness does not, unfortunately, wait upon administrative developments, and, bureaucratic inertia notwithstanding, it was very soon after the outbreak of war that psychiatric problems manifested themselves in the Army in this country. "Army reservists had been called back, many of them unstable and many of them psychotic. The Depots at which these men arrived quickly found that they were faced with a number of problems of quite acute psychotic illness, and civilian psychiatrists were called in to help. A few newly joined medical officers were found to be psychiatrists and were pressed into service." [98] *

The nature of hospitals in France rendered psychiatric work essen-

* At the very beginning of the war, several civilian psychiatrists acted as Honorary Consultants to the D.D.s M.S. of various commands (officially or unofficially), and did most valuable work, especially in dealing with psychotic cases, before the Army psychiatrists were available.

INTRODUCTION

tially similar to that of the Army at home, while, as a result of the subsequent evacuation, the cases from Dunkirk were largely dealt with in this country. Evacuated military psychiatric cases, other than gross psychoses, were treated in the United Kingdom in Emergency Medical Service (E.M.S.) hospitals, and in No. 41 General Hospital. The latter, which had been mobilized in the early weeks of 1940 for service with the B.E.F., but did not have an opportunity of proceeding to France before the Dunkirk evacuation, was set up in Sussex.

Had the medical needs of the Army been limited to in-patient treatment and to the assessment of the condition of those about to be discharged, such a civilian service might have sufficed. But it rapidly became clear that the lack of military psychiatrists was having unfortunate consequences: E.M.S. psychiatric centres, for instance, were receiving, on the one hand, many chronic patients who, in spite of prolonged and intensive therapy, would be permanently unfit for further military service, and, on the other, cases where little more was required than advice to a medical officer on the handling of the simplest psychiatric problems.

In April, 1940, a psychiatrist was attached to the Medical Headquarters of each command in the United Kingdom. The function of these Command Specialists in Psychological Medicine, or Command Psychiatrists, was to act as a specialist adviser to medical officers and others in units, and as a consultant to whom out-patients could be referred. Military psychiatric out-patient centres were set up, and these were able to act as a filter for the E.M.S. hospitals, separating out those cases who appeared likely to recover if retained in their own unit under the supervision of their medical officer. The Command Psychiatrists soon found it impossible to deal, by themselves, with such large areas, the considerable number of out-patients and the many other problems that they were asked to solve.

In the latter part of 1940, it became necessary to appoint more military psychiatrists to each command; these were either full specialists, with the rank of major, or 'graded' specialists with rather shorter psychiatric experience in civil life, with the rank of lieutenant or captain. By 1941, there came to be in each command from three to ten, or at times fifteen, Area Psychiatrists whose work was co-ordinated by the Command Psychiatrist at Command Headquarters.

The main task of Area Psychiatrists was to provide an out-patient service for every area where there were troops or military hospitals,

INTRODUCTION

and to visit various units in connection with their clinical and advisory duties. Simultaneously with the development of this outpatient service, facilities were provided in the Army for the care and treatment of psychiatric patients requiring hospitalization. In 1914-18, as has been mentioned, many difficulties arose from the policy of sending direct to civil mental hospitals serving soldiers who were suffering from psychiatric illness. Furthermore, a large number of soldiers in such hospitals were granted pensions which would probably never have been given had it been possible to make a closer investigation of the origin and constitutional basis of their disabilities. A military mental hospital also had the advantage (in the prevailing circumstances), compared with civil hospitals, of being able to detain a patient without any need for certification. In 1940, therefore, it was decided to treat military cases of psychosis, so far as possible, within the Army organization.

The peace-time accommodation at 'D' Block, Royal Victoria Hospital, Netley, was quite inadequate to deal with the number of psychotic soldiers in time of war, and certain civil mental hospitals were taken over, either in part or entirely, by the Army. The first such military mental hospital to be opened was established in a section of the L.C.C. Mental Hospital at Banstead, Surrey, in March, 1940. Military hospitals for psychosis also admitted a large number of airmen, as the Royal Air Force had no special hospitals for such cases.

Until April, 1942, most of the hospital treatment of psychoneuroses was provided by the special Neurosis Centres of the E.M.S., which co-operated fully with the Army, and by No. 41 General Hospital, and later, by the Military (Psychiatric) Hospital, Bishop's Lydeard, Somerset. The latter came into operation following the mobilization of No. 41 General Hospital for the M.E.F., in December, 1941. Inevitably, however, it also became necessary to provide special observation wards or collecting centres for such cases in military hospitals. Subsequently, special Army hospitals were established, for cases of neurosis, of which the largest was the Military Hospital at Northfield, Birmingham, which opened in April, 1942, and provided 200 beds for hospital treatment, and 600 beds in a 'Training Wing' where the rehabilitation of soldiers suffering from psychoneurosis could be carried out, prior to their return to duty.

Owing to the shortage of man-power and the need for utilizing fully every available man, a scheme was introduced in May, 1941,

INTRODUCTION

largely at the suggestion of Professor Aubrey Lewis who was working in the E.M.S. at Mill Hill Hospital, which made it possible for patients to be discharged from neurosis hospitals to duty of a specific type, if necessary in a selected environment. This was known as the 'Annexure' Scheme.

In January, 1942, psychiatrists were permitted to recommend for transfer to employment of a special nature men who were working in jobs for which they were temperamentally unsuitable. This procedure resulted in a great diminution in the number of cases admitted to hospital because of a psychiatric breakdown, and was a notable achievement in vocational selection and psychiatric prophylaxis.

The increasing number of German and Italian prisoners of war in this country gave rise to certain specific psychiatric problems. Psychotic prisoners of war were treated in Talgarth Military Hospital, which was one of the hospitals taken over by the Army for psychotic cases. Psychoneurotic prisoners of war could be admitted to Talgarth Military Hospital, if it was impossible to supervise them adequately in their own camps.

After the first eighteen months of the war, it became increasingly obvious that administrative procedures were fully as important as clinical or purely professional questions in Army psychiatry. It had been recognized at a very early date that the position of a consultant attached to the Royal Army Medical College and with a nominal office and no secretarial assistance in that establishment, was indeed futile. By a gradual process of infiltration the Consulting Psychiatrist, who was soon followed by the Consulting Physician and Consulting Surgeon, penetrated into the War Office, realizing that only thus could any effective help be given in the development of the Army Medical Services. After a good deal of discussion, the Consulting Psychiatrist was given a room, and, with the assistance of Major A. T. M. Wilson, a psychiatrist who was on the strength of one of the commands, began to establish some real contact with psychiatric affairs and organization in the Army.

Eventually, in April, 1942, a Directorate of Army Psychiatry was set up as part of the Army Medical Services (A.M.D. 11), with a regular R.A.M.C. officer as Director (Col. H. A. Sandiford), and three psychiatric specialists (majors) as Deputy Assistant Directors working with him.* The principal aim of the Directorate was to

* In addition, there were originally two Junior Civil Assistants. In October, 1942, the Director was given the rank of brigadier; one Deputy Assistant Director was made

INTRODUCTION

maintain and promote the mental health and efficiency of the Army by every possible means; and, where it failed in this, it was to provide the means of rehabilitation or treatment for men whose military incapacity was due to psychiatric causes. The Directorate was responsible for the development, control and co-ordination of the psychiatric services of the Army at home and overseas, and acted in an advisory capacity within the War Office. It had three branches, with the following functions:

A.M.D.11(A): Psychiatric aspects of morale, discipline, training and equipment.
A.M.D.11(B): Selection, training and allocation of Army psychiatrists.
Psychiatric aspects of recruiting, selection, grading, allocation and transfer of officers and other ranks.
Psychiatric liaison with the Ministry of Labour and National Service.
A.M.D.11(C): Clinical policy and research.
Psychiatric clinics and hospitals.
Psychiatric liaison with the Ministry of Pensions, Ministry of Health (E.M.S.), and Boards of Control.
Psychiatric aspects of discharges and medical boards.

The Consulting Psychiatrist to the Army worked with the Directorate, and was the professional adviser on all psychiatric matters; with the appointment of a Director of Army Psychiatry as the administrative head of the Army psychiatric services, he became free to visit commands more frequently and to undertake the various exploratory and co-ordinating activities which arose. Like the other consultants to the Army, he was an adviser to the Director-General, Army Medical Services.

In March, 1943, the Senior Psychiatrist of the War Office Selection Boards (W.O.S.B.s) was attached to A.M.D. 11, as an Assistant Director of Army Psychiatry (Lt.-Col.) in charge of the supervision of the psychiatric aspects of officer selection. In September, 1943, the Royal Army Medical College's establishment was amended to include a Consulting Psychiatrist to the Army at home (this appointment being assumed at this time by Brigadier G. W. B. James, on his return from the M.E.F.); his headquarters were, however, at A.M.D. 11, so as to facilitate close liaison with the Consulting Psychiatrist to the Army and with the Director of Army Psychiatry. While the Consultant to the Army at home shared many functions (e.g. as a

Assistant Director (Lt.-Col.); and one of the Junior Civil Assistants was replaced by a Staff Captain (graded psychiatrist). Brigadier Sandiford was Director of Army Psychiatry from April, 1942, to July, 1946.

INTRODUCTION

member of War Office Medical Boards, teaching, etc.) with the Consultant to the Army, his duties were especially concerned with supervising the hospital services, advising Army psychiatric units and military general hospitals, and maintaining liaison with the E.M.S. Neurosis Centres.

Apart from the psychiatric arrangements for the B.E.F., which have already been mentioned, psychiatrists were sent to other theatres overseas. A Consultant (Brigadier G. W. B. James) was posted to the M.E.F. in August, 1940; he was followed almost immediately by six psychiatrists, and a restricted out-patient service was set up, together with two Psychiatric Centres (170 beds each). No. 41 General Hospital proceeded to the Middle East in December, 1941, and opened for patients in March, 1942 (600 beds). In October, 1942, a psychiatrist was attached to the Director of Military Training, Middle East, to carry out an investigation into the psychological aspects of training. A Consultant (Brigadier E. A. Bennet) arrived in India in July, 1942; he was followed, in 1943, by ten psychiatrists, three of whom were engaged in W.O.S.B. work, and there were six psychiatrists in India Command at the time of his arrival. A Command Psychiatrist was posted to Gibraltar in January, 1943.

Two psychiatrists were sent to North Africa, soon after the invasion of that area, in December, 1942; of these, one was attached to a Corps Headquarters, and the other to a general hospital at the base. An Adviser in Psychiatry (Lt.-Col. S. A. MacKeith) was sent to North Africa in May, 1943. No psychiatrist was stationed in Malta during the siege, although a medical specialist (Lt.-Col. R. E. Tunbridge), who was O.C., Medical Division, of a general hospital on the island, was given the local appointment of psychiatrist to the command, and did valuable work in very difficult circumstances. A Command Psychiatrist was posted to Malta in July, 1943, and dealt not only with British Army cases, but also with those of the other Services, especially the Royal Navy. A psychiatrist was officially appointed to West Africa Command at the end of 1943, and another served in East Africa from the beginning of 1943.

In February, 1944, an Adviser in Psychiatry (Lt.-Col. T. F. Main) was appointed to 21 Army Group, B.L.A. During the four months prior to the opening of the Second Front, he supervised the training of Army psychiatrists and regimental medical officers in the handling of acute psychiatric casualties, and elaborated plans to meet the anticipated demands of the forthcoming campaign. In July, 1944,

INTRODUCTION

No. 32 British General Hospital opened an Advanced Section (200 beds) to deal with the cases of 'battle exhaustion' in Normandy, and, in August, 1944, two months after D-Day, this was augmented by a Rear Section (400 beds). A Consulting Psychiatrist (Brigadier T. F. Rodger) was appointed to 11 Army Group, S.E.A.C., in October, 1944 (and later, to A.L.F.S.E.A.). The Consulting Psychiatrist to the Army visited the U.S.A. and Canada in October–December, 1943, and October–December, 1944, and thus established valuable, and mutually beneficial, relations with Army psychiatrists in North America.

It has been mentioned that the Southborough Committee stressed the importance of eliminating cases of potential psychiatric disability at the recruiting stage, and that the Committee were convinced that, in the First World War, "a great number of men who were ill-suited to stand the strain of military service, whether by temperament or their past or present condition of mental or nervous health, were admitted into the Army; there is no doubt that such men contributed a very high proportion of the cases of hysteria and traumatic neurosis commonly called 'shell-shock' ".[128] In the Second World War, Army psychiatrists did not, of course, take part in devising the recruiting procedure which was controlled by the Ministry of Labour and National Service.

The clinical handling of many individual cases in the earlier part of the recent war left much to be desired: certainly, acute neuroses occurring in the battle of Flanders were sometimes left to languish for long periods in general hospital beds under an organic diagnosis with no other treatment than a placebo; and it is equally certain that psychiatrists were at times unduly pessimistic in their assessment of a man's potential military fitness. Their pessimism may sometimes have been justified by the difficulty which then existed, of arranging for a man who was only capable of a limited psychiatric adjustment to be transferred to a type of employment or duty likely to give him the best chance of recovering, or at least retaining his relative adjustment to Army life.

After much discussion, the systems of personnel selection which had been commonly employed in civil life (in industry) and in some foreign armies, found expression in the formation of the new Directorate of Selection of Personnel, in June, 1941. The greater part of intelligence testing and procedures to ensure the allocation of the recruit to the most suitable job available was subsequently under-

INTRODUCTION

taken by this Directorate, while assessment of personality and 'misfit' problems of various types constituted an increasing part of military psychiatric work. The introduction of efficient methods for the transfer of the psychiatric misfit undoubtedly played as large a part in the reduction of the rate of psychiatric invaliding as did advances in therapeutic methods.[9]

The Directorate of Army Psychiatry collaborated with the Directorate of Selection of Personnel, on the introduction of the General Service Corps intake scheme in July, 1942. Approximately 14% of the recruit intake were referred for examination to Army psychiatrists consequent upon poor results shown in the selection tests, or following interview by Personnel Selection Officers. In this way, many thousands of recruits were referred to military psychiatrists during their first fortnight in the Army in order that advice might be given regarding their placement in suitable employment.

The Directorate of Army Psychiatry also worked in collaboration with the Directorate of Selection of Personnel in the scientific selection of officers. As a result of experiments begun in July, 1941, by psychiatrists in Scottish Command, an experimental War Office Selection Board (W.O.S.B.) was set up in January, 1942, and eventually W.O.S.B.s were set up in every command at home as well as in various theatres overseas. One or two Army psychiatrists were included in the establishment of each W.O.S.B.

The importance and magnitude of the psychiatric problem in the Army, from the point of view of the Medical Services alone, will be apparent from the fact that psychiatric disabilities were by far the largest cause of medical discharge among military personnel (other ranks) during the Second World War. Thus, in 1943, psychiatric disorders constituted more than one-third, and in 1944 two-fifths, of all discharges with respect to disease.

The extent of the problem of mental backwardness in the Army was shown by the fact that, following the introduction of the General Service Corps intake scheme, it was found that some 8% of all recruits were so dull and backward as to require special conditions of military environment, training and employment, and about 1% was unfit to be entrusted with fire-arms. These men were for the most part absorbed into the Pioneer Corps, whose companies, both armed and unarmed, were notably successful in utilizing the services of thousands of dullards who were quite incapable of assimilating advanced military training.

INTRODUCTION

Finally, it should be mentioned that much specialized work of very great value was carried out by Army psychiatrists, in such various matters as the psychiatric aspects of discipline and morale, psychological warfare and the psychology of the enemy, psychosomatic disorders and the rehabilitation of the physically disabled, and the civil resettlement of repatriated prisoners of war.*

It seems not inappropriate to conclude this brief introductory survey of the development of military psychiatry during the Second World War with a few remarks on the attitude adopted by the Army towards the introduction of psychiatric methods and concepts. It was not to be expected that the Army would react to psychiatry and its implications in a manner very different from that which had characterized the civilian community and civil medicine. Thus, in the Army, from the very beginning of military psychiatry, "the commanding officer and the regimental medical officer were the first to realize the possibilities of this aspect of medicine. Difficulties, however, there certainly were; and many of them will be commemorated in the half-friendly, half-doubtful nickname of 'trick-cyclists', which was bestowed on psychiatrists at an early date." [9] In the more detailed account which follows, some of these difficulties will be only too clearly apparent.

It must, however, be recorded that British Army psychiatry was fortunate indeed in having two very great allies in Lt.-Gen. Sir Ronald F. Adam and Lt.-Gen. Sir Alexander Hood. With the invaluable support and far-sighted policy of General Adam, who became Adjutant-General to the Forces in 1941, it was possible to introduce into the Army a scientific system of selection of personnel and officers: "His vision and courage led to the development, not only of selection procedures of various kinds in the Army, but also of a great number of other sociological experiments ... and his deliberate contribution to social medicine and social psychiatry as well as to winning the war is difficult to overvalue." [97] And it has rightly been said that when General Hood became Director-General, Army Medical Services, in 1942, he "did more ... than perfect a mechanism inherited from his predecessor: he enlarged its scope. His innovating quality is revealed most clearly, perhaps, in the support he gave, often against advice, to the development of

* It is not within the 'terms of reference' of the present work to consider in any detail the technical aspects of war-time developments of Army psychiatry. A comprehensive technical bibliography of published works on British Army psychiatry and allied subjects is provided, for further reference, at the end of this volume.

INTRODUCTION

psychiatry at a time when this had to contend with opposition not only from powerful military authorities but also from powerful members of our profession." [10]

It may be noted, incidentally, that the Expert Committee which was appointed in September, 1942, by His Majesty's Government to investigate and appraise the work of psychologists and psychiatrists in the Services, in their Report to the War Cabinet in February, 1945, already provided a full vindication of all those whose labours in the fields of psychology and psychiatry contributed so much to the national war effort and received so little recognition or favourable publicity.[91]

The considerable importance and positive nature of the work of psychologists and psychiatrists in the Army is indicated by the following excerpts from the Report of the Expert Committee:

"Service psychology has the positive aim of making the most effective use of human resources. Service psychiatry is more concerned in preventing human waste; hence, it gives first place to preventive measures.* In both spheres of activity, the starting point is the fact of individual differences, for there is considerable variation in all human traits. The object of psychology and psychiatry alike is to ascertain these individual differences so that the unfit can be detected and the fit placed where they can function in a way most useful to the Service and satisfactory to themselves. Hence, the quality of men and women is as important as their quantity; in modern warfare it is no longer a question of 'measuring Guardsmen by the yard'. . . . The Services are not only anxious to recruit mentally and physically sound personnel, but also to maintain health and morale and to prevent breakdown. While they cannot afford in wartime to devote effort to the treatment of individuals likely to be

---

* Official recognition was subsequently given to the importance of preventive psychiatry in the Army, by the publication, in July, 1948, of a most enlightened and progressive Army Council Instruction: this stated that mental health had now been included in the scope of hygiene, and it was intended that psychiatric specialists, working in close co-operation with hygiene officers, should give the necessary training to officers and selected N.C.O.s of all arms in the application of the new methods of promoting mental hygiene in the soldier's way of life. (Cf. A.C.I. 605/48, § 4.) This conception of the co-operation of psychiatrists and hygiene officers in promoting mental health is entirely in agreement with the opinion expressed, in their Report (published two years later), by the Expert Committee on Mental Health of the World Health Organization, "that the most important single long-term principle . . . in the fostering of mental health is the encouragement of the incorporation into public-health work of the responsibility for promoting the mental as well as the physical health of the community. . . . Public-health officers must provide the generalship for preventive mental health work." [44]

INTRODUCTION

physically or mentally disabled for a prolonged period, they are very much concerned to use all available measures at their disposal to reduce the incidence of mental breakdown. This is the essence of the psychiatrist's contribution. Whilst the psychologist estimates the degree of technical aptitude demanded of Service personnel by the complexity of modern weapons and equipment, the psychiatrist assesses their stability in the face of stress produced by the peculiar hazards of modern warfare." [91]

Criticism and opposition are reactions which cannot, in all truth, be said to constitute an unfamiliar or novel experience in psychiatric practice, whether civilian or military.* Indeed, it may be said that criticism was expected by Army psychiatrists, and that it was encountered, and expressed in various quarters in no uncertain terms.† There has been placed on record a personal minute addressed by Mr. Winston Churchill to the Lord President, in December, 1942, in which the Prime Minister referred to the use made of psychologists and psychiatrists in the Fighting Services, in the following terms:

"I am sure it would be sensible to restrict as much as possible the work of these gentlemen, who are capable of doing an immense amount of harm with what may very easily degenerate into charlatanry. The tightest hand should be kept over them, and they should not be allowed to quarter themselves in large numbers upon the Fighting Services at the public expense. There are, no doubt, easily recognizable cases which may benefit from treatment of this kind, but it is very wrong to disturb large numbers of healthy, normal men and women by asking the kind of odd questions in which the psychiatrists specialize. There are quite enough hangers-on and camp-followers already." ‡

* "... It was the doctor who created the speciality of psychiatry. He did it uninvited and against terrible odds, against the will of the public, against the will of established legal authority, and against the will of a variety of established religious faiths. ... The process of opposing psychiatry has not lost its impetus and the conquest of the field of mental disease by medicine is far from complete." (G. Zilboorg, *A History of Medical Psychology*, New York, 1941, p. 25.) "... No other speciality of medicine has had to rescue its patients from persecution, live with them in social ostracism, restore their capacities and then return them to an environment both exigent and suspicious." (A. Gregg, 'A Critique of Psychiatry', *Amer. J. Psychiat.*, 1944, 101: 285–91.)

† Cf., for example, an article by H. J. C. J. L'Etang, 'A Criticism of Military Psychiatry in the Second World War'.[69] The opinions expressed and statements made in this article will serve as well as any to illustrate the misconceptions, misrepresentations, and uninformed generalizations, not uncommon among an appreciable section of the medical profession, as indeed elsewhere.

‡ Prime Minister to Lord President of the Council, 19 December, 1942. Cf. Winston S. Churchill, *The Second World War*, Vol. 4, London (Cassell), 1951; Appendix C,

INTRODUCTION

The position of the psychiatrist in relation to the Army in the Second World War has been well described. Thus, in 1944, Dr. Ernest Jones stated:

". . . One did, it is true, hear stories of how various authorities were determined to purge the Army of the psychological nonsense that had crept in during the last World War and to put all psychiatric illnesses on a proper basis of organic neurology as they had been in the good old days of the Boer War. However this may be, there is little doubt . . . that progress in psychiatry had considerable opposition and prejudice to overcome, a trouble which I understand American military psychiatry has also not been entirely spared. . . . We know that this proceeds from the general dread of mental depths, from aversion to psychological insight, and that it is strongest among those whose mental integrity, often of a very successful order, has been built on defences against those depths. It is therefore to be expected especially in the apparently stable personalities of those who have achieved prominence, political or otherwise, in life. . . .

"Actually the liaison work between the psychiatrists in the Army and both the staff and regimental medical officers is on the whole very satisfactory. . . . The medical officers cannot escape seeing the visible results of psychiatric 'commonsense' on the all-important matters of man-power and morale, and are therefore co-operating with psychiatrists to a very gratifying extent." [66]

Similarly, in 1945, Dr. J. R. Rees wrote as follows:

"Earlier in this present war we were often told that psychiatrists were the fifth-columnists of the Army, and this because they were advising the discharge of men who were obviously too dull or too unstable to soldier. The administrator who has to produce the 'bodies' and is quite out of contact with real live men is critical, and much opprobrium has come to Army psychiatrists because there has necessarily been a high discharge rate from psychiatric causes. The fighting soldier is in no doubt at all as to what kind of man he wishes to have with him. The further you get away from the front line the tougher become the comments, the more hints there are that everyone is trying to evade service, and that is and always has been a common experience of armies. . . . Any suggestion of change may

pp. 814–15. The Prime Minister's scientific adviser and his physician were both strongly sceptical and suspicious of psychiatric activities, and methods of personnel and officer selection.

INTRODUCTION

arouse anxiety and so aggression, which the psychiatrist has to appreciate and counter, treating the situation clinically. Patience, tolerance, infiltration tactics, and skill in counter-attack, which psychiatrists learn through conditions like these, are of some value for the future.* We cannot tolerate the retention of sickness and inefficiency in society just because we wish to avoid tiresome opposition and criticism of ourselves. It is very striking how few of the really intelligent and valuable leaders fail to appreciate the contribution of psychiatry, but we have to beware of those who become 'converts' and thus lost their capacity to help us with real criticism." [97] †

* These aspects of the psychiatrist's work have been admirably discussed by J. A. M. Meerloo in his paper, 'Contribution of the Psychiatrist to the Management of Crisis Situations'.[77]

† It should perhaps here be noted that many Army psychiatrists (and especially, Command Psychiatrists) mentioned in the following pages, originally held the rank of Major, and subsequently that of Lt.-Col. On this point, chronological accuracy has been sacrificed in the interests of consistency and the avoidance of unnecessary confusion.

II

PERSONNEL SELECTION

> Besides, there is no king, be his cause never so spotless, if it come to the arbitrement of swords, can try it out with all unspotted soldiers. — SHAKESPEARE, *King Henry V*

IT HAS BEEN WELL STATED by Dr. J. R. Rees, that "The main opposition to selection procedures is based on the fact that the average man rather dislikes to have his phantasies destroyed. The commonest of all human daydreams is the Cinderella motif or, translated into military terms, the idea that every soldier has a Field-Marshal's baton in his knapsack. Selection hits at this because it implies that someone can demonstrate that this is in most cases not true. Many people object strongly to facing this reality even though it may be pointed out to them how much better it is to make full use in the best possible way of whatever intelligence and capacity they have got." [97] *

It has already been noted that, as early as 1922, following a careful appraisal of the evidence of medical witnesses and combatant officers concerning their experience in the First World War, the Southborough Committee reached the unequivocal conclusion that adequate selection of personnel was an important and potent weapon in preventing and combating the occurrence of psychiatric illness in fighting men.

---

* Such opposition may also arise from certain political or ethical ideologies (and, indeed, misconceptions), based on the utopian assumption that all men have an absolute, fundamental, and innate equality in their potentialities. "While it is clear that all men are equal in their possession of emotional needs, however much these may vary individually, we are indeed forced to accept the fact that they are not identical in their capacity to learn and to acquire skills." [97]

PERSONNEL SELECTION

The Southborough Committee stressed the importance of an adequate and thorough medical examination and grading of recruits, particularly in the event of the introduction of compulsory military service, and stated in this connection: ". . . We are of the opinion that the adoption of the measures we have recommended would result in the admission into the fighting services of a much smaller percentage of recruits mentally and nervously unsuitable for military service than was the case in 1914–18; such men are unlikely to become efficient soldiers, and likely under the strain of war to become the subjects of the different types of hysteria and traumatic neurosis commonly called 'shell-shock'. The occurrence of these conditions militates against the efficiency of the Army, swells the sick returns, increases the amount of hospital accommodation and transport required, and absorbs the time and attention of medical personnel. Eventually a large number of men are returned to civil life, a burden to themselves and the country, requiring prolonged and costly treatment, necessitating a greatly increased pensions list, and extremely difficult to re-establish in civil life. As far as it is possible to foresee the conditions of any future war on a large scale, it seems probable that the circumstances are likely to make even greater demands upon the mental and nervous resources of the personnel of the fighting services than the events of 1914–18. If this should prove to be the case, appropriate measures designed to admit into the services only those who are possessed of at least an average degree of mental and nervous health and stability will be a factor of prime importance in the successful conduct of the war." [128]

If it were characteristic of human nature to learn from the experience of others and from past events, this statement and the early history of the First World War might have been accepted as ample evidence of the need for an active and comprehensive policy of personnel selection in the British Army. During the first three years of that war, as a result of the lack of any thorough medical examination or selection of recruits, "a great number of men who were ill-suited to stand the strain of military service, whether by temperament or their past or present condition of mental or nervous health, were admitted into the Army; there is no doubt that such men contributed a very high proportion of the cases of hysteria and traumatic neurosis commonly called 'shell-shock' ". In fact, the Southborough Committee were of the opinion that the Army would have been better off without these men.[128]

PERSONNEL SELECTION

In spite of this evidence, and that provided by the experience of the armies of other countries, and in particular the experiments in the United States Army in 1917, it was not until April, 1939, that a fairly complete scheme was suggested for the selection of men to be called up for the militia in Britain prior to the outbreak of war. A significant 'Memorandum on the Possibility of Improved Efficiency of Training and Conservation of Man-Power by Group Psychological Testing of Recruits and Improved Psychiatric Facilities during Early Training' was at that time submitted by Dr. J. R. Rees and Mr. Alec Rodger to the medical authorities at the War Office. This report drew attention to the results of research in industrial psychology,* and to the value of special aptitude tests in vocational selection for technical work (e.g. engineering);† as also to the past experience of the fighting services in this country, and the United States Army. It suggested with great moderation, that a preliminary experiment might be conducted to determine whether any good results could be obtained in improving the speed and quality of training of conscripts by the following methods: psychological group tests for intelligence and special aptitude; improved facilities for the psychiatric assessment of certain recruits; and reassessment of recruit rejects, particularly in view of experience that many physiological symptoms and signs which might cause rejection were, in fact, the result of mild psychological disorders.

For reasons which are not clear, the scheme was rejected completely, but it is, perhaps, not without significance that, when eventually systematic selection was introduced into the Army some two years later, it was at the instigation of the administrative side and did not come within the field of the Army Medical Services.

Objections to scientific selection, based on a complete failure to understand its function in social medicine, were also advanced by those responsible for the civilian recruiting boards in Great Britain.[97] It is possible that there was insufficient understanding and inadequate co-operation between the medical officers who served on the

---

* Industrial Health Research Board investigations showed that psychological disorders constituted the largest single factor in incapacity of over one month's duration (cf. M. Smith and M. A. Leiper[117]). More recently, it has been shown that neurotic illness caused between one-quarter and one-third of all absence from work due to illness, in a random sample of some 3,000 factory workers (cf. R. Fraser[48]).

† Examples were quoted of the successful use, and superiority over previous methods, of intelligence and special aptitude tests in the selection of aircraft apprentices (R. H. Stanbridge[120]), Borstal boys (A. Rodger[108]), and entrants to junior technical schools (E. P. Allen and P. Smith[5, 6]).

PERSONNEL SELECTION

recruiting boards and those in the Army. "At times there has certainly been a feeling in the minds of some of the medical officers in the Ministry of National Service that the Army's standards were too high and that, in consequence, too many of the men they had passed in were being boarded out and sent back to civilian life. . . . It is certain that, in recruiting, a penal attitude, such as occasionally has emerged in the statement that 'no one must be allowed to get away with it', is not likely to produce the Army we should all like to see."[96]

One of the most important reasons for the accumulation within the Army, in the absence of selection, of men whose mental background was questionable was that the man-power of this country was so organized that very large numbers of intelligent and able men were reserved in industry; the Royal Navy and the Royal Air Force had a priority of choice; and the Civil Defence Services claimed a great many men. "The Army comes last in the list, and consequently a large proportion of what has been called 'the psychopathic tenth' of the country's man-power finds its way into the Army if the mesh of the recruiting boards is too wide. The Army has therefore to deal with very considerable numbers of dull, neurotic, and unstable men who have got on reasonably well in civil life, whenever employment was plentiful."[96]

There can be no doubt—as pointed out by Brigadier Rees in 1945—that as a result of the delay in introducing selection in the recent war, "many horses were out of the stable before the door was shut. It is sad but true that no force has yet gone overseas from Great Britain, every man of which has gone through selection procedures."[97] The magnitude of the psychiatric problem in the three Services provides an index of the need for thorough selection, and may be illustrated by the number of psychiatric cases that had to be discharged: about 118,000 such cases (men and women) were discharged between September, 1939, and June, 1944. Between one-third and one-half of all medical invalids, men and women alike, were discharged from the Services on psychiatric grounds. About one-quarter of the Army cases had served less than one year. It is clearly desirable, therefore, that recruits should be closely examined at entry.[91]

It has already been noted that, in September, 1939, in addition to the scattered half-dozen regular R.A.M.C. officers with some psychiatric experience, the only psychiatrists recruited for the British Army were two Consultants, one with the B.E.F. in France, and one in Great Britain, so that the amount of psychiatric work, whether therapeutic or prophylactic, that could be undertaken was strictly limited. When the first Command Psychiatrists were appointed, in April, 1940, they were inevitably faced with large numbers of unsuitable and inadequate men, and had to begin combing them out. Many of these men had to be discharged as unfit for service; some could be better placed or more usefully employed in their own or other arms of the Service. Various intelligence tests were brought into use by the different psychiatrists, each using those procedures with which he was most familiar. All the early selection procedures had to be operated by psychiatrists since there was no one else to do this work. On their own account psychiatrists also organized experiments in group testing.

Starting in April, 1940, the Command Psychiatrist, Northern Command (Lt.-Col. G. R. Hargreaves), carried out experiments at No. 11 Depot, R.A.M.C., Leeds, with the invaluable assistance and advice of Dr. J. C. Raven. They used the Penrose-Raven Progressive Matrices test, which was devised to measure innate intelligence and was not an assessment of literacy. Tests of literacy were subsequently introduced as well, as it was obviously necessary to detect those men who were semi-literate or illiterate. The intelligence tests were given to intakes within a few days of their admission to the Depot, and all men who showed abnormal test results were examined individually by the Command Psychiatrist. Later, in the course of these experiments, the Army test F.H.3 was also used, but was discarded after a short while since it was found to be unsatisfactory in various respects. These tests were also used in an attempt to indicate the group of men in each intake, in which potential officers and N.C.O.s were likely to be found, and were given to men applying for commissions or admission to O.C.T.U.s.

As a result of one year's trial, Col. Hargreaves concluded that the Penrose-Raven Matrices provided a readily and easily operated intelligence test, and that its use had speeded up and improved training in the Depot by rendering possible the early elimination of recruits who were unsuitable because of mental defect or low intelligence, and the best utilization, as N.C.O.s and instructors, of men above average intelligence. As early as August, 1940, in a preliminary report to the D.D.M.S., Northern Command, the Command Psychiatrist was able to state that this test had proved most successful in achieving the purposes for which it had been introduced; he strongly recommended its routine application to all recruits at intake centres before the commencement of training.

Simultaneously, Professor Godfrey H. Thomson co-operated with the Command Psychiatrist, Scottish Command (Lt.-Col. T. F. Rodger), in an experiment on men undergoing training at No. 2 Depot, R.A.M.C., Edinburgh. The verbal M.H. test was given to large groups of soldiers, and those who were found to be in the lowest grades of intelligence were referred to the psychiatrist for individual interview.

As a result of these early experiments, Army psychiatrists came to the conclusion that, at that time, about 4% of all intakes were never likely to be efficient in any combatant unit, and that probably another 5% were fit only for the less skilled combatant duties, i.e. the use of the rifle in self-defence.

They were also aware of the fact that highly skilled men, capable of undertaking specialized technical jobs, were being employed in unskilled occupations. They estimated that 20% of infantry intakes and 50% of Pioneer Corps intakes were capable of efficient service in a more skilled arm than that to which they had been posted; and that 50% of every Tank Regiment intake and 20% of every infantry intake had not the degree of innate intelligence necessary for full efficiency in the corps to which they had been posted.

The psychiatrists were—necessarily, at that time—primarily and more immediately concerned with this state of affairs as an important factor in the causation of neurotic illness in the Army. It was, however, all too clearly realized that the lack of adequate selection also entailed a very considerable and serious loss of effective man-power.

Sufficient evidence of the absence of satisfactory methods of selection and allocation, and the consequent inevitable wastage of manpower, in the Army in 1940–1, is provided by the series of inadequate and ineffective Army Council Instructions introduced at that time, which were intended to ensure, to a moderate degree, the satisfactory utilization of skilled tradesmen and men in low medical categories.

Thus, the purpose of A.C.I. 216/40 (March, 1940), on 'Transfers of Tradesmen', was to enable officers commanding units to regulate the employment of their personnel so as to ensure the proper utilization of tradesmen essential to the Army, while avoiding, so far as possible, interruptions in training such as would result from transfers on a large scale. A.C.I. 399/40 (April, 1940), on 'Transfers of Soldiers between Corps at Home', authorized such transfer in the case of certain specified groups of men: it was thereby open to commanding officers, not only to transfer men in their unit who had been incorrectly appointed on enlistment or who, after trial, proved unsuitable, for medical or other reasons, for the corps in which they were serving; but also (assuming, it is to be supposed, that they were necessarily aware of their presence), those with professional or specialist qualifications or abilities liable to be of value in a particular arm or corps—(i.e. commanding officers might, if so inclined, transfer some of their more intelligent and skilled men to other, more suitable, units*).

In the absence of a *general* scheme for the selection of personnel, which alone could lead to the satisfactory allocation of *all* recruits, it was not to be expected that such limited provisions as these, however thoroughly and conscientiously they might have been applied, could solve the existing man-power problems; consequently, the Army's difficulties rapidly became acute, as shown by the publication of the somewhat more positive and forceful A.C.I. 1298/40 (October, 1940), on the 'Testing, Training and Disposal of Potential Tradesmen now in the Army'. This A.C.I. emphasized the fact that, in view of the severely restricted supply of skilled men available from civil life, the Army would have to undertake an immediate comprehensive survey of its own resources of skilled personnel.

Psychiatrists were inevitably faced with the problem of the disposal of men who had developed neurotic symptoms as a result of having been employed in less skilled occupations than their innate ability and civilian attainments warranted. The only course open to them, in such cases, was to suggest to the commanding officer that action be taken in accordance with A.C.I. 399/40, but these provisions were of very limited applicability, and some organization was clearly required, which would have the task of allocating men, from the moment they were recruited, on the basis of their abilities.

While Army psychiatrists had early become convinced of the need for scientific selection, they had been able to make but little progress

---

* Alternatively, they might, no doubt, prefer to retain such men; or else, continue to ignore their specialized potentialities. Cf. the incident in Alan Hackney's novel, *Private's Progress*: " 'You two men,' said a voice behind them.—It was the orderly sergeant with a notebook.—'You any trades?' he asked, pencil hovering.—'Electrical fitter, me,' said Cox promptly.—'I was at a university,' said Stanley.—'Names?' said the orderly sergeant. 'Double away, then, to Company stores for buckets and brushes and get all that old distemper off the A.T.S. Rest Room. Come on! Should be there by now!' "

PERSONNEL SELECTION

against opposition in the matter of introducing group-testing on a large scale. This opposition arose from the fact that many senior officers held the view that dull men made the best soldiers, and that, in this respect, the modern Army was in no way different from former armies; that intelligence tests had, in any case, no validity in the selection of men; and that the psychiatrist's opinion was wrong, and the men discharged on psychiatric grounds had merely successfully deceived the psychiatrist in order to return to civilian life where they might earn large sums of money. On the other hand, commanding officers and regimental medical officers, with few exceptions, supported the psychiatrists. Moreover, among the public there was widespread expression of dissatisfaction at the arbitrary methods employed by the Army in allocating personnel, and complaints were made in the press and in Parliament.*

From the early days of the war, the Director of Military Training had been urged to employ intelligence testing as an aid to the rapid classification of recruits. Towards the end of 1939, tests devised by the Cambridge Psychological Laboratory had been introduced in anti-aircraft training units, with the purpose of selecting the specially skilled men required for A.A. gun teams. In December, 1939, the Director of Military Training proposed to carry out some limited experiments, with the co-operation of the Industrial Health Research Board, in order to ascertain whether any psychological tests might be of practical value in helping officers at training centres to find a short way to selecting suitable men for particular duties.

In July, 1940, the Army Council decided to introduce without delay selection tests into establishments and field units receiving direct intakes of recruits, in all home commands. It was emphasized that these tests, which were of established value in contributing to the selection of specialists and the acceleration of training, were intended to assist commanding officers but in no way to interfere with the exercise of their own judgement. Through the Director of Military Training and the Army Education Corps, Mr. Eric Farmer of the Cambridge Psychological Laboratory, assisted by Mr. Alec Rodger, introduced into these training centres and field units the

---

* The matter had been raised as early as 1940, and the Secretary of State for War stated that it was not considered practicable, in present conditions, to adopt a system of testing the mental capacity of recruits (*Parl. Deb.*, 5th ser., Commons, 359: 27; 2 April, 1940). Early in 1941, it was stated that any soldier with technical qualifications could now apply for trade testing, and that thousands of applications had been received (*ibid.*, 368: 1202–3; 11 Feb., 1941).

PERSONNEL SELECTION

testing of intakes by means of a verbal test, the F.H.3 (later, the F.H.R.) test. The testing was carried out by regimental officers,* and the distribution of test material and collection of results was effected by Army Education Officers.

In October, 1940, Brigadier Rees, after consultation with the Director of Military Training and Mr. Eric Farmer, made arrangements to ensure that men who obtained low scores in the tests would be examined by the Command Psychiatrists, who were thus able to interview most of the dull and backward men in the intakes.

The General Officer Commanding-in-Chief, Northern Command (Lt.-Gen. Sir Ronald F. Adam, later Adjutant-General), reported to the War Office, in October, 1940, that he was impressed by the selection tests for direct intakes, which had now been introduced throughout his command, and felt that it was important that the Army, as the greatest single employer of labour, should appreciate the value of these tests, in the same way that industrial undertakings and the Ministry of Labour had done in recent years. He also made certain suggestions for the improvement of the efficiency of the testing scheme.

These various measures obviously fell far short of requirements. In particular, it was necessary to bring about a fundamental change in the methods of allocating men to units. At that time, the allocation was carried out by the Ministry of Labour, advised only to a slight extent by Military Advisers at the Recruiting Centres, and, except in the case of tradesmen allocated to certain specialized units, was more or less haphazard.

In a memorandum, 'Notes on the Efficient Use of Man-Power', submitted in January, 1941, to the G.O.C.-in-C., Northern Command, the Command Psychiatrist (Lt.-Col. G. R. Hargreaves) recommended that both testing and disposal of recruits be placed under the control of the Adjutant-General, and that a special department be set up at the War Office to direct and administer these activities. He emphasized that the allotment of personnel should be based on the principle that no man was to be employed on work which was either definitely above or definitely below his ability, and that any other method was wasteful of ability, or destructive of unit efficiency; and that this principle was being flouted at the time in every training centre and every field unit of the British Army.

* The German Army, on the other hand, as far back as 1936, had 87 whole-time specialist officers doing this work.

PERSONNEL SELECTION

Referring to the work carried out in the selection and training of recruits in the U.S. Army during the First World War, and its very considerable development in the German Army subsequently, Col. Hargreaves observed that we, in this country, not only had ignored it during the first nine months of the Second War, but were still not in sight of the point where the Americans had left off.*

This memorandum formed the basis of further representations to the War Office, in January, 1941, concerning the serious wastage of man-power, by General Adam who pointed out that, if we were to win the war rapidly, it was essential to overhaul at once the whole system of selection and allocation, and urged that measures be adopted, such as had been recommended by Col. Hargreaves.

On this occasion, sufficient interest was aroused—it may be, with the added stimulus of the by then very serious nature, and the urgency, of the existing man-power situation—for consideration to be given to more detailed proposals, which were the subject of a second memorandum by Col. Hargreaves, in March, 1941, on 'The Selection and Allocation of Army Personnel'. On the basis of recommendations made in this document, and as a result of representations by the Consulting Psychiatrist, an Advisory Committee on Mental Testing was appointed, under the chairmanship of the Director-General, Army Medical Services, consisting of three eminent psychologists (Professor J. H. Drever, Dr. C. S. Myers, and Dr. S. J. F. Philpott).

After making investigations at many training units in the several commands, the Committee issued a preliminary report, recommending that a small number of 'central depots' be set up in each command, where the selection testing of recruits could be carried out by adequately trained staff, and supervised by officers who were specialists in selection work, able to advise and assist in the allocation of recruits to an appropriate arm and training unit. The Committee further recommended, as a matter of great importance, that immediate arrangements be made for the testing, at the central depots, of all men already engaged in Army work which was believed to be either above or below their level of intelligence, in order that they might be reallocated at the depots, for training for suitable duties.

---

* For details of the early work in the U.S. Army, cf. the book by C. S. Yoakum and R. M. Yerkes,[141] published in 1920; and the report on *Psychological Examining in the United States Army* (1921).[92] Accounts of work in the German Army have been given, e.g. by H. L. Ansbacher,[11] C. Burt,[25] P. M. Fitts,[45] J. Galvin[50] and E. Mira.[81] Cf. also P. E. Vernon and J. B. Parry.[125]

PERSONNEL SELECTION

The Committee was also of the opinion, previously expressed by Col. Hargreaves, that the work of selection and allocation which was required in the commands should be directed by a new department of the Adjutant-General's Branch of the War Office:* the Director of Military Training had the power, neither to allocate men to appropriate arms of the Service, nor to effect a rapid discharge of 'impossible' recruits or the transfer of those unsuitably allocated.

The head of this new department should be responsible for appointing the Command Specialists in Selection Tests; control the testing staffs in the various commands; and organize such other activities in this field as might be required: e.g. research into methods of increasing the efficiency and scope of selection tests, for which purpose he should employ the services of the psychologists in each command, as well as those of laboratory staffs in the Universities and elsewhere. The department should be so constituted as to maintain close liaison, both in the War Office and in the commands, with the Directorates of the Army Medical Services (especially, with the Consultants and Specialists in Psychological Medicine), and with those of Recruiting and Mobilization, and of Military Training.

On the basis of all this advisory and exploratory work, it was possible for the Adjutant-General (by then, providentially, Sir Ronald Adam), in June, 1941, to submit a plan of action for consideration by the Army Council; the latter accepted the principle of applying selection tests to Army personnel, including the A.T.S., and requested the Adjutant-General to make the necessary arrangements to give effect to his proposed scheme.

A Directorate of Selection of Personnel was, accordingly, set up, under the Adjutant-General, in June, 1941; its technical work was supervised by industrial psychologists of experience, and a system of intelligence testing, using the Progressive Matrices, was introduced at all recruiting depots. Psychiatrists interviewed all men who, through their poor performance in the tests, were placed in the lowest selection grade (S.G. 5), i.e. those who were mentally dull and backward. A.C.I. 1805/41, dealing with the 'Introduction of a System of Selective Testing in the Army', was issued in September, 1941.

In 1941–2, numerous conversions of units took place (e.g. cavalry regiments to tank battalions, etc.). Among the first of these was the

* It was pointed out, in this connection, that the American Army employed a vocational psychologist in its Adjutant-General's Department, as Director of Personnel Research; and that, in the German Army, some 200 psychologically trained men were actually employed in selection work.

formation of Reconnaissance Corps battalions. The psychiatrists undertook the testing of the men in these converted battalions, in order that those who were considered unsuitable for training in their new duties should be transferred to more suitable units. An appreciable number of soldiers in newly formed armoured units were found to be of too low intelligence to be efficient or reliable in their new duties, but officers were sometimes reluctant to authorize their transfer to simpler duties in another arm.

The purposes of these investigations were not always understood by officers and, at first, psychiatrists encountered not a little opposition and obstruction in their work. The principal reason for this attitude was discussed by a psychiatrist (Major W. R. Bion), in August, 1941, in a report on psychological tests and examinations carried out in an armoured division.

This report emphasized the fact that the tests were concerned with two distinct problems: first, the weeding out of men who were 'below average', a process involving the assessment of a man's military capacity and quality, in which the advice and assistance of combatant officers was invariably sought; and secondly, the detection of those with mental defect or emotional instability, a purely medical question upon which such officers were not competent to form an opinion. Much criticism would be seen to be baseless, if officers did not confuse these two aspects, and realized that the medical decision as to a man's unsuitability on psychiatric grounds did not constitute a critical opinion of the amount of military training he had absorbed, and did not reflect upon the ability or quality of his instructors.

Major Bion pointed out that, sooner or later, a decision would have to be made, as to whether armoured divisions subjected to the stress of active warfare could afford the risk of retaining hard-working and pleasant dullards, who were slower than the average to learn what was required of them, and whose deficiencies might not be clearly apparent in peace-time:* there was, in his opinion, an obvious advantage in employing men of superior intelligence, although their manners might be less docile during the period of training and manœuvres. For new units, it was both important and practicable to select men of higher endowment than those in Selection Groups 4 and 5 who then encumbered, and perhaps endangered, military en-

* Cf. the following statement by the Southborough Committee: "Experience shows that once a man is accepted for service it is in practice impossible to ensure that he will not be employed in the firing line; in periods of emergency military exigencies over-ride every other consideration." [128]

PERSONNEL SELECTION

terprise: the exclusion of the mentally backward and unstable would speed up training and ease the burden of already hard-pressed officers in training units.

With the development of the Directorate of Selection of Personnel, large groups of men whose work in the Army was being changed were subjected to group tests by the Personnel Selection staff, and the psychiatrist interviewed all those who were rated in the lowest selection grade, or whose selection grade was incompatible with the new duties in which it was proposed to employ them.

The psychiatrist's place in selection received official recognition by the publication, in July, 1941, of A.C.I. 1136/41, governing the recommendations of psychiatrists for transfer of men to armed and unarmed companies of the Pioneer Corps, and terminating a period in which commanding officers and psychiatrists alike made recommendations for such transfers. In the course of the next few months, it became apparent that many men had been recommended by C.O.s for transfer to unarmed companies, not because this was the most reasonable or beneficial course in the men's own interest, but because the C.O.s were anxious to get rid of them. Indeed, on re-examination by psychiatrists, after the latter had assumed sole responsibility for recommending such transfers, a large percentage of the men who had been disposed of in this way proved capable of more skilled employment.

As already mentioned, it was on the recommendation of the commanding officer, advised by the psychiatrist, that men of at least average intelligence could be transferred to such employment as was considered most suitable for them, in accordance with A.C.I. 399/40. Eventually, in January, 1942, authority was given (by A.C.I. 84/42) for the transfer or disposal, on the recommendation of psychiatrists, of men who, through mental backwardness or instability, were unfit for their present employment, but likely to become efficient either after hospital treatment or in other employment.

In the winter and spring of 1941-2, the Directorate of Selection of Personnel carried out experiments in intake selection, with the co-operation of Army psychiatrists. As the value of selection work had by then become sufficiently recognized to enable the administrative difficulties to be overcome, these experiments resulted, in July, 1942, in the introduction of the General Service Corps intake scheme.*

---

* An outline of the proposed scheme was given in May, 1942, in A.C.I. 1151/42, on the 'Policy for Selective Testing of Recruits and Common Primary Training for all Arms'.

PERSONNEL SELECTION

All men on entering the Army were now first taken into the General Service Corps where, during their period of basic training, they were subjected to a series of intelligence and aptitude tests, interviewed by specially trained Personnel Selection Officers, and subsequently, wherever possible, posted to the most appropriate duties in the Service. The function of the psychiatrist in General Service intake procedure was essentially complementary to that of the Personnel Selection Officer. Certain classes of recruits were referred to the psychiatrist for advice by the medical officer or Personnel Selection Officer: viz. men in the lowest selection group, stammerers and illiterates, men who had been educated at Special Schools, and those whose placement or assessment proved difficult because of a history of psychiatric illness, presumed psychiatric symptoms or abnormal behaviour, bizarre test results, or apparent lack of 'combatant tendency'.

Some 14% of the total intake were referred to the psychiatrist, who was able to recommend the following several methods of disposal: allocation to a specific type of employment; transfer to a primarily non-combatant arm (e.g. R.A.M.C., R.A.S.C., R.A.O.C., R.E.M.E., etc.), or to an armed or unarmed company of the Pioneer Corps; or lowering of medical category, admission to hospital, or discharge by a medical board, on account of psychiatric illness or disability.

Army selection procedure had been applied to the relatively small numbers of Royal Navy and Royal Air Force personnel who had originally been transferred to the Army in August, 1944. Subsequently, during the spring of 1945, some 16,000 men were transferred from the Royal Navy and the Royal Air Force to the Army. These men were subjected to a selection procedure of a type similar to that used in the General Service Corps intake scheme. They were required in the Army mainly for duties as infantrymen, and certain minimum standards were, therefore, laid down. Some 18% of these 16,000 men were rejected as being unsuitable for service in the particular employment in the Army for which they were required. Of the total, 10% were rejected by medical officers, 4·5% by psychiatrists, and 3·5% by Personnel Selection Officers.

The earliest memoranda on selection prepared by psychiatrists and psychologists had proposed a scheme whereby misfits already in the Army would be referred to special selection centres for disposal. Such Army Selection Centres were instituted early in 1943. A.C.I.

PERSONNEL SELECTION

393/43, issued in March, 1943, specified the types of case for which they were intended.

This A.C.I. referred to the acute man-power situation and the urgent need for employing every man in the Army on work most suited to his medical category and aptitude. In particular, attention was drawn to the fact that men whose medical category had been altered were in many cases transferred with little regard to their individual aptitude or to the man-power requirements of the different arms of the Service; and that the morale of men in low medical categories had suffered as a result of their unsuitable employment, although experience had shown that, appropriately employed and trained, such men could not only render valuable service, but release men of higher categories for more active duties.

It was proposed not only to establish Army Selection Centres, but also to increase the number of physical development centres for the remedial training of men in low medical categories on account of physical disabilities.

The psychiatrist's work in these Army Selection Centres was similar to that in the General Service intake procedure, although the cases sent there presented a very different psychiatric problem. The men referred to these Centres had, on an average, over two year's Army service, many were in the higher age-groups, and the majority were in the lower medical categories. They were all, for one reason or another, difficult to employ satisfactorily, and it was for this reason that their commanding officers transferred them to an Army Selection Centre. The methods of disposal available to the psychiatrist were similar to those in General Service work, and in addition the psychiatrist's recommendation was obtained before a soldier was sent to a Command Labour Company or a Young Soldier's Training Unit (Special Training Unit). Whereas less than 15% of General Service intakes required psychiatric opinion, almost 50% of the men sent to Army Selection Centres were referred to the psychiatrist.

It was suggested by the Directorate of Army Psychiatry, in July, 1943, that Army Selection Centres might also be used for the selection of Commando and Airborne recruits, thus widening their field of activity; it had, in fact, originally been intended that the Centres should deal with all kinds of selection in the Army (apart from that of new intakes). This suggestion was the result of advice sought from the Director of Army Psychiatry by the A.D.M.S., Combined Operations Headquarters, because of the number of psychiatric breakdowns occurring among Commandos in action. It was the opinion of the Director of Army Psychiatry that some four-fifths of such breakdowns could be prevented by adequate selection of recruits. In fact, however, no specific selection procedure was introduced for Commandos. The procedure ultimately adopted in the selection of parachutist volunteers will be referred to later.

It was further suggested by the Directorate of Army Psychiatry, in April, 1944, that all men who left a Convalescent Depot in a medical category lower than that required for their present employment and arm of Service, should proceed *direct* to the nearest Army Selection Centre. This was intended to prevent the deterioration in morale which inevitably resulted from long periods spent in 'Y'-List Depots and from several subsequent temporary postings.

The first Army Selection Centre was opened at Matlock, Derbyshire, in March, 1943. The work increased, and by the summer of 1944 there were four Centres (Matlock, Edinburgh, Croydon and Aberystwyth), with a Central Clearing House at Croydon. In April, 1944, No. 3 Army Selection Centre was allocated to 21 Army Group and thereafter dealt only with men from that formation.

In addition, an Army Selection Training Unit was established at Leeds, in August, 1943. Its purpose was primarily to train men coming from Army Selection Centres for the job in the Army for which they had been recommended; and incidentally, to give them general military training in addition to vocational training, and deal with their welfare problems. Another function of the Army Selection Training Unit was to receive escaped or repatriated prisoners of war, and to assist in their military or civil rehabilitation.

The Army Selection Centre was open to criticism. It was concerned almost entirely with sorting, and training very definitely took second place; indeed it could hardly be otherwise, in view of the diversity of arms and regiments represented in any one intake. It was a temporary attachment, during which time the men belonged to no formal unit, and this necessarily had its repercussions on the morale and the welfare of individual men. The methods employed at the Selection Centre were criticized as being too theoretical, and the desirability of obtaining, in addition, a combatant officer's opinion of the men was stressed by many visitors. Finally, the Army Selection Centres were unable to deal with all the men referred, and additional personnel and accommodation were required.

In the light of all these facts, it was therefore decided to set up a

PERSONNEL SELECTION

formation based on a divisional war establishment, which would undertake this selection, at the same time providing a certain amount of military training, and into which the technical staff would be absorbed. It was thereby possible to increase the number of men dealt with, from 2,200 to 2,650 per fortnight.

Although certain disadvantages of such an organization were foreseen from the technical aspect of selection, it was hoped that these would be more than compensated by the closer liaison between selection and training, and by the improved morale of the men. There was, in fact, general agreement that the incorporation of the Centres within the Division had raised the morale of the men, who felt that they belonged to a unit whose function they understood. Further, it was hoped that selection would be more accurate if a unit Grading Board were established which not only would be in possession of the findings recorded by the Personnel Selection Officer, but would also have the opinion of a man's Company Commander and the results of the military and physical tests of elementary training. The unit was set up as 77 Division, with its Division H.Q. at Darlington. The staff included an Adviser in Psychiatry (Lt.-Col. R. F. Barbour). In November, 1944, the first intake was received, and intakes were admitted weekly until April, 1945, when the divisional units, redesignated as 45 Division, were reorganized in order to deal with all repatriated prisoners of war.*

By the beginning of 1946, the man-power situation had changed, and as a result of the speeding up of the release scheme there was a very considerable and urgent demand for men for certain extra-regimental employments which had generally been carried out previously by older men of low medical category. 45 Division was reorganized to deal with this new situation. Soon afterwards, the Division was disbanded and, in April, 1946, the responsibility for sorting and reallocation of men was undertaken by the Selection Wing of the War Office Selection Centre, at Lingfield, Surrey. This unit was concerned only with selection (including psychiatric examination, when required), and did not undertake any training. Early in 1947, the Selection Wing closed, and its functions were carried out by Senior Personnel Selection Officers of commands (where necessary, in conjunction with medical officers and psychiatrists).†

* The functions and procedure of 45 Divisions were set out in A.C.I. 389/45, in April, 1945.
† The introduction into the Army of the Arms Basic Training Unit system, in March, 1948, placed the responsibility for reallocation on the Senior Personnel

PERSONNEL SELECTION

The selection of the A.T.S. had never been carried out along similar lines to that of soldiers. There was no routine referral of specified cases to Army psychiatrists on recruitment, but a considerable number of recruits were always referred from A.T.S. Training Centres as ordinary out-patients. In March, 1943, the experimental Selection Centre, A.T.S., was set up. The general procedure was similar to that in Army Selection Centres, apart from the fact that the smaller numbers involved allowed the adoption of a board technique, the psychiatrist being a member of the unit board.

In February, 1943, in view of the man-power situation, it was decided to discharge while still at Primary Training Centres men who had been placed in medical category 'C' and who were not employable in clerical duties. The wisdom of this decision was subsequently questioned on several occasions, and eventually, in July, 1944, 78 men who were due to be discharged in accordance with this policy were submitted to a special investigation. Of the 12 men of this number who had been placed in Category 'C' on psychiatric grounds, 10 were unemployable and only 2 were suitable for strictly limited employment. These and certain other investigations confirmed the view that men placed in category 'C' for psychiatric reasons could, in the vast majority of cases, make no useful contribution to the Service; and it was felt that these untrained soldiers, if retained, would not only prove a liability to the Army, but consume valuable general medical and specialist time and man-power, out of all proportion to their usefulness. In July, 1945, it was decided that all recruits found unfit for service except in the Pioneer Corps, or who were capable only of performing simple routine duties, should be discharged at the Primary Training Unit.

In January, 1943, an investigation was initiated by Army psychiatrists, to ascertain whether psychiatric examination and selection of paratroop volunteers could reduce the wastage rate. During this enquiry it was found that, of those accepted by the methods in use at that time, nearly one-quarter (24%) failed during parachute training, and that among those who succeeded in qualifying as parachutists there had been a heavy wastage during collective training in the battalions.

Selection Officer of the arm (cf. A.C.I. 276/48, issued in April, 1948). This new system of basic training, which replaced the General Service intake system, and the simultaneous introduction into the Army, in April, 1948, of the 'Pulheems' system of medical (including psychiatric) classification, naturally brought about certain modifications in selection and psychiatric procedure which, however, are not within the scope of the present work.

PERSONNEL SELECTION

The psychiatrists who undertook the enquiry began by taking the parachute training course and qualifying as parachutists. They then interviewed all volunteers at the Airborne Forces Depot, before these men began their training. As a result of this examination they were able to give a psychiatric 'predictive' grading to each volunteer, but no action was taken on the basis of these gradings, which were not made known either to the men or to the members of the Depot staff. By following up the men during training, it became possible to correct the original psychiatric standards by experience: thus, in due course a 'screening' process similar to that employed by the W.O.S.B.s, comprising a series of written tests and carried out by Sergeant Testers, was introduced, which made it possible to select cases for individual psychiatric interview while dispensing with the necessity of interviewing all volunteers. A few cases in which interpretation of the tests proved impossible were referred for psychiatric interview, as were all men in the two lowest predictive grades.

It was shown that the predictive grades allotted by the psychiatrist after interview had a high correlation with those obtained by the screening process, and the psychiatric gradings showed a high correlation with instructors' assessments at the training centre. Follow-up studies showed that psychiatric grades provided effective prediction of all forms of training wastage other than through accidental injuries. As a result of these experiments it was possible to estimate that, had the men in the lowest psychiatric predictive grade and those considered unsuitable by the Depot medical officers (for physical reasons) been rejected before training, the wastage during training would have been reduced to about 10% and some 80% of the volunteers would have been accepted for training.

A report, at the beginning of 1944, on the results of the new method of selection of paratroop volunteers, showed that this earlier estimate had proved correct. About 20% of volunteers were rejected at the initial selection stage, the great majority of these men being rejected by the psychiatrist and by the medical officer.* About 70% of all candidates arriving at the Depot completed the course successfully, and the training wastage did not rise above 10%. Thus, more than four-fifths (84%) of the total wastage was eliminated from the training period by selective methods, or in other words, occurred at the initial selection stage. It was, therefore, clear that here was yet

* Of those men rejected by the psychiatrist and the medical officer, about one-half were rejected by the former, one-quarter by the latter, and one-quarter by both.

another instance in which the application of scientific selection had proved of very real value and had achieved its purpose.

The training staff were very satisfied with these results and the consequent small training wastage. It was obvious that the right men were being selected for parachute *training*, but it was felt that some effort should be made to obtain evidence that the men who had been selected were equally successful in actual *operational* work. For this purpose, a psychiatrist who had been engaged in the selection work at Airborne Forces Depot was sent to North Africa and Italy in the latter half of 1943. However, although the Airborne Division expressed themselves as perfectly satisfied with the men they were receiving, it was not possible to obtain statistical proof of the success of the selection method: the subjective opinions of N.C.O.s, Platoon and Company Commanders, respectively, as to the value of the individual men obviously showed little or no correlation, depending as they did largely on interpersonal emotional relationships.

The clinical experience of Army psychiatrists suggested that the selection of Army apprentices was by no means sufficiently stringent. This fact was particularly emphasized by the problem which frequently arose of having to decide upon the correct disposal of any apprentices who had developed a neurotic illness or had shown other signs of maladjustment. An investigation into this question was undertaken by an Army psychiatrist (Major A. A. Baker), in September, 1947. Examination of intakes into Army Apprentices' Schools revealed that the actual wastage, through administrative or medical discharge, of apprentices was in the region of 10%. Although the majority of these boys were discharged within one year of entering the Army, a certain number were not discharged until after more than one year's training, and it was noted that the latter had a definite adverse effect on the morale of the other apprentices.

A scheme was suggested, which would make it possible to detect *at intake* those boys who were unsuitable because of low intelligence or temperamental instability. It was recommended that all boys should be tested and interviewed at intake by the Personnel Selection Officer, and that those considered unsuitable or of doubtful stability should be referred to the psychiatrist. Boys found to be unsuitable should be discharged at once. In doubtful cases, they should be retained and re-examined after a few months. The enlistment of boys who appeared to be relatively immature but basically stable, should

PERSONNEL SELECTION

be deferred for one year, at the end of which period they would usually be found to be suitable for enlistment.

The investigation revealed the very great importance of adequate selection of these boys. At one apprentices' training wing, it was estimated that about half the boys in one particular intake were unsuitable. In the great majority of cases where boys developed neurotic symptoms or became disciplinary problems, and were eventually discharged, their unsuitability could have been predicted with reasonable certainty. A few boys had been definitely unwilling to become apprentices; their story was almost identical in each case: the boy came from an unhappy home, had been employed in several civilian jobs and had failed to settle down, and was forced by his parents to join the Army 'as a punishment'.

The report noted that defects in the existing system, by which a boy was only discharged from the Army when he had become a medical or disciplinary casualty, had been emphasized by some recent clinical cases. One lad, of poor personality, intelligence and home background, was eventually discharged on administrative grounds after six months' service which included three visits to a psychiatrist, two spells in hospital, repeated disciplinary offences and a staged 'suicidal attempt'. It was pointed out that it should not be necessary for a boy, unsuited to Army life, to be forced to demonstrate this by such gross behaviour before he could be discharged as unsuitable. Considerable pressure was sometimes brought on the psychiatrist to discharge an unsuitable apprentice on medical grounds 'because administrative discharge would take so long'. The report emphasized yet again that the longer a misfit remains in a unit, the greater the harm done both to his and to the unit's morale.

It was also found that a number of boys entered the Army with very little idea of the nature of the training ahead of them. Indeed, it was surprising how many of them expect an apprentice's life in the Army without any training as a soldier at all. Major Baker commented that the boy with the character of the type the Army requires would not be discouraged by accurate accounts of Army life, but would certainly feel some resentment if he was misled by rosy pictures painted by an enthusiastic recruiting officer. It was manifestly unfair that a boy who had joined the R.A.O.C. because he was told at the recruiting office that, once in the Army, he could apply for a transfer to the real unit of his choice, should then find that this promise could not be kept; as also that his parents should have to

PERSONNEL SELECTION

pay £20 to release him. To solve this unsatisfactory problem, it was suggested that boys who had joined a unit which did not provide the training they required should either be transferred at once (i.e. within one month of entry) or be given the option of discharge without payment on their part. The financial loss from the Army's viewpoint would be negligible compared with that involved in training an unwilling boy at a trade he did not intend to follow, and that resulting from the medical and disciplinary consequences of maladjustment.

In conclusion, the following statement by Dr. J. R. Rees, in 1943, may provide a fitting summary of the aims and ultimate achievements of those engaged in personnel selection in the Army in the Second World War: "The Directorate for Selection of Personnel had undertaken a complete job-analysis of the multitudinous tasks in the different arms of the Service, and as a result was able to lay down the standards of intelligence and other aptitudes necessary for each job, thus providing a basis for the correct posting of men in certain proportions to each type of unit. The accomplishment of this work produced a revolutionary change in the Army's utilization of manpower and has set a standard which will certainly be applied in industry and in social life in the post-war world. The matching of men to suitable work is as valuable a means of psychiatric prophylaxis as anything that could well be devised.

"In this mass selection of men Psychiatry is perhaps the handmaid of Industrial Psychology, whereas in other fields—e.g. officer selection, and with other groups in which temperamental factors must be assessed—Psychology is the handmaid of Psychiatry. In fact, in the Army the psychologists and the psychiatrists work together as a team in the best possible way, and their interdependence is fully demonstrated." [96] *

---

* Complementary to the foregoing survey of the psychiatric contributions to personnel selection in the Army, cf. the comprehensive account of the psychologists' work in this field, by P. E. Vernon and J. B. Parry, *Personnel Selection in the British Forces*.[125] Cf. also T. F. Rodger.[109]

III

OFFICER SELECTION

> ... When a young man, reeking of perfume, came to thank him for promotion in rank, Vespasian turned his head away in disgust and cancelled the order, saying crushingly: "I should not have minded so much if it had been garlic."
> SUETONIUS, *De Vita Caesarum*

"THE CAPACITY FOR LEADERSHIP, the ability, character and insight of the officer are of paramount importance for the happiness and welfare as well as for the efficiency of the men he commands. Far too many men have broken down because of having indifferent officers. Too many units have failed in their task at some vital moment because they were inadequately led and insufficiently knit together as a team." [97] Thus, one of the most important factors in influencing individual and group morale is the quality of the leadership. In peace-time, the Army chose its officers with some care; those who selected them knew the types of young men coming up through certain schools, knew and understood their background, and were, as a rule, reasonably well able to assess their quality. There were, of course, not a few exceptions to this rule.

In the First War, when the need for officers became urgent, men could be judged on the qualities which they had shown as non-commissioned officers in actual battle, and accordingly selected and sent for training as officers. This ideal method of selection was not, however, practicable, except in a small number of cases, in the early days of the Second World War.

The authorities were much concerned, about 1941, at the high rejection rate from Officer Cadet Training Units, and because unsuitable men were being selected for training and then had to be

OFFICER SELECTION

rejected, there was a serious wastage of training time, and obviously, the morale of the O.C.T.U.s was adversely affected by the large proportion of failures. A highly undesirable result of such rejections was that an excellent N.C.O., who had, however, reached the summit of his potentialities, would be sent up to the O.C.T.U., would fail there and return to his unit, a dissatisfied man and no longer a good N.C.O.

Candidates were recommended by their commanding officers, but were selected largely as a result of a ten- or fifteen-minute interview by a small Command Interview Board of senior officers.

It was clear that some unsuitable and unstable men were given commissions. On the other hand, there was reason to believe that not all suitable men found their way to Command Interview Boards and that those who did arrive there were by no means invariably passed to O.C.T.U.s There was no scientific testing: a candidate stood or fell by the first, subjective impression he created, and this procedure was ironically, but aptly, referred to as the the 'magic eye technique'.*

Whatever might be said about such oneiromantic methods of selection, it could not reasonably be argued that they had any objective, scientific validity. Psychiatrists and psychologists were well aware that the decisions of this type of selection board were to a great extent affectively determined and on occasion, no doubt, influenced by a somewhat inordinate, unconscious affinity for $‛οι καλοί$. The position at that time has been well summarized by Brigadier Rees: "Since the supply of young men from the universities and public schools was drying up, the interviewing officers sometimes found themselves rather at sea, since for purposes of rapid assessment they understood too little of the background and outlook of many of the candidates whose civil life experience had been so completely different from anything of which they had previous knowledge. A candidate who could 'sell' himself well might get past, though unsuitable; the diffident candidate, though potentially admirable, might be failed." [97]

* One is reminded of the recruiting advertisement which appeared, some years ago, in the daily press: it shows a young Naval officer, obviously on a visit to the Old School, watching the boys playing cricket; he has turned to speak to the Head, and is pointing with his pipe in the general direction of the cricketers. Under the picture, in large letters, is written: 'Now HE looks a likely lad . . .' Cf. also the statement by Lord Moran: "I remember a member of your Lordships' House . . . once saying to me: 'I know when a man comes through the door if he is my man.' . . . But these men are far too few. . . . Their methods evade definition; they are subjective—they cannot be taught to others" (*Parl. Deb.*, 5th ser., Lords, **155**: 1049–50; 26 May, 1948). No doubt, such men are rare indeed; it is also possible that 'such men are dangerous'.

OFFICER SELECTION

There was, in fact, general dissatisfaction in the Army and throughout the country in regard to the existing methods of officer selection, and this public concern was reflected in the numerous questions on the subject in the House of Commons, from the end of October, 1939, onwards.*

In 1941, when the Army psychiatrists were first asked to undertake experiments in officer selection, the rejection rate at O.C.T.U.s varied from 20% to 50%. Selection methods had already been initiated for other ranks, and it was only logical that their application to officer candidates should be considered in an effort to improve this most unsatisfactory situation.

At this stage of the war, Army psychiatrists had accumulated considerable knowledge of the Army and its personnel problems. They were constantly aware of the fact that psychiatric factors were often responsible for producing inefficiency in officers, and that the rate of psychiatric breakdown among officers was high. A considerable number of officers had been brought back from the reserve although they were, in fact, unfit for military service. Some of these had even been in receipt of disability pensions for neurosis since the First World War; many had clearly been inefficient on psychiatric grounds for some appreciable time before they were sent for a psychiatric interview. In addition, a fair number of men, newly commissioned from the ranks, had a history of psychiatric instability which should have excluded them. It was also evident that neurotic breakdown had often occurred because a man was unable to carry a degree of responsibility commensurate with his increase in rank. In view of these facts it was natural that the authorities should seek advice from the psychiatrists, whose work had shown the usefulness of their training in personality assessment. It seemed certain that psychiatric examination of candidates for commissions would reveal a large proportion

---

* Cf. successive ministerial statements: "Everybody knows that the system for provision of officers ... could hardly be more democratic than it is" (*Parl. Deb.*, 5th ser., Commons, 355: 1005; 12 Dec., 1939). The selection of officers "is based on personality, power of leadership and intelligence" (it was not made clear how these qualities were assessed) (*ibid.*, 356: 355; 23 Jan., 1940). The nature and aims of the new system were outlined: "These tests are being slowly introduced ... for a special reason. They have been in use in the German Army and in the American Army for some time, but we are not Germans or Americans, and we were not sure that the tests of other nations might prove applicable to our own people" (*ibid.*, 377: 1987–92; 19 Feb., 1942). "... It has been decided thoroughly to re-examine the existing methods of selecting officers, ... to ensure that the best possible use is made of the available officer material of the Army. I do not wish to suggest that the present system ... is failing to produce the best men. On the other hand, this is so vital a matter that it is just as well to make quite sure" (*ibid.*, 378: 1150; 11 March, 1942).

OFFICER SELECTION

of those who would be likely to fail, for one reason or another, in their training and service.

It should be emphasized that officer selection was, from the outset, essentially a rejection procedure. The candidates were already selected by their C.O.s, and the function of any selection procedure was to be limited to the rejection of those men who were considered unlikely to succeed. The psychiatrists were asked to investigate methods of lowering the rejection rate at O.C.T.U.s, and were not asked to find means of selecting men from units.*

At the end of June, 1941, at a meeting held at the War Office to discuss the institution of psychological tests for the Army as a whole, the Adjutant-General (Lt.-Gen. Sir Ronald Adam) stated that he was not satisfied with the existing system of selection of candidates for O.C.T.U.s, and asked for the development of a test, possibly on the German model, for officer candidates. It was agreed that intensive research over a period of some three months would be required at one or two O.C.T.U.s, in order to test the suitability of personality tests of the German type. In the meantime, it was suggested, some improvement in the existing system of officer selection might be introduced, and the application of a higher type of group test and possibly of standardized interviews should be considered.

It was first ascertained, by a thorough examination of all candidates by medical specialists (physicians), that the standard physical examinations which the men had received prior to being sent up for training were adequate. Thus, it appeared that the main emphasis was to be placed on the psychiatric aspect of the problem. With the encouragement of the Adjutant-General, various preliminary experiments were started, in July, 1941, to discover possible techniques for the rapid selection of large numbers of candidates.

To aid in selection, psychological tests had been used in the armies of a great many countries in all parts of the world.† The German Army, for example, from about 1926, had used scientific methods of selection of officers and specialists. In June, 1941, at the suggestion of the Consulting Psychiatrist to the Army, the Command Psychiatrist, Scottish Command (Lt.-Col. T. F. Rodger), with the co-operation

* Much of the historical account here given of the early development of the War Office Selection Boards is based on the summary by Lt.-Cols. T. F. Rodger and J. D. Sutherland, in their important and valuable report on 'The Role and Status of the Psychiatrist in the War Office Selection Boards' (September, 1943).

† A useful survey of the methods employed and the results obtained, during the years preceding the Second World War, was made in 1941 by T. W. Harrell and R. D. Churchill.[56]

of a civilian psychiatric research worker (Dr., later Major, E. Wittkower), had already begun unofficial experiments designed to test the value of psychological methods in the assessment of officer candidates. Professor F. A. E. Crew (later Brigadier, Director of Medical Research, Army Medical Department) placed at their disposal his laboratory in the University of Edinburgh.

Routine intelligence testing, as it became available throughout the British Army, gave a rough indication of the group from which potential officers should be chosen, i.e. those men with an intelligence above average. It was, of course, realized that intelligence alone did not fit a man to be an officer. Personality, character and temperament were of equal importance, and to test these, special methods were evolved. In other words, it was intended through these unofficial experiments, to estimate the value of psychological methods applied to personality testing. From a study of such methods as had been employed elsewhere, it was decided that, in order to gain insight into a candidate's personality, it was necessary to adopt an approach in which the technique of the individual personal interview (by highly skilled interviewers) and the test methods of the psychological research worker were combined with observations of the individual's performance of practical tasks.

A procedure of this sort was devised, and as a first experimental trial, with the co-operation of the G.O.C.-in-C., Scottish Command, the two psychiatrists studied a group of some 50 officers attending the Company Commanders' School in Edinburgh. This School provided advanced training for officers who had already had experience in the Army as junior officers. A good deal was, therefore, already known about the officer qualities of the students when they joined the course.

An assessment of officer quality was made on the basis of a group intelligence test, a short questionnaire, and a psychiatric interview which lasted about one hour. Some effort was made to reproduce and try out the German Army methods of officer selection. To reveal temperamental and personality factors, laboratory tests were provided. It was then possible to compare the opinion formed on each candidate by the psychiatrist, on the basis of assessment procedure lasting about 2–3 hours, with that formed by the Commandant and staff of the School on the basis of their own experience and close observation during five weeks.

The results of these experiments were very encouraging, since there

OFFICER SELECTION

was agreement in some 80% of the cases between the psychiatric opinions and those of the staff of the school. It was found that in nine-tenths of the candidates about whom there was disagreement, there were underlying personality deviations which had escaped the attention of the Commandant. In some cases the psychological abnormality was severe. In a memorandum on this first experiment, issued in September, 1941, the psychiatrists reached the following tentative conclusions: (i) A psychological interview, provided that the results of an intelligence test were taken into account, gave an accurate assessment of the qualities of an officer. (ii) The time employed in this procedure was too long, necessitating as it did, for each candidate, the individual attention of a skilled psychiatrist for one hour. (iii) The auxiliary tests employed would give a rough indication of the defects and potentialities of the candidate, and it was reasonable to assume that, if the results of these tests were available prior to the interview, the latter could be shortened (to a period of, say, $\frac{1}{4}$ hour) and still give valuable results. (iv) The accuracy of the indication provided by these auxiliary tests would be increased if more tests could be devised and employed. (v) The examiner could undertake a further, longer examination in cases where he was left in doubt after the shorter interview suggested.

A second group of officers, studied in the same way, gave even better results; agreement between the psychiatric opinions and the School reports rose to 90%, a fact which was attributed to the mutual education of the Commanding Officer and the psychiatrists in the significance of the personality characteristics relevant to officer quality.

The study of the two groups, comprising a total of nearly 100 officers, demonstrated that psychiatrists could, on the basis of intelligence tests and a one-hour interview, reach an estimate of officer quality which had a high correlation with that made by experienced Army officers after four or five weeks' close contact with the subjects under the working conditions of the School. In the study of the second group of officers, the psychiatrists were assisted by a psychologist in conducting the laboratory tests.

As a result of these preliminary investigations, a conference was held in Edinburgh in December, 1941, at which the tests used were demonstrated to the Adjutant-General, the Director of Selection of Personnel, and the Army Commander in Scotland. The psychiatrists concerned pointed out that their initial experiments demonstrated

OFFICER SELECTION

that the only successful technique so far achieved was an assessment based on the intelligence test and psychiatric interview. The experiments carried out with the laboratory tests had not yet reached a stage where any specified testing procedure of this kind could be recommended, but the importance of pursuing investigations along these lines, with the collaboration of psychologists, was stressed. Various possible organizations were discussed, and it was agreed that the selection unit should take the form of a board. The president of the Board should be an experienced senior regular officer who would interview each candidate. Specially selected regimental officers, to be known as Military Testing Officers, would observe the candidate in military situations and provide the Board with common-sense judgements on his military value. It was decided to set up an experimental unit, and, if this proved successful, other Boards would be established.

In order to corroborate the findings of Lt.-Col. T. F. Rodger and Major E. Wittkower as a result of their preliminary experiments, a further investigation was carried out, between January and August, 1942, on a series of over 200 officers attending the Company Commanders' School in Edinburgh. On the basis of their interviews and the scores in intelligence tests, the psychiatrists were able to confirm that their opinion on the officer quality of the students agreed with the opinion of the C.O. and staff of the School, on an average, in some 90% of cases. It was found that, provided experience and training were adequate, the psychiatrist in his interview could achieve a high degree of reliability when estimating officer quality. In the cases of divergence of opinion between the psychiatrists and the School, it was found that there were differences in estimations of intelligence, in the interpretation of personality, or due to discovery of latent psychiatric disability, in that order of frequency. About half of the divergent opinions were reconciled after discussion.

The experimental Board was formed in January, 1942, in Scottish Command, and became No. 1 War Office Selection Board (W.O.S.B.). It consisted of a president, a Military Testing Officer, two psychiatrists, one psychologist and two Sergeant Testers (of the Personnel Selection staff). After some preliminary discussions and trials of the tests, the first batch of officer candidates was examined in February. A medical specialist was also attached to No. 1 W.O.S.B. at its inception.

From the results of the experimental trials at the Company

OFFICER SELECTION

Commanders' School, the Adjutant-General decided that each candidate would be interviewed by a psychiatrist, and the testing procedure was designed to include an interview with the president, and military and psychological tests. A programme of military tests was devised, and the Military Testing Officer and president made separate and relatively complete reports on each candidate. Originally, each member of the Board was regarded as filling an independent role, and the separate reports of each were brought together for the first time at a final conference. From the start, the work of the psychologists and the psychiatrists was closely integrated, and was largely directed towards the development of a satisfactory battery of written tests. The first psychologist of the Board (Lt.-Col. J. D. Sutherland) was, in fact, a psychiatrist as well, and throughout this experimental phase contact was maintained with an experienced psychologist, who later came into the Army as Senior Psychologist (Lt.-Col. E. L. Trist). The psychiatrists, psychologist and Sergeant Testers constituted, in effect, the technical department of the Board. Various types of personality test were at first used experimentally, but most of these had to be abandoned on account of the time required for either their interpretation or their administration.

By March, 1942, a technique for the selection of officers had been developed to the satisfaction of the War Office, and it became possible to establish permanent W.O.S.B.s in every part of the United Kingdom and, later, with the Forces overseas. Within a year of the formation of the first experimental W.O.S.B., every candidate for an emergency commission was appearing before one of these Boards. In addition to the W.O.S.B.s in this country, there came into being at various periods of the war, from the middle of 1943 onwards, and according to the requirements of particular theatres of operations, one W.O.S.B. each for B.N.A.F., Gibraltar, C.M.F. and B.L.A., three Middle East Officer Selection Boards for M.E.F., five Service Selection Boards for India Command* and one for A.L.F.S.E.A. The staff of each Board at first consisted, as a rule, of a president and a deputy president (senior regular officers), three Military Testing Officers (line officers of some experience), one or two psychiatrists, a psychologist and Sergeant Testers.

* The Consultant Psychiatrist to India Command (Brigadier E. A. Bennet) at first encountered not a little opposition to the proposed introduction of W.O.S.B. procedure in India: he was, however, subsequently able to confer on the subject with General Wavell, then C.-in-C., who was satisfied as to the potential value of the new methods of officer selection.

OFFICER SELECTION

The experimental Board eventually became the Research and Training Centre,* which had the function of carrying out research into the selection techniques, with a view to determining their value, and improving and developing the tests, and of training specialist staff to carry out the practical testing at W.O.S.B.s. This function was later taken over by No. 25 W.O.S.B.

After the introduction of the General Service intake scheme in July, 1942, men who were regarded as potential officer material, on the basis of tests and interview by the Personnel Selection Officer at a Primary Training Centre, were given 'Officer Rating 1', which was recorded in their documents. These men, and any others recommended by their C.O., were sent to W.O.S.B.s. Having been passed by a W.O.S.B., officer cadets proceeded for training, in the case of infantry to a Leader Training Battalion, and in the case of other arms to a Basic O.C.T.U. Those who passed at the Leader Training Battalion or Basic O.C.T.U., if intended for a non-fighting arm, such as R.E.M.E., were commissioned direct into that arm, and if intended for a fighting arm, were sent to the O.C.T.U. for their particular arm, where they might pass or fail.

It is now proposed to survey in more detail the development of the work of the psychiatrist and the psychologist at the W.O.S.B.s. At an early stage, certain practical considerations had to be faced, which determined the trend of future developments. The first of these was the large number of officer cadets required by the Army in the course of the year following the introduction of the Boards, and the second was the shortage of adequately trained psychiatrists and psychologists.

It was, therefore, necessary to abandon the investigations dealing with more refined tests for the assessment of the individual, and to replace these by procedures which could deal adequately with large numbers. The scarcity of psychologists made it impossible at the time to preserve the original pattern of the Boards, as at No. 1 W.O.S.B. The new Boards could not each have a psychologist, and could have only one psychiatrist who was unable to interview all candidates at sufficient length to permit a comprehensive appraisal. To meet this situation Psychological Departments, amalgamating the work of the psychiatrist and psychologist, were established at the Boards, and consisted of the psychiatrist (in charge), and specially trained Sergeant Testers acting as psychological assistants.

* This had originally been given the unsatisfactory designation, 'Control and Development Centre'.

OFFICER SELECTION

After some experimental trials, a battery of written group tests was evolved, which provided, as well as a measure of the candidate's ability, a 'personality pointer', the function of which was to direct the psychiatrist's attention to certain features requiring investigation in his interview. That is to say, the written test battery was to be used primarily as a 'screen' for separating candidates into three groups: candidates in the 'doubtful' group required careful assessment in a more lengthy psychiatric interview, whereas for those in the 'poor' and 'good' groups, the interview could be shortened considerably without loss of efficiency. Care was taken to avoid having all the long interviews consecutively, so that candidates would not be aware that they had been singled out for special psychiatric investigation.

As a result of the establishment of Psychological Departments, psychiatrists' reports at final Board conferences came to include all the findings of the psychological tests as well as those of the interview.

Simultaneously, the pressure of work on the president gave rise to the question, whether a form of 'screening' could similarly be provided for his use. It was to meet this need, in the first place, that Major W. R. Bion developed the so-called 'Leaderless Group' method.[19]

Major Bion has summarized the development and technique of the Leaderless Group tests as follows: "When the War Office Selection Boards were set up it was believed by many that both the supply and the quality of officers were falling off and must continue to fall off as the war went on. There was certainly very little doubt that the belief was true in so far as it referred to the past. But as the senior psychiatrist called in to advise on selection and methods of selection, I pointed out that there was no reason why this statement should be regarded as an axiom. It could be maintained that in a nation at war the supply of leaders could be made to increase and their quality, thanks to the compulsion of national need, could be made to improve.... The proposals put forward to bring this state of affairs to pass, over the whole field of selection and not merely at the War Office Selection Boards, were rejected.... It became necessary to confine our activities to the selection of candidates from among those who appeared at the Boards.

"The essence of the technique which was evolved, and which has since become the basis of selection techniques in many different fields, was to provide a framework in which selecting officers, including a psychiatrist, could observe a man's capacity for maintaining personal relationships in a situation of strain that tempted him to disregard the interests of his fellows for the sake of his own. The situation had to be a real life situation. The situation of strain, and the temptation to give full rein to his personal ambitions was already there; the candidate arrived prepared to do his best and get himself a commission and, naturally, he feared the possibility of failure. Furthermore this was a real life situation. The problem was to make capital of this existing emotional field in order to test the quality of the man's relationships with his fellows.

"This was done by a method so simple and so obvious, when it has been propounded, that its revolutionary nature can easily be lost sight of. The man found he was not entered in a free-for-all competition with other candidates. Instead he found himself the member of a group and, apparently, all the tests were tests, not of himself, but of the group. In concrete terms, a group of eight or nine candidates ... was told to build, say, a bridge. No lead was given about organization or leadership; these were left to emerge and it was the duty of the observing officers to watch how any given man was reconciling his personal ambitions, hopes and fears with the requirements exacted by the group for its success. That, in brief outline, is the basic principle of all the Leaderless Group Tests.

"A little consideration will show that the situation thus created is very closely parallel with countless other emotional situations in an officer's life, not even excluding action. For though the emotional tensions in this situation are low compared with those in battle, they are nevertheless sufficiently powerful to make all candidates feel that their time at a War Office Selection Board has been a heavy strain despite the interest of the experience and the apparently easy programme. It was found that if the testing officers watch what they are meant to watch they have no difficulty in matching what they have found out about a man's personality with what they know will be the sort of job with which he will have to cope as an officer.

"... It is important to insist that the actual task of the test is merely a cloak of invisibility for the testing officers who are present; an artificiality intended to explain, and therefore to explain away, the presence of the testing officers. It is not the artificial test, but the real life situation that has to be watched—that is, the way in which a man's capacity for personal relationships stands up under the strain of his own and other men's fear of failure and desires for personal success." [19]

The Leaderless Group tests were not intended to replace all other tests, but to shed light, so far as possible in isolation, on certain important qualities of personality affecting inter-personal relationships, and this they achieved to a greater extent than any other test hitherto elaborated.

Not only did this method of investigation provide the president with a useful form of screening, but also it enabled each member of the Board to obtain a far more complete and integrated picture of the candidates' personality and character, and consequently it was invaluable as a means of reconciling discrepant opinions in cases where, formerly, the one-sided and independent approach of the several members might have led to disagreement at a final Board conference, when each compared his assessments with those of his colleagues for the first time. For implicit in the Leaderless Group method was the concept of the observer team in which the three Board members (president, Military Testing Officer, and psychiatrist) shared, at an early stage in the Board's proceedings, a common experience of the candidate, to which each could subsequently refer the findings of his own special investigations. Thus, differences of opinion could be resolved through the process of investigation rather than merely by argument at the conclusion of the proceedings.

The Leaderless Group technique, and its corollary of the observer team, provided the psychiatrist with a second method of screening, the results of which could be compared with the findings of the personality pointers. On the basis of these two methods of sorting, he could be reasonably certain as to which candidates might safely be given only a short interview, and which of them would require a longer one before a final judgement could be made. Despite these screening procedures, however, many psychiatrists still felt that their opinion on candidates whom they had not interviewed at length, was not of the same value as that which they could form as a result of a full interview. They were aware of a lack of knowledge of the pattern of the candidate's psychological development, which such interview alone could give them.

From the start, the psychiatrist had two main functions at the W.O.S.B. As technical adviser, he was expected to give an expert opinion on the psychological aspects of the military tests, a function which he carried out in co-operation with the psychologist on the Board, and the technical staff of the Research and Training Centre. As medical examiner, he originally interviewed every candidate, and

OFFICER SELECTION

was, therefore, in a position to assess personality and stability in each case.[46]

Because of the large numbers of candidates and the short supply of psychiatrists, it became impossible to maintain the original policy, in spite of the psychological tests which were designed to shorten the interview. When only one psychiatrist was available on the Board, it was necessary to alter the procedure so that he interviewed only the 'doubtful' cases. Consequently, a system had to be introduced whereby the president and Military Testing Officer could refer to the psychiatrist candidates about whom they felt uncertain, even if such cases had not been singled out as 'doubtful' by the personality pointers. In the case of those candidates whom he could not interview, the psychiatrist did not feel that he was in a position to provide the president with technical information other than intelligence test results. One consequence of this was that some presidents, faced with the position of having an incomplete technical report, wished to have access to the rough data of the personality pointers. This course was opposed on the grounds that the rough data required psychiatric interpretation, and that some of the tests had been given on the understanding that they were confidential to a medical man. It was the view of psychologists and psychiatrists that reports based on the personality pointers and read at the final Board conference, should be the responsibility of the psychiatrist, as senior technical adviser, or, in his absence, of the psychologist.

When the Selection Boards were first organized, it was believed by some of the senior officers concerned that the original work had been so successful that all that was necessary to ensure adequate selection was a psychiatric interview and intelligence tests. In fact, it was often thought at that time that the non-technical members of the Board served no other purpose than to provide 'cover' for the psychiatrist. However, "from very early days it became obvious that they were not just there for the sake of respectability but that the three lines of approach to the candidates, when fused, were likely to produce the fairest and best ultimate result. . . . The task of the doctor and the psychiatrist is to advise on physical and mental fitness, but the final word and assessment should be given by a man experienced in the particular job for which the candidate is being selected, in this case a senior Army officer." [97]

It was, of course, to be expected that many objections would be raised to the psychiatric contribution to officer selection. A very

OFFICER SELECTION

senior regular officer who was of the greatest assistance in the development of these special Boards had, before the recent war, the distinction of being the only serving British officer to have seen the German Army officer selection work in progress. His suggestion, on returning to this country, that similar methods might be introduced into the British Army was firmly rejected with the words: "X—you're the bloody Freud of the British Army!" [97]

For reasons which were primarily political, presidents of Selection Boards were instructed, in March, 1943, that the duties of psychiatrists should be confined to interviewing cases referred by the president, which must not comprise more than 50% of the candidates. The value to the Board of the psychiatrist as medical examiner was consequently almost entirely stultified. As a result of this policy, a very considerable proportion of candidates were dealt with by the Boards without an effective third opinion. Unfortunately, such a procedure also inevitably encouraged the misconception, already current among external critics, that the psychiatrist only interviewed 'abnormals', and rendered more apprehensive and critical, in this respect, those who felt that they had been singled out for a more searching test.

A certain number of complaints were made about the tactlessness of psychiatrists in their interviews. In particular, questions on sex and religion, asked by psychiatrists in individual cases for specific technical reasons, were taken out of their context and gave rise to distorted generalizations, on the tenuous basis of highly coloured statements by a few rejected candidates. Some of the criticism was, however, justified: one or two psychiatrists were inclined unnecessarily to ask embarrassing questions which were resented by the candidates, and, as soon as this became known, were removed from the Boards. In introducing a revolutionary procedure and adapting it to meet the immense and urgent demands of a war-time army, it was inevitable that mistakes would be made, but this did not reflect on the basic soundness of the procedure itself.

As a result of pressure at a high level, instructions were issued early in 1943, that no questions on these subjects would be asked by psychiatrists at W.O.S.B. interviews. It should, however, have been clear to all but the most prejudiced, that it was of the greatest importance for psychiatrists, as medical men required to assess emotional maturity and stability of personality, to enquire in appropriate cases into so significant an aspect of the human mind, behaviour and

OFFICER SELECTION

social adaptation, as sexual adjustment. Similarly, it should have been obvious that, in dealing with religion, psychiatrists were not concerned with a candidate's views on transubstantiation or parthenogenesis, that they might advise his rejection on grounds of heresy: rather were they attempting a fundamentally sociological evaluation of a man's attitude to established authority, and the manner in which he reconciled his own views and convictions with those of other sections of the community.

The complaints which had most frequently been made about the old Selection Boards had been allegations that candidates were asked at interview about their school, their father's occupation and income, and so on. After the introduction of W.O.S.B.s, the public required reassurance that the new methods of officer selection were fair and 'democratic', and therefore welcomed the information given by the Secretary of State for War, in the House of Commons, that, from three representative samples totalling nearly 5,000 candidates accepted for O.C.T.U.s in 1943, approximately one-quarter had been educated at public schools, and three-quarters at grant-aided secondary schools and elementary schools.*

It is, perhaps, hardly necessary to add that the new methods of officer selection did not apply to the Brigade of Guards, who suffered no such unseemly interference in their well-tried ways.†

It was a very common experience at all W.O.S.B.s for visiting senior officers to arrive at the Board in a critical frame of mind and, knowing little or nothing of the procedure, under numerous misapprehensions. Few, however, who remained at a Board long enough to attend the final conference, went away critical, and many became enthusiastic.

In general, the role of the psychiatrist in W.O.S.B.s was criticized on the alleged grounds that he had too much influence in selection procedure; that he recommended the rejection of suitable candidates; and that any possible merits of his interview were outweighed by the damaging effects of the considerable resentment which it aroused in candidates.‡

These criticisms were not difficult to refute. In the first place, it would have been a very serious criticism if the psychiatrist had not

---

* *Parl. Deb.*, 5th ser., Commons, 397: 1435; 1 March, 1944.

† Cf. *Parl. Deb.*, 5th ser., Commons, 383: 2133–4; 22 Oct., 1942—and *ibid.*, 436: 211–12; 29 April, 1947.

‡ Characteristic of such criticism were the views expressed in a book by Lt.-Gen. Sir Giffard Martel.[76]

OFFICER SELECTION

occupied an influential position, as the only member of the Board with adequate scientific training and experience in the assessment of personality. Secondly, it was demonstrated beyond doubt that psychiatric methods had, in fact, greatly reduced the rejection rate of potentially suitable candidates: follow-up investigations on O.C.T.U. cadets who had been selected during the period from May to September, 1942, when new and old Selection Boards were working simultaneously, proved that the new Boards increased by 50% the number of cadets rated 'above average', whereas the old system was extremely wasteful, in that it rejected at least one out of three of the best candidates appearing before the Board.

Finally, a few facts should be noted concerning the attitude of candidates in general. In the summer of 1942, candidates at several W.O.S.B.s, replying anonymously to a questionnaire, had expressed unanimous enthusiasm about the new testing as a whole and, almost without exception, had commented favourably on the psychiatric interview. In December, 1946 (after the decision to remove psychiatrists and psychologists from W.O.S.B.s), the Director-General, Army Medical Services (Lt.-Gen. Sir Alexander Hood), stated that the majority of candidates who had a psychiatric interview felt reassured about their abilities and capacities, and those who had heard distorted rumours about this interview could be relieved of their misapprehensions by a psychiatric examination: if *all* candidates were interviewed, there would be no suspicion in the minds of those referred, as had been alleged, that their 'mental health and adjustment were in question'. General Sir Ronald Adam (formerly Adjutant-General), speaking in 1948 as Chairman of the National Institute of Industrial Psychology, observed: "We well knew with what suspicion the soldier looked on the old type of selection board which had consisted of two or three officers. When the new type War Office Selection Board had been working for six months in one command, the number of applicants for commissions rose by 25%." [3]

Indeed, it may be said that all available evidence suggests that the Army as a whole approved overwhelmingly of the new procedure, on account of its manifest fairness: to relinquish the scientific attributes of the new procedure was to relinquish the very parts of that procedure upon which the conviction of fairness was based.

W.O.S.B.s- only selected candidates for emergency commissions. In January, 1943, it was decided by the War Office that psychologists and psychiatrists on the staffs of W.O.S.B.s would be co-opted to special Boards interviewing officers with emergency commissions who applied for commissions in the Regular Army. Army psychiatrists and psychologists specializing in W.O.S.B. work held a meeting at the War Office to discuss the technical aspects of the selection of officers for regular commissions. The psychologists and psychiatrists working with the Regular Commissions Board acted as technical advisers to the president; the psychiatrist interviewed applicants, and the psychologist administered special intelligence tests and interpreted the test results. A special questionnaire was also devised, with a view to eliciting facts of psychological significance.

In interviewing candidates for regular commissions, an attempt was made in every case to deal with minor maladjustments in so far as the limited time would allow, and the candidates invariably expressed their gratitude for the help given. In some instances these expressions of gratitude were reiterated before the final Board, and more than once, time was found to accede to a candidate's request for a second interview. Even were the fact not already known to military psychiatrists, experience with this group alone provided a very obvious indication of the prevalence amongst officers of that type of mild psychiatric condition which, although not producing gross disability, is yet responsible for a very real loss in military efficiency.

In August, 1943, it was decided by the War Office, partly, no doubt, because of the limited number of psychiatrists available, that the latter would no longer be employed in the selection of officers for regular commissions. At least two senior officers with appreciable experience of the work of Regular Commissions Boards expressed their disagreement with this decision, and drew particular attention to the risk, in the absence of psychiatric advice, of selecting an unstable candidate or, alternatively, of rejecting a stable one on suspicion of mental instability unconfirmed by expert opinion. Psychologists were still employed by the Boards for the purpose of administering and interpreting intelligence tests, and summarizing the results of a new questionnaire which was introduced.

Gradually, it also became necessary to adapt the W.O.S.B. techniques to other purposes. For example, it was found that a number of officers, after receiving treatment in psychiatric hospitals, were fit for further military duty provided that certain modifications were effected in their employment. Administrative arrangements were,

OFFICER SELECTION

therefore, made in July, 1943, enabling medical boards in the hospitals concerned to recommend that such cases be referred to No. 25 W.O.S.B., in order that the capacity in which they would be of greatest use to the Service might be determined. The Selection Board's technique was suitably modified to deal with these officers, who attended in small groups of six or eight. The Board included a psychiatrist, who reviewed every case, and War Office representatives from the Military Secretary's Department and from the branch (A.G. 12) responsible for the extra-regimental employment of officers. The Personnel Branch endeavoured to place the officer in suitable employment, according to the Board's recommendation: only if all efforts in this direction failed, did it become necessary to request him to relinquish his commission.

A somewhat similar modification of the W.O.S.B. technique was introduced to deal with cadets who had broken down during their O.C.T.U. training and required treatment in a psychiatric hospital. When these cadets became fit to return to duty, arrangements were made through the War Office for their attendance at No. 21 W.O.S.B. The Board was requested to state, in each case, whether the candidate was suitable for further training in his present arm, or in some other arm, or whether he was altogether unfit to continue O.C.T.U. training. It was found that the very large majority of such cases were in the last category.

No. 21 W.O.S.B. also re-examined all cadets who, having been passed by W.O.S.B.s, subsequently failed at Leader Training Battalions, Basic O.C.T.U.s, or O.C.T.U.s. If the Board confirmed that a cadet was unsuitable, they could recommend either that he be given another chance, often in another arm of the Service, or that he be returned, as definitely unsuitable, to his original unit. In this way, No. 21 W.O.S.B. acted as a second filter for a few cases of a doubtful nature.*

A modified W.O.S.B. procedure was also used in selecting candidates for commission in the A.T.S. In 1943, two Boards, on which women psychiatrists were employed, were set up for this purpose.

In India, W.O.S.B. procedure was adapted to the special requirements of Selection Boards for the Indian Air Force, Royal Indian Navy, W.A.C. (India), Military Air Raid Service Battalions, Veterin-

---

* It was decided by the War Office, towards the end of 1946, that No. 21 W.O.S.B. should be disbanded, on the recommendation of the Crocker Committee that cadets should not be re-examined by this procedure.

OFFICER SELECTION

ary Corps, and I.A.M.C. cadets, and similar methods were used in interviewing Indian Army officers under adverse reports or unsuitably employed, and all candidates failing at the O.T.S.*

The Directorate of Army Psychiatry was also approached on several occasions by the civil authorities, with requests for assistance in the selection of candidates for the Civil Service (which led to the development of the Civil Service Selection Boards), and Civil Defence officers, by a modified W.O.S.B. technique including personality tests and psychiatric interviews. Thus, in 1943, a group of some 30 National Fire Service officers was interviewed each month by the W.O.S.B.s. In July, 1943, an experiment was made along similar lines, in the selection of key personnel who were required to investigate the methods and organization of the Civil Service. In July, 1944, the Indian Government requested the loan of a psychiatrist familiar with W.O.S.B. technique, to assist in the development of scientific methods of selection of candidates for the Indian Civil Service, and a psychiatrist was accordingly sent to India for this purpose for a period of ten months or so.

Psychiatrists on W.O.S.B.s co-operated also in the selection of Psychological Warfare personnel for S.H.A.E.F., in 1944. The methods employed were found by S.H.A.E.F. to be so successful that a psychiatrist familiar with these techniques was sent to the United States, for some months in 1944, to assist in the setting up of similar Boards in America

One important field in which little was done was that of N.C.O. selection. Intelligence alone is neither a sufficient nor an adequate guide, but short of a complex system such as was employed by the W.O.S.B.s, no technique was suggested. It was felt, however, that the development of screening techniques, in conjunction with practical outdoor tests similar to those used by the W.O.S.B.s, might in time provide a method specifically applicable to the selection of N.C.O.s.

The technical staff of the Research and Training Centre had long

* In a foreword to an explanatory pamphlet, published in 1945, on the new system of officer selection in India, General Auchinleck, C.-in-C. in India, wrote as follows: "I have spent my life as a soldier trying to gauge the character, personality and efficiency of leaders of all grades and I have seen many methods of selection.... As a result of my experience I have no hesitation in saying that the methods of selection described in this pamphlet are immeasurably superior to any system of competitive examination or selection by interview previously known to me. I hope that all who are interested in the subject will read this description of these modern methods of selection, which are the result of much care and thought, and the elimination of error by systematic thorough trial over a long period." [127]

recognized the need to obtain more data on the reliability and validity of W.O.S.B. tests and interviews, and on the contribution to the final decision of the Board made by each part of the procedure. Such data could not be obtained, on any large scale, from the work of the ordinary operative W.O.S.B.s, for various technical reasons: e.g. that Board programmes had never been standardized, systematic reporting had never been instituted, there were variations in Board personnel, and it was difficult to estimate the degree of influence which members of the Board exerted upon one another. At the beginning of 1945, the Adjutant-General (Sir Ronald Adam) also requested that the Research and Training Centre devise and validate a testing procedure for the use of the post-war Army, with a view to the selection of candidates for both permanent and temporary or militia commissions. It was clear that the general investigation desired by the Research and Training Centre, and the specific enquiry requested by the Adjutant-General, could be carried out simultaneously. For this purpose, it was necessary to design and validate a standardized procedure and programme of tests and interviews. This research, planned in May, 1945, was undertaken at No. 14 W.O.S.B.

The standard W.O.S.B. programme devised as a result of the experiments at No. 14 W.O.S.B. required the services of a psychiatrist, a commissioned psychologist who interviewed candidates, and two Sergeant Testers. It was realized that, unfortunately, owing to a shortage of specialists, few Boards would have their full complement of psychological staff, and indeed, in December, 1945, it was necessary to issue instructions to W.O.S.B.s embarking on the new standard programme, providing for modifications of procedure which the situation rendered essential.

Already in March, 1945, the Senior Psychiatrist at the Research and Training Centre (Lt.-Col. J. D. Sutherland) had been warned to expect a reduction in the number of psychiatrists available to W.O.S.B.s, and that it was possible that none would be left for work on the Boards dealing with the general run of candidates. Col. Sutherland consequently felt obliged, at that time, to state his conviction that the withdrawal of psychiatrists from the Boards, should it occur, would inevitably result in a considerable loss of efficiency in selection, which could only be compensated by developing an 'interview role' for the best and most experienced of W.O.S.B. psychologists. Failing such an alternative, officer selection could no

OFFICER SELECTION

longer claim scientific status: it would become an entirely lay procedure, with the only addition of intelligence tests.

In August, 1946, two committees were appointed by the Army Council, to enquire, respectively, into the system of selection for regular commissions of emergency commissioned officers (Ritchie Committee), and into the work of W.O.S.B.s (Crocker Committee).

The psychiatrists on the Regular Commissions Boards having already been disposed of, it was presumably now decided to complete the job commenced in 1943, and the Ritchie Committee recommended that the psychologists should be removed from these Boards, and that the intelligence test should be eliminated. The War Office, however, compromised, in November, 1946, by accepting the first, but not the second, recommendation.

The Crocker Committee, in its turn, recommended that psychiatrists and psychologists should no longer act as permanent members of W.O.S.B.s, which advice was also accepted by the War Office: instructions were consequently issued, in December, 1946, that all such experts be withdrawn from these Boards. At the same time, the Directorate of Army Psychiatry was informed that consultation with psychiatrists by W.O.S.B.s was 'still desirable in some cases', and was requested to continue the system which had been in operation for some time, whereby Area and Command Psychiatrists were available for advice on such cases as might be referred to them by presidents of the Boards. It was also stated that the technical advice of the psychiatrist attached to the War Office Selection Centre was still required, and it was therefore requested that this appointment be retained.*

With regard to the Crocker Committee's recommendation that psychiatrists and psychologists were no longer considered necessary as permanent members of W.O.S.B.s, the Director of Army Psychiatry (Brigadier A. Torrie) commented that the inception and development of W.O.S.B. procedure was due to these experts and that their presence on the Boards was necessary if that procedure were to be carried out adequately; the main advance of W.O.S.B. procedure was to substitute for the interview board an assessment from three angles, and it could be said without exaggeration that the assessment from the psychological angle was not the least

* This decision of the Army authorities, on the removal of psychiatrists and psychologists from officer selection boards, was questioned in the House of Commons (cf. *Parl. Deb.*, 5th ser., Commons, 431: 959-60; 10 Dec., 1946).

important of these, and to discard it was clearly a retrograde step. Brigadier Torrie further made the observation—highly relevant and pertinent in its implications—that, obviously, the fact that psychiatrists and psychologists were no longer available in sufficient number could not be disputed, and some modification of W.O.S.B. procedure must, therefore, necessarily take place; but that it should be made clear that this modification arose solely from lack of specialized personnel, and *that it was regarded as a temporary measure and not a deliberate policy.*

In December, 1946, the D.G.A.M.S. submitted to the Adjutant-General (Lt.-Gen. Sir Richard N. O'Connor) his comments on the decision to remove psychiatrists and psychologists from the W.O.S.B.s. In General Hood's opinion, psychiatrists, when available, should be present as advisers to W.O.S.B.s for several specified reasons, among which were the following: first, the role and function of the psychiatrist was to pass candidates who would otherwise fail for lack of scientific assessment, a fact which was confirmed by follow-up investigations; secondly, while the subject of psychiatry was a scientific one, it was still developing, and for this reason it was essential that the scientific worker should be in continual contact with day to day development, and this he could not do unless he were always available as an adviser to the Board; and thirdly, assessment of psychological fitness and of capacity to bear strain was essentially a function of the psychiatrist since, through his professional training and experience, he was concerned with the stresses which caused breakdown and with their psychological mechanisms.

The Adjutant-General did not agree fully with the remarks of the D.G.A.M.S., and considered that the strength of feeling in the Army against psychologists and psychiatrists was such that, at this stage, it was advisable to withdraw them from the Selection Boards. It may, however, be noted that, from what has already been said, there would appear to be no evidence in support of this view. It seems clear that opposition in the Army came, if not exclusively, at least preponderantly, from certain senior officers and administrative quarters, whose influence eventually brought about a reversal of the progressive policy which had so successfully been introduced and developed under Sir Ronald Adam, during the crucial years of the war.

The Adjutant-General suggested that the terms 'psychologist' and 'psychiatrist' be decently concealed beneath such a title as 'special selection officer'. It had, indeed, already been proposed in December, 1942, that the psychiatrist on a W.O.S.B. should change his name, but on that occasion he was to be allowed the title of 'medical officer'. Rejecting any such proposal, Brigadier Rees had then observed: "Experience in civil life, as well as in the Army, shows that greater difficulties arise from the camouflaged psychiatrist than are ever likely to arise when he sails under his own colours. It is a mistake to go on trying to make psychiatry 'respectable', labelling it 'neurology' as in the last war or calling the psychiatrist just a medical officer. We are getting nearer the time at which the gulf between the so-called physical and the so-called mental disorders will be adequately bridged and when it will be as natural for the ordinary man to seek general specialist advice about his personal or environmental emotional stresses or his dis-ease, as it now is for him to enquire about the vitamins in his diet."

Evidence as to the value and effectiveness of W.O.S.B.s in practice, was provided in May, 1948, in the course of a debate in the House of Lords concerning the Civil Service Selection Boards (C.S.S.B.s) which, as already mentioned, made use of techniques, suitably modified, which had been developed by the W.O.S.B.s. It may be mentioned, incidentally, that this debate provided occasion for much misinformed and destructive criticism of C.S.S.B.s and W.O.S.B.s alike.*

In the course of this lengthy debate, Lord Piercy, who had been associated with the National Institute of Industrial Psychology, stated that it had been possible during the Second World War to compare, on a scientific basis, the results of selection by the W.O.S.B.s (which dealt with a very large number of men) with those of selection by traditional methods. In one large sample of men who had been selected for the O.C.T.U.s by the respective methods, the figures representing their comparative ranking when they passed out of the O.C.T.U.s were as follows:

Grading of Candidates	Old Methods	W.O.S.B.s
Above average	22·1%	34·5%
Average	41·3%	40·3%
Below average	36·6%	25·2%

* *Parl. Deb.*, 5th ser., Lords, **155**: 1034–95; 26 May, 1948. Cf. in particular the strongly expressed views of Lord Moran and Lord Cherwell, who were, respectively, physician and scientific adviser to Mr. Winston Churchill during the recent war. The whole of this debate, however, is worthy of study: in spite of much obscurantism, it is illuminating.

These figures illustrated two points: first, that none of these systems as at present devised could be 100 per cent. perfect; and secondly, that in those conditions and for those purposes for which they were employed, the W.O.S.B.s did their work of selection with an impressive margin of superiority over the ordinary, traditional methods.*

The selection Research and Training Unit (which replaced the Research and Training Centre) published, in 1948, a significant report of an investigation into the validity of the work carried out by one W.O.S.B. during the first few months of 1946. The salient feature of this investigation was the statistically significant evidence of satisfactory selection, as shown by the correlation of the Board's gradings with subsequent O.C.T.U. gradings, in the case of 76 candidates who had been interviewed by a psychiatrist highly experienced in W.O.S.B. technique, and its contrast with the lack of any such evidence with regard to 76 candidates who did not have a psychiatric interview. The first group of candidates did not differ in any systematic way from the second group. The report stated that the results of this investigation were consistent with the view that, for the candidates interviewed by this particular psychiatrist, here was an instance of the functioning of a W.O.S.B. as originally intended, i.e. with a psychiatrist drawing the attention of the non-technical members of the Board to relevant aspects of the candidates, and generally assisting them to form, in the light of their military knowledge, a judgement of the candidates comparable with, and sometimes superior to, his own. On the other hand, there was a complete absence of any evidence of transmission of efficiency to these same non-technical members in the selection of candidates not interviewed by this psychiatrist.

It is relevant here to quote the conclusion reached in 1949, from a critical survey of the validation of W.O.S.B. procedure, by Vernon and Parry: "The conclusion that appears to follow from this review is that W.O.S.B. methods, applied haphazardly according to the whims of the staff are only of slight value, but that when standard techniques are evolved and applied uniformly by trained and experienced personnel, a satisfactory reliability may be obtained. Only under such conditions can good validity be expected, and a great deal more, admittedly difficult, research is needed to prove the value of the contributions of the various parts of the procedure. A number of such investigations are now under way." [125]

In an investigation, carried out in 1944–6 (and reported in 1948),

* *Parl. Deb., ibid.*, **155**: 1064–6.

of a considerable number of officers who had been passed by W.O.S.B.s and subsequently, during their commissioned service, developed a psychiatric illness requiring hospitalization, Major H. Harris was able to show that psychiatric breakdown was far more common among those in the lower ranges of 'officer intelligence rating', and those whose educational standard was below that which they should have attained in view of their innate intelligence. The importance and wide applicability of these findings is demonstrated by the fact that 58% of such cases came from no more than 7·5% of all candidates who passed. Major Harris pointed out that, with a single index based on the combined assessment of intelligence and education (as normally measured in objective terms by the W.O.S.B.), and of the relation between the two, it was possible to isolate this small group of accepted W.O.S.B. candidates; and that, by the use of the index, it should be possible to refer to the psychiatrist a considerably larger proportion than hitherto of potential cases of psychiatric breakdown.

It is important to record the fact that, in the course of 1948, a disquieting number of cases of psychiatric breakdown, enuresis, or with other evidence of instability, occurred at O.C.T.U.s. There was also one suicide which, it was felt, might very well have been avoided had there been a psychiatric interview at the W.O.S.B. After the removal of psychiatrists from the W.O.S.B.s, presidents could only be advised to refer to a psychiatrist any case where they were in doubt as to a candidate's mental stability.

In view of these disturbing developments, and the recent investigation outlined above, the Chief Psychologist (Col. B. Ungerson) recommended, in October, 1948, that more positive instructions be issued to the presidents of W.O.S.B.s, concerning the use of psychiatrists in the more difficult and doubtful cases; and in particular, as to the advisability of referring to the psychiatrist candidates within a specified lower range of 'officer intelligence ratings' and educational standards. The Chief Psychologist was aware that some, at least, of the presidents would receive such instructions sympathetically, since they had previously expressed their lack of confidence in judging the future development of young and immature candidates. While he realized that it would inevitably raise emotional resistance in some quarters, he felt obliged to put forward this recommendation, if such unfortunate tragedies as the O.C.T.U. suicide were to be avoided in future.

OFFICER SELECTION

After the somewhat melancholy, but, it is hoped, instructive, account of opposition, retrograde action, and disintegration, 'that ends this strange eventful history' of the vicissitudes of personnel and officer selection, it is perhaps desirable to view in perspective the significance and limitations of scientific selection, in the light of the following observations: "It is of some importance to remember, in thinking of selection, whether it be of men in large groups, or specialists where the procedure can be in greater detail, that in the Army one is selected for specific martial roles and that it would be disastrous if gradings or rejections made for these purposes were to cling in any way to the future life and reputation of the men so graded. The man in the lowest selection group, S.G. 5, may have a limited value to the Army, but he may be a first-class man in his particular niche in civil life. The officer who lacks the kind of qualities to make him a leader of fighting men may be one of the great men in his own subject. . . . We must never make the mistake of confusing the results of selection for some specific task with the assessment of a man's potential contribution to life as a whole." [97] *

* For a detailed, but extremely individual, account by a psychiatrist of methods used for officer selection, cf. the book by H. Harris, *The Group Approach to Leadership-Testing*.[57] A comprehensive survey of the psychological aspects of officer selection is given by P. E. Vernon and J. B. Parry.[125] Cf. also T. F. Rodger.[109]

IV

MENTAL DEFECT AND DULLNESS

BECAUSE OF THE LIMITED MAN-POWER available in Great Britain, and the considerable and urgent demands made on these resources, in the Second World War, by the fighting services, civil defence and industry, it was necessary to make the greatest possible effective use of men of low intelligence. A very great problem was, however, created by the introduction of such men into the British Army.

There may possibly have been some truth in the popular tradition, in the past, that the dull man made a good soldier, with lengthy and careful training in relatively simple duties under peace-time conditions. The position was, however, very different in the presence of the stresses and increased tempo of modern warfare, and the duties of the modern infantryman, which demand a technical knowledge of a number of specialized weapons and the mastery of many skills, require an average degree of intelligence and present an impossible task to the dull man. Whereas he may have been capable of carrying out some simple job in a restricted, protective environment in civilian life, the dullard, placed amongst men of relatively higher intelligence in the Army, often became maladjusted and developed feelings of inferiority and anxiety. Being slow to learn, he held back the squad or class during training, aroused antagonism and impatience in his comrades and instructors, and himself became frustrated.

It was not long before this maladjustment of men of low intelligence in the Army began to manifest itself in many different ways.* It led

---

* Already in 1917, intelligence tests carried out in the U.S. Army had clearly demonstrated that men of low intelligence preponderated in the groups designated,

MENTAL DEFECT AND DULLNESS

to 'malingering', mental instability and breakdown. Mental dullness was also found to be a frequent cause of military delinquency, and particularly absenteeism; and the dullard often became a disciplinary problem in his unit through failure to understand the nature of regulations and the reason for them. Investigations showed that the incidence of venereal disease, scabies and pediculosis, and the general sickness rate were appreciably greater among dullards than among men of average intelligence.

As a result of intelligence tests carried out during 1940 in Northern Command, it was found that 50% of every Tank Regiment intake and 20% of every infantry intake had not the innate intelligence required for full efficiency in the corps to which they had been posted. The Command Psychiatrist (Lt.-Col. G. R. Hargreaves) reported that at least 4% of all intakes would never become efficient in any military capacity: they would be liable to results of maladjustment and inadequacy such as have been mentioned, and would prove incapable of looking after themselves even in minor emergencies. As civilians, however, they would be capable of making a useful contribution to the war effort, e.g. in simple repetitive tasks in industry. He estimated that, in the field units, some 4% of the men were unlikely to become efficient in any corps and, at the very least, another 5% were only suitable for service in less skilled employment.

Experience has shown, therefore, that the misplaced dullard becomes in modern war a consumer of man-power and a general liability to the Army. Some of the evidence, which was already impressive in the early days of the war and which further accumulated during subsequent years, of the military inefficiency of men of low intelligence is reviewed below.

Lt.-Cols. T. F. Main and A. T. M. Wilson carried out an investigation in Western Command, in August, 1941, in an attempt to discover how far misfits and untrainable men were concerned in repeated absence without leave. It was found that, of 300 soldiers under sentence for A.W.O.L., one-half had the intellectual capacity found in the least intelligent quarter of the population, i.e. this group of men contained twice the number of dullards and defectives usually found in homologous conscript groups. Of these delinquents, about one man in seven (15%) was entirely unsuited for any form of military service on account of a severe degree of mental dullness or

respectively, as disciplinary cases, 'ten poorest privates', 'men of low military value', and 'unteachable men'.[141]

MENTAL DEFECT AND DULLNESS

defect, an assessment which was confirmed by their military records. Similarly, during a period of six months in the second half of 1942, the Command Psychiatrist in Northern Ireland examined some 50 disciplinary cases, of which number nearly three-quarters were charged with A.W.O.L. or desertion: he found that no less than 50% of these men were either mentally defective or dull and backward.

In a study of nearly 1,000 deserters in B.A.O.R. in 1944–5, Lt.-Col. J. C. Penton noted that the tendency to desert appeared to be greatest amongst men of relatively low intelligence: some 50% of deserters were in the lower half of the intelligence rating scale, as compared with some 35% of a control group consisting of a random sample of non-delinquents.*

The actual figures are given in the following table:

Intelligence Rating	Frequency % Deserters	Controls
G1	2·6	5·7
G2	10·9	19·8
G3	9·8	11·9
G4	10·3	11·7
G5	14·1	13·2
G6	16·7	14·7
G7	15·8	9·6
G8	11·4	7·9
G9	6·7	4·8
G10	1·7	0·7

In 1944, an analysis of over 1,200 consecutive reports on disciplinary cases referred to psychiatrists prior to trial showed that more than one-quarter of the men examined were mentally dull or defective; of these dullards, it had been recommended that one-fifth be discharged on medical grounds, one-quarter be transferred to the Armed Pioneers, and one-third be transferred to the Unarmed Pioneers, on completion of sentence.

From December, 1944, all men admitted to Group 'C' Military Prisons and Detention Barracks (i.e. recidivists and those considered to have an undesirable influence in ordinary Military Prisons and Detention Barracks) were examined by psychiatrists. Of the first 500 consecutive admissions, 30% were already in the Pioneer Corps (and 3% more were recommended for transfer to that Corps), and 50%

* The intelligence rating scale Gl-10 was a 10-point scale used in the B.L.A. before the invasion of France, covering the same range as the 6-point (S.G. 1–5) scale now in general use for other ranks. The lower half of the scale is from G6-10.

MENTAL DEFECT AND DULLNESS

were in the two lowest intelligence-groups, S.G. 4 and 5 (as compared with 30% in a random sample of soldiers).*

In an investigation, in Western Command, of reports by military psychiatrists on 450 men under arrest and awaiting trial during the year 1945, Lt.-Col. D. L. Mackenzie found that 23 cases had six months' service or less; of these, 15 men (i.e. two-thirds) were in the intelligence-groups S.G. 4 and 5, 5 men (i.e. one-fifth) were already in the Pioneer Corps, and 5 more had been recommended for transfer to that Corps. The Director of Army Psychiatry reported that, during a tour of B.A.O.R. in September, 1947, he saw 25 soldiers under sentence who were chronic offenders; of these, 17 men (i.e. two-thirds) were in the groups S.G. 4 and 5, and 10 men (i.e. two-fifths) were in the group S.G. 5. From the records of these delinquents it was clear that most of them had given little effective service in the Army.

Finally, an investigation, in April, 1948, of the educational standard and intelligence level of nearly 450 soldiers under sentence in the Military Prison, Shepton Mallet, and the Military Corrective Establishments, Colchester, confirmed earlier findings. It was found that among the military prisoners, there were five times as many men of the lowest (markedly backward) educational standard, and twice as many men of the next lowest standard (those who do not reach the top form in elementary schools), as occur in the Army as a whole. Similarly, among the military prisoners there were twice as many men of the two lowest selection groups, S.S.G. 4 and 5, as in the Army as a whole—i.e. nearly twice as many in S.S.G. 4, and nearly three times as many in S.S.G. 5, as in the total Army population.

The actual figures for the various intelligence-groups are given in the following table:

S.S.G.	Frequency %	
	Prisoners	Army Population
1	0·9	10·8
2	2·9	16·4
3+	12·5	20·0
3−	22·5	23·2
4	41·6	22·7
5	19·6	6·9

* In selection procedure, the range of scoring for each of the several tests (Progressive Matrices, Verbal, Arithmetic, etc.) is divided into six grades known as 'Selection Groups' (S.G.), numbered S.G. 1, 2, 3+, 3−, 4 and 5; these are standardized to

MENTAL DEFECT AND DULLNESS

The relative proportion of men from the Pioneer Corps among military prisoners was five times that which would have been expected in relation to the Army as a whole.

These data provide sufficient evidence of the high incidence of delinquency in the Army among men of low intelligence.

In the early months of the war, many men suffering from psychiatric breakdown were found to be mentally defective, and dullards formed a fairly high proportion of the psychiatric cases evacuated from France and admitted to psychiatric hospitals.

When the first Command Psychiatrists were appointed, they found that a very large number of the men referred to them from units were mentally defective, but these cases were usually not sent for examination until they had developed symptoms of instability superimposed on their mental defect. Many had gross hysterical symptoms, collapsed on the parade ground, or developed aphasia, marked tremor, or morbid anxiety with fits of crying. These reactions had usually been induced by training programmes which were beyond the capacities of the dullards who, whereas they might have been able to carry out the simpler training required of an infantry soldier in former wars, were quite unable to master the more complex drill required for such weapons as the Bren gun.

An investigation in B.A.O.R. in 1948 similarly showed that, among the cases of psychiatric illness referred to psychiatrists, there was a preponderance of men of low intelligence: twice as many soldiers as would have been expected (in proportion to their number) in the group S.G. 5, and one-half (50%) more than expected in the group S.G. 4, developed psychiatric disabilities.

It was also found, as a result of another investigation in B.A.O.R. in 1948, that there was a higher incidence of venereal disease in soldiers in the lower intelligence-groups: one-third more than would have been expected in the group S.G. 5, and one-half more than expected in the group S.G. 4, contracted V.D.

The actual figures for B.A.O.R. are given in the table overleaf.

Statistical evidence obtained in 1948 also demonstrated that the hospital admission rate in the Army among the lowest

represent the highest 10% (S.G. 1), the lowest 10% (S.G. 5), and the intervening groups each of 20%, of the military population. While intelligence levels have frequently been recorded, on the basis of the Progressive Matrices test alone, as S.G. 1–5 it has been found more useful for practical purposes to formulate a 'Summed S.G.' (S.S.G.) based on the combined S.G. ratings of five of the different tests. The S.S.G. ratings are similarly distributed on a 6-point scale.

MENTAL DEFECT AND DULLNESS

intelligence-group (S.S.G. 5) was 14%, as compared with a sickness rate of 6% for the Army as a whole.

S.G.	Frequency % of various S.G.s		
	V.D. Cases	All Soldiers	Psychiatric Cases
1	4·2	10·2	6·9
2	9·8	17·7	12·1
3+	19·7	22·5	17·2
3−	26·3	23·8	21·5
4	33·5	21·0	32·8
5	6·5	4·8	9·5

Col. Hargreaves carried out an investigation, in 1940, into the incidence of parasitic infestation (scabies and pediculosis capitis) among Army and A.T.S. recruits, respectively, according to levels of intelligence. It was found that the incidence of these conditions was appreciably higher among the two lowest intelligence-groups, a fact which must be correlated with the relative standards of personal cleanliness of recruits of various intellectual levels. It was found that the incidence of scabies and pediculosis increased progressively in inverse ratio to the degree of intelligence. Amongst Army recruits, twice as many as would have been expected in the group S.G. 5, and one-half (50%) more than expected in the group S.G. 4, suffered from scabies. Amongst A.T.S. recruits, one-half more than would have been expected in the group S.G. 5, and one-third more than expected in the group S.G. 4, had pediculosis capitis.[97]

The actual figures are given in the tables (a) and (b) opposite.

Apart from the immediate problems so far discussed, resulting from the presence in the Army of maladjusted dullards, Army psychiatrists were faced with two other problems, in this connection, which were essentially dependent upon the availability or lack of adequate administrative provisions: first, how best to employ those dullards whom it was necessary—or indeed, in view of the manpower situation at that time, essential—to retain in the Army; and secondly, how to get rid of those who were too unstable, or of too low intelligence, to be anything but useless and a source of inefficiency from the military viewpoint, but might, in a number of cases, be suitably and usefully employed, in a selective environment and limited capacity, in civilian life. The first of these problems requires to be considered in relation to the development of the Pioneer Corps; and the second, in relation to administrative difficulties. A corollary to these two problems was the urgent need to eliminate

MENTAL DEFECT AND DULLNESS

at intake unstable dullards, and men of such low intelligence as to be unsuitable for any kind of military employment, by the introduction of an adequate system of personnel selection.

It is, therefore, relevant to survey briefly the history of the development of the Pioneer Corps, in so far as it concerns the employment of men of low intelligence in the Army.

(a) Of 37,330 Army recruits in consecutive intakes, 435 (1·2%) had *scabies*:

S.G.	Frequency % of various S.G.s		% Infested in each S.G.
	Infested Recruits	Total Recruits	
1	4·6	10·6	0·5
2	14·3	18·7	0·9
3+	24·1	25·1	1·2
3−	19·6	22·4	1·1
4	27·2	17·6	1·9
5	10·2	5·6	2·2

(b) Of 1,576 A.T.S. recruits, 442 (28%) had *pediculosis capitis*:

S.G.	Frequency % of various S.G.s		% Infested in each S.G.
	Infested Recruits	Total Recruits	
1	0·0	1·5	0·0
2	2·7	10·9	7·0
3+	11·1	17·0	18·3
3−	17·9	22·1	22·7
4	41·2	31·9	36·3
5	27·1	16·8	45·5

The United States Army demonstrated, in the First World War, that the worst soldiers were often the best diggers, and this fact was once more convincingly proved in the British Army in the recent war. Psychiatrists were faced, at an early date, with the problem of the employment in suitable occupations of the considerable numbers of stable but backward men entering the British Army. It was realized that the various difficulties in which dull men became involved, and the morbidity to which they were subject, were but manifestations of a low personal morale, itself the result of the inherent inability of these soldiers to attain the standards expected of them and to absorb training as quickly as their fellows, and the consequent frustration which they must necessarily experience.

In a half-hearted attempt to deal with this situation, the authorities at first allowed some of these backward men to find their way, by

MENTAL DEFECT AND DULLNESS

somewhat devious administrative routes, into labour companies of the Auxiliary Military Pioneer Corps.*

In these early days of the war, the Pioneer Corps contained not only dull and backward men, but a number of aliens and men in low medical categories; and, in addition, not a few 'intelligent undesirables' were transferred to the Corps by commanding officers who—to borrow an official euphemism—had "interpreted the term 'dull and backward' too widely". The Pioneer Corps, therefore, comprised ordinary armed companies, special Agricultural ('N') Companies which were originally intended for the rehabilitation or restricted employment of neurotic patients discharged from military hospitals, and special unarmed companies in which dullards and others were employed as unskilled labourers.

Psychiatrists attempted to deal with the problem of the employment of dull and backward soldiers by obtaining their transfer to these unarmed companies, which were variously if unimaginatively known as 'B', 'B.M.' or 'M' Sections; the first two abbreviations were commonly interpreted as 'Batty' and 'Bloody Mental' respectively, and consequently, as the Consulting Psychiatrist later observed, neither was very suitable to be applied to a group of men who were already feeling inferior and sometimes unwanted.

In November, 1940, in a memorandum to the D.G.A.M.S., the Consulting Psychiatrist suggested that, in order to utilize to the full the services of dull and backward men, there should be set up as soon as possible in each command a special Training Depot, which might be called an 'Army Training Depot' so as to avoid confusion with an Infantry Training Centre (I.T.C.) while at the same time giving no indication to the men themselves that they constituted an 'inferior group'. Brigadier Rees pointed out that the A.M.P.C., to which a number of such men had been transferred at the beginning of the war, had recently been armed and, therefore, it was no longer possible to make such transfers.† Moreover, a backward, untrained recruit transferred to the A.M.P.C. was likely to have a 'raw deal' from his fellows, and was as liable to break down as if he had gone into an ordinary I.T.C. In consequence, it

* The title of the Corps was changed, in November, 1940, to 'Pioneer Corps'.

† As a result of the fact that some companies of the A.M.P.C., sent to France as labourers, had been armed in an emergency and had fought off a German attack, the authorities decided, in July, 1940, to arm *all* British members of the Corps (cf. *Parl. Deb.*, 5th ser., Commons, 363: 1149; 30 July, 1940). Only 25% of the men in the A.M.P.C. serving with the B.E.F. had been armed (cf. *ibid.*, 358: 1654–5; 18 March, 1940).

MENTAL DEFECT AND DULLNESS

was necessary to discharge from the Army a very large number of dullards who might otherwise have been employed in simple duties.

It was suggested that the Training Depot should be organized in the same way as an I.T.C., but that training should take place at a slower pace, the use of firearms should not be taught, and appropriate forms of special training should be introduced. Various types of men might be placed in different companies, and those who subsequently proved unsuitable could be discharged. During the course of their training, the men would be graded according to the jobs for which they were most suitable; the majority would probably be trained for labouring work and eventually form special companies of the A.M.P.C., while others might be trained for certain simple routine duties in ordinary units.

In conclusion, Brigadier Rees expressed the view that the establishment of such Training Depots would increase the efficiency of all regular training units by relieving them of the men who wasted instructional time, demoralized recruits, and hindered progress. At the same time, many of these misfits could, by skilled training and careful placement, render good service to the country, while entailing almost no additional expenditure.

The administrative procedure devised, in November, 1940, and January, 1941, for the transfer of men to the Pioneer Corps could not, in the opinion of Army psychiatrists, solve the problem of dealing with the dullards, not only because the selection of cases to be transferred was primarily the responsibility of the C.O. of the unit and was, consequently, for the most part arbitrary and unsatisfactory, but also because it had been officially decided that, although arms would in future be drawn only for 25% of the strength of the Pioneer Corps, all Pioneers would still be expected to be capable of using them.

The procedure eventually introduced in July, 1941, by A.C.I. 1136/41, for the transfer of dull and backward soldiers, including those in Young Soldiers' Battalions, was a definite improvement from the psychiatric point of view. This A.C.I. provided that transfers of such men to the Pioneer Corps would be carried out only on the recommendation of the Command or Area Psychiatrist, and that soldiers who, because of mental dullness, were unfit for any form of military service, were to be discharged from the Army.

In August, 1941, the D.G.A.M.S. recommended to the Director of Labour the formation of special companies of the Pioneer Corps

MENTAL DEFECT AND DULLNESS

(to be called 'Mobile Labour Companies'), to which dullards could be posted who were not fit for service in ordinary armed companies: and thus, in September, these special unarmed companies were re-established.*

In November, 1941, at a War Office meeting of Deputy Directors of Labour, Lt.-Col. A. T. M. Wilson defined the two categories (later incorporated in A.C.I. 84/42) of men who were of low intelligence but *emotionally stable*: i.e. those who were so dull and backward that they were not fit to bear arms; and those who had a capacity to learn which was much below average, and who therefore could not benefit by advanced training, although fit to bear arms.

With the introduction of adequate selection of men to be transferred to the Pioneer Corps, and as a result of the general personnel selection procedure which, from July, 1942, rendered possible the posting of recruits in the lowest intelligence-groups from the Primary Training Centre direct to the appropriate section of the Pioneer Corps (or, in some cases, to domestic and simple administrative duties in other arms), it was found that the morale and performance of dullards so employed showed considerable improvement, with a corresponding decrease in the incidence among them of neurotic instability, 'malingering' and minor illness, delinquency, and venereal disease. Living and working together with men of like capability, and with the benefit of special assistance in matters of education and welfare, they were better adjusted to their environment, were more efficient, and caused less trouble than when distributed throughout the Army. Nevertheless, the Pioneers remained a greater liability to the disciplinary and medical authorities than other units.

Army psychiatrists became aware at an early date that there were certain cases of mental dullness in which there was some doubt as to the man's suitability for employment in the Pioneer Corps. It was felt that it would be of considerable assistance in assessing the future performance and military usefulness of doubtful cases if, instead of transferring them directly to the Pioneer Corps, they could be sent

---

* They were at first named by the authorities, with a regrettable if by now familiar lack of imagination, 'Q' Sections. The Consulting Psychiatrist was obliged to write to the D.G.A.M.S.: "This, I am afraid, is too obvious. There are not many words beginning with Q, but 'queer' is one which springs to the mind, and though it is a very small point I hope you will urge that this terminology shall be discontinued forthwith. I have already had protesting letters . . . about the matter from various parts of the country." The Command Psychiatrist, South-Eastern Command (Major E. A. Bennet), suggested the designations, 'Unarmed' (instead of 'Q') and 'Armed' Companies, which were eventually adopted for the Pioneer Corps.

for preliminary observation to special units, where they could be partially trained and educated. In March, 1941, the Command Psychiatrist in Northern Ireland (Lt.-Col. J. D. W. Pearce), with the co-operation of the D.D.M.S., the Assistant Director of Labour, and 'A' Branch, B.T.N.I., established an unofficial, experimental unit, known originally as B.T.N.I. Training Detachment, and subsequently as the Pioneer Training Pool. It was decided that, where a man was not considered suitable for immediate, permanent transfer to the Pioneer Corps because he appeared somewhat unstable, or of too low intelligence, or both, but not to such a degree as would justify his immediate discharge as permanently unfit for any form of military service, he would be recommended, with the approval of the Command Psychiatrist, for attachment on trial to the Pioneer Corps for a period not exceeding 28 days.

The first 65 men recommended for 'attachment on trial' were collected from 15 different units, and a four-weeks' training syllabus was worked out. On examination of this first batch of men, it was apparent that treatment very different from the usual Army routine would have to be adopted. Many of them were in possession of kit, clothing, etc., which was in a very bad condition. Enquiries elicited the information that the majority had, because of very low mentality, been employed permanently, in their original units, on sanitary and cookhouse fatigues, and that it had not, therefore, been considered worth while to exchange their kit for them; this fact had obviously contributed to their bad reaction towards Army life. Many had family troubles which had not previously been investigated. A large majority were unable to read or write, and experienced much difficulty in understanding such matters as rates of pay, etc. During the period of four weeks, an attempt was made to give basic education to illiterates, to deal with welfare problems, and to train the men both physically and mentally.

The majority of the men sent to this unit showed a very marked improvement in adjustment and morale, which made it possible to reach a more accurate decision, at the end of the period of training, as to each man's disposal. It was possible in this way to retain for general labouring duties in the Army hundreds of men, most of whom would otherwise almost certainly have required to be discharged, as a result of their original psychiatric examination (before rehabilitation), as permanently unfit for further military service in any form. During the two years of its existence, the Pioneer Training

MENTAL DEFECT AND DULLNESS

Pool dealt with 579 men 'attached on trial'. Of these, 500 men (86%) were found, after four weeks' training, to be suitable for permanent transfer to the Pioneer Corps, and only 79 men (14%) proved to be unsuitable for further service, and were eventually discharged from the Army. It was considered essential, however, to place the men who had been successfully rehabilitated in special sections under special N.C.O.s, if they were not once more to deteriorate, and become maladjusted and inefficient.

Unfortunately, in spite of this significant achievement, it was not possible to obtain the necessary support of the non-medical authorities at the War Office, to enable such units to be generally established on the pattern of the experimental Training Pool in Northern Ireland, and the latter was disbanded in March, 1943.

In July, 1941, the authorities decided (in A.C.I. 1253/41) to establish 'Convalescent Observation Depots', with the expressed intention of avoiding the heavy losses of man-power then resulting from the discharge from the Service (by medical boards) of men with physical disabilities, and also (on the recommendation of psychiatrists) of dull and backward men who were unsuitable for the Pioneer Corps. All such men, physical cases of certain types and unstable dullards alike, were to be sent to these Depots for 14 days, after which period a decision would be made as to their disposal (reallocation or discharge), and psychiatrists were to discontinue recommending men for discharge from the Army on account of mental dullness.

In a memorandum to the D.G.A.M.S., on 'The Situation with regard to Mental Defect and the Disposal of Dull and Backward Men', the Consulting Psychiatrist expressed not only his disagreement with this proposed policy, in so far as it applied to dullards, but also a wider concern about the needs of the Army and the war effort, and the social problem involved. He drew attention to the financial burden and wastage of man-power, and other problems which, directly or indirectly, were caused by soldiers of low intelligence in the Army; and further, to the many suggestions that had been advanced for the better management of this problem group, e.g. his own proposal, in November, 1940, for special Training Depots.

Brigadier Rees pointed out that, in spite of the introduction, at the instigation of the D.G.A.M.S., of Unarmed Sections in the Pioneer Corps, to which reasonably stable dullards could be transferred, and which had proved of outstanding value, these Sections

MENTAL DEFECT AND DULLNESS

had been abolished on a recent instruction from the Director of Labour—which referred to the up-grading of these men, as if their grey matter could be increased by administrative fiat—so that it would once again be impossible for psychiatrists to transfer many suitable defectives to the Pioneer Corps. While combatant units were anxious to dispose of the dull men from their intake, psychiatrists appeared to be obstructed at home in their unremitting efforts to make the optimum use of this section of poor material which came into the Army.

Finally, it was stated that it was unfair to the Army and to the soldier that a specialist recommendation as to disposal should be subject to review by those with no specialized knowledge; and that the retention in the Army of emotionally unstable dullards would be detrimental to the morale of the Pioneer Corps. The Consulting Psychiatrist also recommended that all dullards with more than six months' service appear before a medical board, that all obviously unstable defectives be discharged administratively, and that those whose degree of stability was in doubt be sent to special Training Wings in Pioneer Corps Depots (according to the previously proposed scheme for special Training Depots, and the Northern Ireland experiment), where, in the course of training, they might be observed and graded under working conditions, and a decision reached (with psychiatric advice) as to their disposal.*

Another experiment which may be mentioned was the formation, in October, 1943, of a special unit, known as No. 1 Pioneer Training School, near Ipswich, in Eastern Command, with the primary object of assessing the fitness to bear arms of certain men in the Unarmed Pioneer Corps. Men from unarmed companies were selected for the four weeks' course by a psychiatrist and in this way a certain number of men were found to be fit for transfer to armed companies. It was suggested by the psychiatrists concerned, that all men who were considered for transfer from unarmed units might with advantage first be passed through this unit, in order to determine their suitability or otherwise for the proposed method of disposal, but it was, of course, realized that the total number of men concerned was, in any case, very small.

In assessing a man's suitability for an armed or an unarmed unit

* In October, 1941, A.C.I. 1253/41 was cancelled, and replaced by A.C.I. 2148/41, which provided for 'Medical Examination Centres' with the purpose of avoiding unnecessary invaliding from the Army for physical disabilities, but specifically excluding dull and backward soldiers and all other psychiatric cases.

of the Pioneer Corps, psychiatrists had to bear in mind the fact that men in Armed Sections were considered to be fit for service overseas, whereas men in Unarmed Sections were regarded as fit only for home service.

In the early stages, the authorities brought considerable pressure to bear in an attempt to employ Unarmed Sections in unsuitable duties. The fact that many stable dullards had made a good adjustment under the favourable conditions of the Pioneer Corps was erroneously interpreted as an indication that these soldiers were fit for routine infantry duties, and numerous efforts were, therefore, made to induce psychiatrists to place dull men in a higher category which would permit their employment in this capacity. It eventually became obvious, however, even to the authorities concerned, that dullards who had been placed, often by error, in unsuitable and more complex occupations subsequently almost invariably broke down and deteriorated, with the result that it was necessary to discharge them from the Army on psychiatric grounds.

Of a group of 86 men from the Unarmed Pioneer Corps who were referred by their C.O. to one psychiatrist, in November, 1943, as suitable for armed companies, 62 men (72%) were found to be hopelessly unfit to bear arms; the remaining 24 men (28%) were recommended for No. 1 Pioneer Training School, with a view to subsequent upgrading if they proved suitable on the course. Many of the soldiers referred had, in addition to their mental deficiency, not only obvious signs of neurotic instability, but minor physical defects.

In February, 1943, 19 volunteers for the infantry were recommended by various psychiatrists for transfer to the Pioneer Corps because of mental dullness, having been examined within a fortnight of entering the Army, as a result of selection tests. The authorities decided, as an experiment, to allow these men to proceed, after completion of their basic training, to normal infantry training, and to call for reports by the C.O.s of the Infantry Training Centres. After a follow-up of 4½ months, it was found that 13 (68%) men had received unfavourable, and 3 (16%) had received favourable, reports; in the other 3 cases, no definite report could yet be given. As a result of this experiment the executive branch concerned decided that recommendations for the transfer of infantry volunteers to the Pioneer Corps would be implemented at the end of basic training, and that such men would not in future be posted for infantry training.

MENTAL DEFECT AND DULLNESS

In 1944, nearly 2,000 men were transferred from the Pioneer Corps to an infantry division for training. About half of this number had originally been posted to the Pioneer Corps as a result of psychiatric recommendations, and half of them had been posted to that Corps before the introduction of the General Service scheme or in order to make up deficiencies. These men had been selected for transfer, as the 2,000 men of the *highest* physical and mental standard in the Armed Pioneer units in Northern Command, at a time when the man-power situation was very grave. After ten weeks' training, it was found that more than 50% were suitable only for employment in the Pioneer Corps; only 3% were considered fit for infantry duties; some 7% were fit only for domestic and simple administrative duties within the division; and less than 40% were regarded as possibly employable on garrison duties. Similarly, when, in April–May, 1945, a thorough search was made throughout the Armed Pioneer Corps in the U.K. for infantry trainees, not more than 400 potentially suitable subjects were found. From these data, it was clear, as the Director of Selection of Personnel pointed out in July, 1945, that the Pioneer Corps was not a source of infantry reinforcements and should be excluded from further consideration in this respect.

These various examples provide sufficient evidence of the futility of attempting to employ on more skilled duties men who, as a result of selection tests and psychiatric examination, have been found suitable only for service in armed or unarmed units of the Pioneer Corps. Any move to allocate large numbers of men in the selection group S.S.G. 5 to normal fighting arms is very quickly found to be deleterious to morale and efficiency in those arms.*

It may be mentioned that illiteracy and semi-illiteracy among recruits gave rise to various administrative and educational problems in the Army. Illiteracy occurred in about 1%, and semi-illiteracy in some 20–25% of recruits.† As a general rule, the illiterate soldier proved to be of very little use in a modern army, but his prospects

---

* After September, 1946, there occurred for a while, for a number of reasons, a lowering of standards applied to the drafting of men into the infantry and other arms. Within a year, the unequivocal results of this change were manifest, and the Director of Army Psychiatry reported, in September, 1947, on the unduly large number of dull and backward men in B.A.O.R., and drew attention to the high incidence among them of V.D., delinquency, psychiatric and other illness (figures confirming this impression have already been given).

† For figures relating to various periods, cf. *Parl. Deb.*, 5th ser., Commons, **395**: 1550; 15 Dec., 1943; **426**: 144; 30 July, 1946; **430**: 89; 19 Nov., 1946; and **434**: 1523–5, 1580–1; 13 March, 1947.

of effective service depended on the extent to which the condition was caused by lack of educational opportunity, as opposed to mental dullness. It was obvious that the majority of such cases were of low mental capacity and, after July, 1945, it became the usual policy to discharge such men at intake. In March, 1944, six-week courses in basic education were introduced by the Army educational authorities, and courses were subsequently held regularly for illiterates who were considered by Army psychiatrists and Personnel Selection Officers to be likely to benefit by such education.

It would be both tedious and unprofitable to discuss in any great detail the complex administrative aspects of the vicissitudes of Army policy in relation to the disposal of men with mental defect or dullness. However, a few of the more relevant administrative developments which have not already been mentioned may briefly be summarized.

Before the war, it was possible to discharge mental defectives from the Army either by medical board, or by certain general, routine administrative procedures.* After the outbreak of the war, however, such cases could only be discharged by medical board, with the unfortunate result that, through administrative rigidity and official casuistry, it became necessary for all dull and backward men to be dealt with, on discharge, in accordance with the regulations applicable to 'soldiers of unsound mind' or 'mental cases'; i.e. much as if, in civilian practice, it were necessary, say, to deal with borderline defectives in the same manner as certified psychotics.†

Thus, it is not surprising that much unnecessary distress was caused to the men concerned and their families, in cases where dullards who had been satisfactorily employed and adjusted in civil life and had been accepted for military service, were subsequently discharged from the Army in the circumstances described. Representations to the authorities, in this connection, were initiated in February, 1940, by the O.C., Military Hospital, Edinburgh (Lt.-Col. F. A. E. Crew), who suggested that medical boards and psychiatric specialists be authorized to report on such men as being unlikely to profit from military training, and that they thereafter be discharged gently and

* Cf. *King's Regulations*, 1935, § 383, (xvi) (*a*), (*b*); and § 383, (vi) (*a*), and (xviii) (*a*).
† These regulations provided that a harmless soldier of unsound mind (accompanied by an 'unarmed conducting party') could be handed over to the care of relatives or friends, who must first sign a certificate to the effect that "The nature of his disease and the fact that he may possibly be dangerous has been explained to me, but I am willing to accept full responsibility for him in every way." Cf. *King's Regulations*, 1935, §§ 403 (*a*) and 406; and *Regulations Med. Services Army*, 1938, § 546 and App. 20.

MENTAL DEFECT AND DULLNESS

sympathetically, encouraged to return to their former occupations and so serve the country to the best of their ability. The Consulting Psychiatrist pursued the matter and suggested that such men might be discharged, as before the war, by simple administrative procedure (on the recommendation of a psychiatrist).

As a result of these representations, certain instructions were issued by the War Office, in March and May, 1940: consequently, the method of discharge from the Army of mental defectives and dullards which was available in April, 1940, to the newly appointed Command Psychiatrists, was to forward to the War Office, for consideration and approval, a recommendation supported by reports by the C.O. and medical officer of the man's unit. This procedure was extremely unsatisfactory to all concerned, in that usually several weeks, and not infrequently several months, elapsed before recommendations for discharge were implemented, and during this time emotionally unstable dullards often broke down, or their condition deteriorated, with the result that it was necessary to admit them to hospital for treatment.*

In September, 1940, the War Office authorized the discharge from the Army of men, over 41 years of age and having voluntarily enlisted, who were either mentally defective, or habitual criminals. The official document, somewhat curiously phrased and conceived, stated that representations had been made from time to time that young soldiers particularly disliked having to associate with older men who had a bad criminal record, or who were of very low mentality, and so unaccountable that they were dangerous to the unit in a crisis; and that C.O.s of units had also suggested that these types of men should be discharged, as they were regarded as a menace and a source of trouble.†

In addition to the difficulties and delays in discharging unstable and low-grade dullards, the situation was, at the same time, aggravated by the fact that, in the absence of any adequate selection of

* Authority for the discharge of these cases was eventually delegated to G.O.s C.-in-C., Commands, in November, 1940. In a sample analysed in December, 1940, 59% of the men discharged in Northern Command for congenital mental defect had over 3 months' service *before* they were sent for examination by a specialist; 34% had over 6 months' service.

† Although this decision certainly did not run the risk of being too widely applicable, it was further specified that such discharges would not exceed two per thousand, and, after 1st November, 1940, one per thousand, of the strength of each command.—In November, 1940, the sheep were officially separated from the goats, and separate instructions were issued by the War Office, dealing, respectively, with the disposal of dull and backward men, and that of habitual criminals.

recruits at intake, large numbers of dull and backward individuals were still entering the Army. The complete failure of the authorities concerned to realize the importance of this fact is illustrated by their decision at that time to 'comb out' agricultural labourers for the Army. As pointed out by Col. Hargreaves in January, 1941, such a decision was farcical: as a group, these men were of very low intelligence; they could not, therefore, be expected to learn new skills in adult life, and could make little contribution to the work of modern armies, whereas, in their present agricultural employment, they had work which was both within their capacity and of vital importance to the community.

In March, 1941, the Command Psychiatrist, Northern Command, outlined a scheme for the selection and allocation of Army recruits, and suggested that men who were found, as a result of preliminary tests at the Ministry of Labour's recruiting examination, to fall into the least intelligent 25% of the population, should be sent to special Mobilization Depots, where further group tests, and, where necessary, individual testing and psychiatric examination, would be carried out. In this way, it was suggested, it would be possible to discharge rapidly those men who, because of mental defect or dullness, were unsuitable for military service, and to determine which men were suitable for employment in the Army in simple duties and in the Pioneer Corps.

In this connection, it may be mentioned that, in July, 1941, Brigadier Rees stated, in his memorandum on 'The Disposal of Dull and Backward Men', that the psychiatrists' attempts to deal efficiently with the problems of mental defect in the Army had brought little but hostile criticism from the Medical Services—a situation which also occurred in the First World War, in our own and in other armies. He drew attention to a leading article in *The Lancet*, which spoke of our "tardy recognition . . . of the fact that the soldier's mental qualities are at least as important as his physical, in estimating his efficiency, or placing him in the job where he will be most useful", and which referred to the organization being set up in the United States on the general principle that "the Army needs men sound in mind and body, it is not to be considered a corrective institution for psychopaths",* with the comment that this "is

---

* The American article to which *The Lancet* referred, stated: "The common fallacy that 'the Army will make a man of Johnny' has no place in the present system. The Army is an organization for the defence of the nation and is not to be considered a corrective institution." [126]

MENTAL DEFECT AND DULLNESS

flouted by those misguided patriots among examining doctors who can't see why 'a bad hat should get away with it' ".7

It was not until January, 1942, that an Army Council Instruction (A.C.I. 84/42) was issued, which dealt not only with the disposal of soldiers who were dull and backward, but also with others who for psychiatric reasons were unlikely to become efficient in their present military employment. This A.C.I. introduced certain important modifications in the methods of disposal of dullards, and constituted a very considerable advance in the administrative aspects of military psychiatric practice.

This A.C.I. reclassified dull and backward soldiers in relation to procedure for their disposal, and included the following provisions: soldiers whose mental backwardness rendered them permanently unfit for any form of military service would be brought before a medical board, with a view to their discharge from the Army on medical grounds; those who were emotionally stable, but so dull and backward that they were not fit to bear arms, though fit for routine manual work, would be transferred to an unarmed unit of the Pioneer Corps; and those who were emotionally stable, but had a capacity to learn which was much below average and were therefore unlikely to benefit by advanced training, though fit to bear arms, would be transferred to an ordinary armed company of the Pioneer Corps. Soldiers who were considered, either on the basis of their military service, or on medical examination in the unit, or as a result of selection tests, likely to fall into one of these categories, would be referred by their C.O. to a psychiatrist, who would recommend such action as might be necessary according to the provisions of the A.C.I.*

In July, 1942, with the introduction of the General Service intake scheme and the application of selection procedure to all recruits, it became possible to post men of low intelligence from the Primary Training Centre direct to suitable employment in the Pioneer Corps or elsewhere, and to detect at an early date unstable dullards who were not fit for military service.

In December, 1941, instructions were issued by the War Office, providing for the psychiatric examination, either before or after trial by court-martial, of soldiers suspected of low intelligence which

---

* A.C.I. 84/42 was amended, in June, 1944, by A.C.I. 904/44—A.C.I. 1493/44, issued in November, 1944, provided for the after-care of certain classes of soldiers discharged from the Army because of mental backwardness.

would not have been detected or recorded because of their enlistment before the introduction of selection testing, and whose unsatisfactory conduct might possibly be due to the fact that they were mentally backward and were serving in an unsuitable unit. The purpose of these instructions (which, in January, 1942, were incorporated in A.C.I. 137/42) was to ensure that these men, if proved to be dullards, would in due course either be transferred to an appropriate unit of the Pioneer Corps, or discharged from the Army, according to their mental capacity and stability.*

* Further instructions were subsequently issued, in February, 1942, and June, 1943, and in A.C.I. 1483/44 (November, 1944), concerning the psychiatric examination and report in disciplinary cases, which applied not only to dullards but to all psychiatric cases.

V

DISCIPLINARY PROBLEMS

> Men's thoughts are much according to their inclination: their discourse and speeches according to their learning and infused opinions; but their deeds are after as they have been accustomed.
> FRANCIS BACON

IT IS CERTAIN THAT, with regard to the problem of 'military crime', the Army psychiatrist is in a difficult position. As is the case with 'criminal' acts in any particular community or social organization, 'military crimes' consist in the transgression of a specific and rigid code of behaviour. The psychological and social adjustment of the civilian recruit to that code obtaining in the Army obviously constitutes a definite and important problem. Lt.-Col. N. Copeland has rightly pointed out that, in relation to the community as a whole, military crime is not necessarily anti-social conduct. Certain forms of behaviour which in a civilian setting might well be regarded as socially desirable and commendable, in the Army would essentially be regarded as a serious military crime: for example, the soldier who absents himself without leave from a draft for overseas service in order to visit his sick wife. In this connection, it may thus be said that in not a few instances it is, in a sense, the law and not the individual which has created the crime, and the words of De Quincey will be recalled: "By the law I came to know sin." The civilian recruit, the conscript, will tend to act 'after as he has been accustomed'.

Another difficulty may result from the sudden removal of the dullard or neurotic from the restricted civil environment to which he may have made a relative, if somewhat precarious, adjustment, and his transfer to a totally different environment requiring a considerable degree of readjustment even on the part of a reasonably stable and mature individual. The dullard or neurotic may, therefore, be incapable of acting otherwise than 'after as he has been accustomed'. This aspect of the problem and its consequences were, of course, far more pronounced before the introduction into the Army of an adequate system of personnel selection. The mechanization of the Service, intensive training and the tempo of modern warfare, very soon showed that one of the Army's main problems was the 'military misfit'. Such 'misfits' could be recognized at all stages of their military career—at intakes, training centres, medical units, and in Military Prisons and Detention Barracks.

The work of Army psychiatrists in relation to military delinquency, and to disciplinary problems and procedure, was necessarily governed by the practical limitations imposed by the general urgent demands of the national emergency and conditions of war, the restricted number of psychiatrists and specialized personnel available, and the nature and administrative rigidity, *ipse per se*, of the military organization.

In consequence, it may be said that military psychiatry had, in this respect, two principal objects. The first of these was stated by Brigadier Rees as follows: "Military crimes are easy to commit, and especially is this so for the dullards and the neurotics. We have aimed at avoiding conflicts of opinion, waste of psychiatric time through appearance at courts-martial, and the undertaking of legal procedure in psychiatric cases, where no good purpose was likely to be served either for the group or for the guilty individual." [96]

In addition, as specialists became available both in the field of psychiatry and in that of personnel selection, it gradually became possible to attempt to formulate a more rational classification of delinquents, which could serve as a basis for practical psychiatric work in relation to such cases and to the disciplinary problems that arose. As a result, the methods subsequently evolved were directed, more often than had previously been the case, towards the investigation of causative factors, with a view to the prevention of further crime, and towards the effective reintegration of the delinquent within the military social field.

It is relevant first to review some of the developments which eventually led to the introduction of the more recent administrative provisions for the psychiatric examination and disposal of military de-

DISCIPLINARY PROBLEMS

linquents of certain types, and the function of Army psychiatrists in relation to these cases.

The soldier who is referred for psychiatric examination, whether because of present or past delinquencies, presents many problems both clinical and administrative. The need for co-operation between psychiatrists and the military authorities, in dealing with disciplinary cases, had long been recognized by the more enlightened Army officers, both medical and non-medical, and had been clearly stated, as early as 1920, by Dr. Stanford Read. It was Dr. Read's opinion that "all frequent offenders, and certainly a large proportion of court-martial cases, should be mentally examined in order to get at the basic root of their anti-social acts, and so treat the offender and not the offence".[95]

As a result of the extensive mobilization, following the outbreak of the Second World War, of conscripts of all grades of mental capacity and stability, from many totally dissimilar socio-economic strata, there was a marked increase in the incidence of military offences. The urgency and complexity of the problems occasioned thereby, and the gradual development and increasing realization of the importance of psychiatry in the Army, were largely responsible for the introduction of administrative procedures designed to deal with some of the medico-legal questions arising in disciplinary cases.

At the beginning of the war there existed only the various general statutory and administrative provisions, regarding the medical examination of a soldier before or after trial by court-martial, and medical evidence during trial, where there was a question of insanity, or some doubt as to his mental condition.*

Officers considering the suspension and review of sentences awarded by courts-martial, under S. 57A of the Army Act (cf. *Army Act, 1955* S. 120), were instructed to direct special attention in all cases to the question, "whether the soldier was at the time subjected to any special stress, fatigue, disability or temptation". It was pointed out that "On active service additional considerations may arise. For example, some men . . . may commit grave military offences through momentary loss of control over their nerves and without any real wrongful intent." †

* *Army Act*, S. 130 (cf. *Army Act, 1955*, S. 116); *Circ. Memo. on Field Gen. Courts-Martial on Active Service for use in the UK.*, 1940, §§ 56, 57, 58 (*c*); *King's Regulations*, 1935, § 678 (*c*); 1940, § 691 (*c*).
† *Manual of Military Law*, 7th ed., 1929, pp. 796–8.

DISCIPLINARY PROBLEMS

As already mentioned in the chapter on Mental Defect, instructions were issued by the War Office in December, 1941 (and later incorporated in A.C.I. 137/42), concerning the psychiatric examination and disposal of certain delinquent soldiers suspected of mental backwardness.

The need had long been recognized for specific instructions clarifying the Army psychiatrist's position in relation to medico-legal procedure in *all* psychiatric examinations in disciplinary cases. Eventually, the several authorities concerned agreed to the publication of a Memorandum submitted by the Consulting Psychiatrist to the Army, which was issued in February, 1942, to all commands at home, and consisted of explanatory notes for psychiatrists. Part of the Memorandum which summarized the duties of unit medical officers with regard to the medical examination and, if necessary, the reference to a psychiatrist, of soldiers awaiting trial or commission to prison or detention, was circulated separately for the information of medical officers. It was the purpose of these instructions to ensure that the fitness to plead and 'criminal responsibility' of a soldier awaiting trial would be the subject of full and informed consideration by the convening officer, rather than that it should be raised in court for the first time by the defending officer. The Memorandum also set out the form of report to be used by psychiatrists, and defined their general function in disciplinary cases.

In March, 1943, the Judge Advocate-General's Branch raised the question of the misuse of psychiatrists' reports in court-martial cases. The principal difficulty was caused by defending officers who obtained psychiatric reports (particularly in cases of psychiatric disability not amounting to legal 'insanity'), which they produced in court, usually after the findings had been promulgated and in plea of mitigation of sentence. The court was, as a rule, not competent to interpret the report.

It was, therefore, considered advisable, in June, 1943, to issue another Memorandum clearly defining the function of Army psychiatrists in such cases, and the use which should be made of their reports. It was hoped thereby to obviate the hitherto frequent misunderstandings, and to ensure the adoption of the same procedure and form of report in all cases. It was thus intended that the Army psychiatrist should act, in every instance, in his proper function of expert adviser, briefed neither by the prosecution nor by the defence. It was felt that this was a significant advance, compared with

DISCIPLINARY PROBLEMS

civil legal procedure where medical witnesses did not act as expert advisers to the court but were called as witnesses by the prosecution or the defence. The Memorandum also revised the form of psychiatric report to be used in disciplinary cases. It was found that, where the procedure laid down in the Memorandum was followed, there were no difficulties in connection with the psychiatric issues.*

By defining the specific functions of psychiatrists in disciplinary cases, the administrative procedures outlined above formed, to some extent, a basis for more general confidence in the validity and reliability of psychiatric opinion, and were effective in disposing of accusations that psychiatrists were interfering with the proper administration of justice. These regulations were, therefore, generally welcomed by psychiatrists and by legal and executive officers alike.

The importance of ensuring that adequate facilities were available for the psychiatric examination of soldiers before trial, was clearly demonstrated by the remarkably constant findings in an analysis of the specialist reports in several large groups of such cases, at different periods between 1942 and 1945 inclusive. Of all the cases examined, about 80% were suffering from some demonstrable form of psychiatric illness. Most of these were psychoneurotics or psychopaths, but one-eighth to one-quarter of the total number examined were mentally defective, and some 3% to 6% were suffering from psychosis. It must, of course, be remembered that these cases were referred to psychiatrists prior to trial, because someone other than a psychiatrist or the accused considered a psychiatric opinion advisable; in other words, it was as a rule the most obvious cases, which could be picked out even by non-specialist medical officers or laymen, which were referred for psychiatric examination.

An Army Council Instruction (A.C.I. 373/42), issued in February, 1942, dealt with the methods of disposal, in various circumstances, of soldiers who had been found on medical examination to be permanently unfit for any form of military service, and were awaiting trial on a charge of desertion or absence without leave.†

Even during the latter half of 1942, considerable difficulty was still being experienced by psychiatrists in some areas, notably in Northern Ireland, in obtaining the appropriate disposal of disciplinary cases

---

* This document was incorporated, with a revised version of A.C.I. 137/42, in A.C.I. 1483/44 (issued in November, 1944).

† This A.C.I. was replaced, and its provisions extended to all disciplinary cases recommended for discharge on medical grounds, by A.C.I. 156/43, published in January, 1943.

DISCIPLINARY PROBLEMS

who were psychiatrically unfit. Over a period of six months, the Command Psychiatrist in Northern Ireland examined some 50 disciplinary cases (about three-quarters of this number being charged with A.W.O.L. or desertion): of the total number, he recommended that 50% be discharged from the Service on account of mental defect or other psychiatric disability, and that another 20% be transferred to the Pioneer Corps, but for various reasons, only one-third of the former, and one-fifth of the latter, were in fact disposed of according to his recommendations.*

In the early years of the war, considerable difficulty was experienced in disposing of soldiers of 'habitual bad character', chronic delinquents who gave no useful service in the Army, and whose influence on their units was deleterious to morale and military efficiency. Constantly involved in disciplinary procedure, and spending the greater part of their Army life in Military Prisons or Detention Barracks, these men were a considerable burden on the financial resources and man-power of the Army at this critical time. The principal difficulty in disposing of such men was administrative, and arose from the fact that discharge from the Army under certain relevant provisions of King's Regulations † had, unless in very exceptional circumstances, been in abeyance since the outbreak of war.

Another difficulty in the disposal of these cases was that they not infrequently presented a medical, psychiatric problem as well as an administrative, disciplinary one. Although a number of persistent military offenders were of the 'chronic criminal' type, i.e. recidivists of long standing in civil life, many others, such as those frequently absent without leave, came into the group of 'unwilling soldiers'. The latter have always been a problem in conscript armies, and include many different types of individual: some have developed in early childhood an anti-social, paranoid attitude towards the community and towards authority; others are easily discouraged, have stronger loyalties to their home and family, and are of low individual morale; many are mentally unstable and emotionally immature individuals of poor basic personality, low intelligence, or a psychopathic constitution.

* Representations resulted in the publication, in February, 1943, of a local Routine Order directing that, in future, the provisions of A.C.I. 156/43 would be strictly observed, and there was, subsequently, a great improvement in the general position with regard to the disposal of such cases.
† Viz., *King's Regulations*, 1940, § 390, (xi) (*a*), (*b*); (xii) and (xiii)—authorizing the discharge of soldiers for civil conviction of felony, on military or civil sentence of penal servitude, for misconduct, or after sentence to be discharged with ignominy.

DISCIPLINARY PROBLEMS

Army psychiatrists frequently pointed out that such individuals were not only useless to the Army and inefficient in themselves, but also a source of low morale and a danger to their comrades in battle, and these views received the support of many experienced combatant officers and others. The reluctance of the authorities to discharge these men was in part due to a belief that the serious man-power situation would not permit the Army to dispense with the 'services' of even the most inefficient and subversive individuals, though the latter spent most of their time in detention or absence and consumed, in the course of disciplinary procedure, much useful man-power which could ill be spared. It was also feared that large numbers of soldiers would be encouraged to commit frequent delinquencies in order to obtain their discharge, if it became known that this policy had been reintroduced. Furthermore, the psychiatrists were accused of seeking to enable delinquent men to evade military service, of attempting to 'get them off' and allowing them to avoid responsibility for their actions, and just retribution and condign punishment for their misdeeds.*

The psychiatrists, however, held the view that quality was of more importance than quantity, that the general effect on morale and fighting efficiency was a prime consideration, and that there was little to be said in favour of regarding the Army as a penal colony or forced labour camp.† It is interesting to recall that psychiatrists were also frequently accused of enabling 'malingerers' to evade military service, either by rejecting them at intake or by obtaining their medical discharge on the grounds that they were suffering from psychiatric illness.

In September, 1940, the War Office issued instructions concerning the 'discharge of soldiers considered mentally unfit and habitual

---

* Even as late as 1945, a Member of Parliament asked the Secretary of State for War if he would "keep a careful watch on these psychiatrists, bearing in mind that it would be highly improper if men got relief quicker through the 'glass house' than by any other means", and received the assurance, "I have been doing what my hon. Friend exhorts me to do, for some years past" (*Parl. Deb.*, 5th ser., Commons, **410**: 2259; 15 May, 1945).

† These views, which reflected the concern of Army psychiatrists about the selection of personnel and the state of morale in the Service as important aspects of psychiatric prophylaxis, and were shared by a number of experienced combatant officers and even by a few administrators, were by no means new. In 1879, in the Commons debate on the Army Discipline and Regulation Bill, Mr. Parnell stated: ". . . What was the punishment proposed by the clause? It was that a soldier guilty of desertion should serve longer in the Army. . . . If . . . a longer period of service was held out as a punishment to soldiers, the Army would be made objectionable to those persons desirous of enlisting" (*Parl. Deb.*, 3rd ser., **248**: 732; 26 June, 1879).

DISCIPLINARY PROBLEMS

criminals', which applied only to voluntarily enlisted men over 41 years of age.* There was no suitable method of discharge for younger men of the chronic delinquent or anti-social psychopathic type.

Thus, in the first years of the war, psychiatrists could recommend the discharge of chronic delinquents on purely medical grounds, only in those cases where there was definite evidence of gross psychiatric disorder, or in accordance with the various regulations gradually introduced concerning the disposal of dullards, in those showing definite evidence of mental defect. The large majority of chronic delinquents and unstable anti-social psychopaths could be discharged neither on administrative, disciplinary grounds, nor in appropriate cases, on psychiatric grounds. In particular, much difficulty was experienced in dealing with a number of soldiers whose chronic delinquency and military inefficiency was the result of a deepseated and long-standing disorder or defect of character, associated with emotional instability and immaturity, of the type known as 'psychopathic personality'.

The problem of the disposal of these 'psychopathic delinquents' was discussed by the various departments of the War Office concerned, in the summer of 1942. It was considered by the medical authorities, and in particular by the psychiatrists, that there were many practical and administrative reasons which made it impossible or undesirable to deal with all cases of this type through purely medical channels. In September, 1942, at the suggestion of the Director of Army Psychiatry, it was agreed that chronic delinquents showing evidence of lifelong anti-social psychopathic traits should be discharged by an administrative procedure,† and not in the same manner as other psychiatric cases.

It was not until January, 1944, however, that instructions were issued by the War Office to the headquarters of all commands at home, Home Forces and 21 Army Group—(and in October, 1944, to all commands overseas)—authorizing the discharge of 'psychopathic delinquents', whose disability was partly a medical and partly a disciplinary problem, by the above mentioned administrative procedure. These provisions were also applicable to patients of this type in military psychiatric hospitals, who had been found after investi-

---

* These instructions have been mentioned in the chapter on Mental Defect. In November, 1940, separate provisions were made for dull and backward men in this limited category, and the earlier instructions were restricted to habitual criminals over the age of 41 years.

† Under *King's Regulations*, 1940, § 390, (xviii) (*a*).

DISCIPLINARY PROBLEMS

gation not to be amenable to medical treatment or disciplinary measures. It must be admitted that, from the psychiatric point of view, it is not quite clear to what extent an individual who is acknowledged to be suffering from a 'disability' may be said (as in these instructions) to show 'an obvious unwillingness to overcome' its effects. In January, 1945, these provisions were extended to 'psychopathic delinquents' under sentence in Military Prisons and Detention Barracks, and those serving in Labour Companies, Special (Young Soldiers') Training Units, or 45 Division. It was decided that men of this type and in these units would not in future be sent to military psychiatric hospitals for observation except in cases of clinical necessity, but all applications for discharge as 'psychopathic delinquents' would be submitted only on the recommendation of a psychiatrist, and accompanied by a psychiatric report.

In July, 1945, a War Office Memorandum reintroduced the administrative discharge, under the provisions of King's Regulations which had been in abeyance, of soldiers of 'habitual bad character' who gave no useful service and were a harmful influence in their units, but could not be disposed of by existing procedures. It pointed out that there was, at that time, no satisfactory method of discharging men of this type below 41 years of age, unless they were in a low medical category or could be classified as psychopathic delinquents.

In December, 1945, all existing regulations concerning the discharge of habitual bad characters and psychopathic delinquents were incorporated in an Army Council Instruction (A.C.I. 1469/45).* The latter provided that *all* applications to the War Office for discharge of such men, whether for misconduct or as psychopathic delinquents, would be accompanied by a recent psychiatric report. It was thus finally possible for the Directorate of Army Psychiatry to ensure in every case that a man whose chronic anti-social behaviour was primarily due to definite psychiatric disability would be brought before a medical board, with a view to his discharge from the Army on medical grounds; or, that a man whose delinquency was primarily due to a psychopathic personality defect but whose disposal on purely medical grounds was not considered justifiable or practicable would be discharged accordingly. In cases where it was considered that there was no psychiatric disability, discharge was carried out on administrative, disciplinary grounds.

* This was replaced in June, 1946, by A.C.I. 650/46.

DISCIPLINARY PROBLEMS

Whatever the limitations, deficiencies and difficulties which, from the psychiatric point of view, were inevitably inherent in such a medico-legal, psychiatric-administrative compromise, it is certain that, from the pragmatic aspect of administratively efficient expedience, the measures embodied in A.C.I.s 1469/45 and 650/46 proved to be fully justified. Not only did they greatly facilitate and accelerate the disposal of these difficult cases, but at the same time, by requiring the psychiatric examination of nearly all men who were to be discharged from the Army on disciplinary grounds, they ensured so far as possible that any psychiatric disability would be detected and taken into account in determining the method of such a man's discharge and that in consequence, so far as possible, he would not suffer any injustice in this respect.*

Although these A.C.I.s were described by some critics, with more bitterness than truth, as 'the last nail in the coffin of military discipline', in fact they were generally welcomed by Army psychiatrists, disciplinary authorities and all others whose task it was, in their several spheres of action, to maintain and strengthen the morale, and hence the discipline and efficiency, of the Army. The men who could thus be discharged had been a burden to the Service, and had exerted an influence deleterious to military morale, discipline and efficiency, out of all proportion to their actual number. On an average, some 20 soldiers were discharged each month as psychopathic delinquents, under the provisions of one of these two successive A.C.I.s.

It remains to be noted that a preliminary psychiatric survey of a number of cases of psychopathic personality, who had been discharged either on medical grounds or as psychopathic delinquents, strongly suggested that at least some 50% of such men, who had subsequently proved such a liability to the Service, could without doubt have been detected at intake by a reasonably careful examination and case-history. Many had lifelong histories of maladjustment at home, at school and at work, of delinquency, neurotic symptoms, etc. Many showed evidence of mental dullness or instability.

From the very large number of disciplinary cases examined by

---

* Cf., however, the critical discussion on these methods of disposal of chronic and 'psychopathic' delinquents, in the report by Majors R. H. Ahrenfeldt and P. R. A. May, 'Practical Considerations on the Disposal of Delinquents in the Army' (September, 1949), part of which is reproduced in Appendix A.

DISCIPLINARY PROBLEMS

Army psychiatrists, it became clear that such military delinquents could conveniently be classified into five principal groups: young delinquent soldiers, recidivists or 'habitual bad characters', psychopathic and neurotic personalities, dullards, and psychotics. It was consequently possible to develop specific measures for the disposal and treatment of each particular group.

In the case of the first two groups, certain interesting sociological experiments were carried out in the Army for a limited period during the recent war; and although psychiatrists, largely because of their many other urgent commitments and the shortage of specialized personnel, were unable to play as important a part in these experiments as would have been desirable, they nevertheless were able to act in an advisory capacity, and contributed to the success of the schemes by assisting in the selection of the men to be rehabilitated. These experiments were the Special Training Units for young delinquent soldiers, and the Command Labour Companies for older, habitual offenders. Lt.-Col. R. F. Barbour, while acting as Psychiatric Adviser to 45 Division, was also adviser to the Director of Army Psychiatry on problems relating to Special Training Units and Command Labour Companies.

From the outbreak of war, there was an influx into the Army of volunteers under the age of 18 years, and these were formed into Young Soldiers' Battalions. The high incidence of delinquency (particularly, absence without leave) in these battalions presented a serious problem to the military authorities. The reasons for this state of affairs are complex, and may here be discussed.

Because of the lack of any scientific selection or allocation of recruits at the beginning of the war, a certain number of the young volunteers who were accepted for military service were for various reasons unsuitable. Not only were a number of dull and backward, and psychiatrically unstable men passed as fit for service, but the Army also attracted many individuals with questionable motives and poor personalities. The latter included, for example, aggressive and anti-social psychopaths, neurotics over-compensating for their inadequacy and weaklings compelled by social pressure or anxious to prove to themselves and to others their 'toughness', young chronic delinquents escaping from difficulties in civil life or seeking further adventure, and those who for diverse psychiatric reasons could not settle down to any job and were of the 'ne'er-do-well' type. Another important factor, in these young volunteers, was their chronological

DISCIPLINARY PROBLEMS

and emotional immaturity.* It is also true that these adolescents, as a group, were or had been subjected to the influence of the manifold causes of the increase in juvenile delinquency which was then occurring throughout the country.

Nevertheless, that these were not the main causes of the difficulties in the Young Soldiers' Battalions was clearly shown by psychiatric investigations into conditions in five 70th Battalions in Northern Command, and one 70th Battalion in Scottish Command, in July and September, 1941, respectively. These reports revealed that the basic problem in the young soldiers' units was one of low morale, and that this constituted as always a most suitable 'culture medium' in which the relatively small number of criminal, psychopathic, dull or unstable individuals necessarily exerted a maximal influence.

It is of obvious significance that the different detachments in one battalion showed striking variations in attitude and morale. Officers who had failed to build up good unit morale were ready to place the blame for unsatisfactory conditions on the alleged presence of large numbers of young criminals (ex-Borstal lads, etc.) and dullards, although they were unable to produce records to substantiate their statements. Some officers were uninspired, and a large number of N.C.O.s were too old for this type of unit, had no interest in the work, and were inadequate and unsuitable types who had been transferred because they were those least wanted by their original units. As one psychiatrist observed, there were reasons for supposing that it was the N.C.O.s rather than the men who were the poorer material at the outset.

One of the psychiatrist's reports clearly demonstrated the importance of the factor of immaturity in the lowering of these young soldiers' morale. Their ideas of what they expected from Army life when they volunteered were often of a highly-coloured adolescent type. More than half of them had quite certainly enlisted for reasons of pure patriotism. They were thus, at their age, more readily disillusioned by unnecessarily repetitive training, by long hours of hard duty under poor hygienic conditions, by the petty injustice to be found in small isolated detachments, by irregular leave, and by the lack of inspiring leadership in some parts of the battalion. Very many of them had joined other units for what were, to them, very

* An investigation by Lt.-Col. J. C. Penton in 1945–6 showed that a high proportion of deserters were in the lower age-groups, and that there were more than twice as many young volunteers among the deserters as in the Army population as a whole.

DISCIPLINARY PROBLEMS

strong reasons. They had chosen these units for reasons of local or family affiliation, and because they saw themselves as good Seaforths, Gordons, Camerons, etc. After a period of service with their senior relatives and with older men from their own locality, to be sent to a 'Boys' Battalion' was a great disappointment. They were unable easily to transfer their esprit de corps to the new unit. Thus demoralized, they were, on account of their age, more easily led by subversive talkers than would have been older, more mature men. Many, when they found that their spontaneity and early enthusiasm went unappreciated, learned gradually to order their lives to avoid punishment rather than to become good individual soldiers. The doctrine of the regular soldier, that it is unwise to volunteer or to make oneself conspicuous, was presented to them in extreme form by N.C.Os. many years their senior. Such an attitude was obviously inconsistent with the normal way of thinking of a man of 18.

These men were, for the most part, employed on monotonous and arduous aerodrome duties. This practice prevented real military training and the formation of esprit de corps when it was most needed. The young soldiers were probably the keenest recruits, but in this most unproductive job, many of them protested that they had not enlisted to be labourers. Further, they were always at a disadvantage to the R.A.F. personnel. There was a very marked and constant correlation in the rise and fall of the crime rate (and particularly, A.W.O.L.) when the unit took over and relinquished these aerodrome duties.

In many cases, young soldiers of hitherto excellent behaviour had in this way, on transfer to a Young Soldiers' Battalion, become demoralized and consequently delinquent: once their record was spoilt, they became resentful and discouraged, and developed a typically adolescent 'I won't play' attitude. They became involved in a vicious circle of absence, detention, no leave, and absence again. They made such statements as: "I have gone from bad to worse, I don't care what happens now"; or, "I don't care how long my crime sheet is, I would rather be in detention than here; I would soldier in a proper unit."

As early as November, 1940, following a discussion with the Assistant Director of Training who was much concerned about the problem of delinquency among young soldiers, Major G. H. Gilbey, W. Yorks., put forward a 'Salvage Scheme for Youths' and suggested the formation of a special battalion for the difficult cases. It

DISCIPLINARY PROBLEMS

was realized that the routine methods of military punishment not only were unlikely to have either deterrent or beneficial effects on these young soldiers, but could in fact be harmful. Major Gilbey commented that there were only two alternatives to his plan: to discharge all those who were not responding to Army training, and to refuse to recruit youths of 'bad character'; or to leave them where they were in the hope that they would eventually become good soldiers. For obvious reasons, neither alternative was desirable. Although the scheme was supported by the Army Commander, it was deferred as higher authority remembered the reactions to 'penal battalions' in the First World War. However, the problem remained, and Major Gilbey persevered, with the result that, in September, 1941, the Northern Command Young Soldiers' Training Camp was established at Pontefract, Yorks., as an experimental measure.

Instructions were accordingly issued to units in Northern Command, informing C.O.s that the training at this camp would be specially organized with a view to reclaiming young soldiers from a career of crime and converting them into good soldiers. All soldiers under 21 years of age who would normally be awarded a sentence of detention or a long period of C.B. might, at the discretion of their C.O., be sent to the Training Camp; and the sentences of all soldiers under 21 years who were at that time undergoing detention with their units, would be remitted and the men despatched to the Camp.*

The age limit for retention in the Young Soldiers' Training Units was officially set at 20 (later 21) years, and the normal period of training was three (later four) months. The programme of training included all general military subjects, and the organization and staff were, so far as possible, planned in such a way that the fullest attention might be given to the study of individual character. While attending a course at a Y.S.T.U., a soldier was subject to ordinary military discipline. It should be noted that intakes to these units eventually included a number of young conscripts as well as young volunteers.

It soon became apparent that many unsuitable cases were being sent to these units. An investigation was, therefore, carried out by a

* The scheme was officially recognized by the War Office and, in May, 1942, the Camp became No. 1 Young Soldiers' Training Unit (Y.S.T.U.). Two more Y.S.T.U.s were established, at Lowestoft, Suffolk (June, 1942), and Redhill, Surrey (September, 1942), respectively. In October, 1943, these units were renamed 'Special Training Units' (S.T.U.s). The policy and administrative procedure for Y.S.T.U.s were described in A.C.I.s 1371/42 (July, 1942), 192/43 (February, 1943), and 1486/43 (October, 1943).

DISCIPLINARY PROBLEMS

Personnel Selection Officer, a psychiatrist and a combatant officer, in the course of which every soldier in the S.T.U.s was subjected to a battery of intelligence and aptitude tests, and was individually interviewed. The data so obtained made it possible to sort out and appropriately dispose of unsuitable cases, such as dullards and neurotics, and the psychiatric interviews revealed that some of these soldiers were hopeless military material, and their discharge from the Army the only solution.

This investigation led to the introduction of a more scientific method of selection of cases to be sent to S.T.U.s. A War Office Memorandum, issued in April, 1944, attempted to provide, in general terms, criteria for the classification of young delinquent soldiers in the three broad groups, to be sent, respectively, to the three S.T.U.s: those with no record of serious military or civil delinquency, who showed an unsatisfactory attitude to authority and military discipline, but were of reasonable intelligence and emotional stability and regarded as redeemable; those with a record of detention in the Army or delinquency in civil life (or both), whose conduct in the Army was unsatisfactory, but who were still regarded as potentially redeemable; and those with a history of delinquency in the Army or in civil life (or both), and of several periods of detention, who were considered relatively unlikely to prove redeemable, in view of their history and personality.

A feature of some significance in this Memorandum was the recognition of the importance of emotional, rather than chronological, age in the selection of cases for S.T.U.s; and it was thus stated that, in exceptional circumstances, very immature men whose prospect of redemption was really good might be admitted to a S.T.U. up to the age of 24 years. The Memorandum also made it clear that no definite objective criteria could be laid down for the selection of these various types of delinquent: the prospect of redemption and probable response to disciplinary measures could not be determined in terms of psychological tests or the number of entries on the Field Conduct Sheet, but only by careful psychiatric assessment of the history and personality. It was further decided that C.O.s should no longer be authorized to transfer young soldiers direct to S.T.U.s, and that all cases recommended for such transfer would first be examined by selection teams (including psychiatrists) at Army Selection Centres, who would make the final decision.*

* Cf. A.C.I. 691/44 (May, 1944), replacing A.C.I. 1486/43.

DISCIPLINARY PROBLEMS

All S.T.U.s had been disbanded by August, 1945, so ending an important and promising experiment in social rehabilitation, which was only in its early stages.* Summarizing the work of the S.T.U.s, Col. Barbour concluded that, with the average offender, these methods worked excellently; with the more complex anti-social individual, rehabilitation by this system was not so easy. It should be added that it was in the treatment of these more complex cases, as well as in the selection of trainees, that psychiatrists, had they been available, could have made a valuable contribution to the experiment. In spite of certain limitations, however, it was estimated that over 75% of the trainees made a good adjustment on returning to their units.†

In the First World war, 'penal battalions' were formed to 'deal' with the problem of persistent offenders and troublesome individuals —the so-called 'habitual bad characters' and 'unwilling soldiers'. At the beginning of the recent war, because of the shortage of manpower and for various other reasons, the Army also decided to retain these soldiers, and considerable difficulties were at first experienced in attempting to discharge them from the Service. As might have been—and by some, had in fact been—anticipated, the problem created by these men, in consequence of this policy, had by 1942 become acute, and it was decided that it was necessary to segregate persistent offenders in special units.

In November, 1942, the War Office authorized the formation of Command Labour Companies for habitual bad characters who, because of their age-group, could not be discharged from the Army. As an experimental measure, two unarmed Labour Companies were formed in January, 1943, in Scottish and Northern Commands re-

* As a result of the more stringent selection of cases, and with D-Day and the mobilization of 21 Army Group, intakes into S.T.U.s decreased to one-quarter of their former size. By the autumn of 1944, the units were only half-full and were receiving very small intakes. One S.T.U. was therefore closed in October, 1944, and following V.E.-Day and consequent reductions in home establishments, both remaining units were disbanded in August, 1945.

† According to their follow-up reports, it would appear that some 80% of men sent to No. 2 S.T.U. were successfully rehabilitated for military service. For further information on the work of the S.T.U.s, cf. the book by J. Trenaman, *Out of Step*.[122]

It may here be noted that, in September, 1952, Dr. J. C. Penton presented a paper on 'The Juvenile Delinquent in the Forces', to the Psychology Section of the British Association for the Advancement of Science. Research into the military careers of juvenile delinquents when called up for service showed that about one-half made satisfactory soldiers; one-fifth, tolerable soldiers; and the remaining 30% were a liability. Of a control group, 90% made good soldiers, and 4% were a complete liability. (Cf. *The Times*, 10 Sept., 1952.)

spectively, and were employed on long-term unskilled work.* It should be made clear, however, that these units were not intended to be penal battalions, and the importance of their reformatory aspect was emphasized by the authorities. The selection of men for transfer to the Labour Companies was left to the discretion of G.O.s C.-in-C., Commands, and for this purpose, civil and military crime records were to be taken into account. From the outset of the experiment, the Director of Army Psychiatry pressed for the introduction of some form of psychiatric 'screening' of soldiers who were to be sent to the Labour Companies, as the experience of Army psychiatrists showed that many quite unsuitable men, such as recidivists and mental defectives on licence, were being recruited into the Service and it was feared that not a few of these individuals would be transferred to the new companies.

The scheme worked relatively satisfactorily, but it soon became clear that better results would be achieved if the Companies were graded, and the men to be sent to them were more carefully selected in the first place. A number of dullards and a few psychotics, among other unsuitable cases, had, as anticipated, been posted to the Labour Companies on the direct recommendation of C.O.s, and this necessitated a continual sorting of intakes by psychiatrists. Examination, in March, 1943, of the first 120 men sent to No. 2 Labour Company showed that one-quarter were unsuitable for such training, and in 23 of these cases transfer to the Pioneer Corps was advised. In view of these findings, it was agreed by Northern Command that all men from that Command should be examined by a psychiatrist before being sent to a Labour Company.

In December, 1943, the War Office directed that men who had been selected by their C.O. for transfer to a Labour Company, would first be sent to an Army Selection Centre, where a full selection team (medical officer, Personnel Selection Officer and psychiatrist) would decide whether they were, in fact, suitable for such transfer or whether they should be reallocated to another unit or arm, or disposed of through medical channels. Those men who were finally selected for Labour Companies were to be classified in three groups: 'redeemables', who were considered likely to become satisfactory soldiers after a course of special treatment; 'doubtfuls', who could not yet be classified as wholly 'incorrigible'; and 'incorrigibles',

* Nos. 1 and 2 Labour Companies, at Edinburgh and Tadcaster, Yorks., respectively.

DISCIPLINARY PROBLEMS

hardened criminals who remained unaffected by any kind of special treatment. In order that these groups might be segregated, and dealt with in different ways, two more Labour Companies were formed, in January, 1944, in Western and Scottish Commands respectively.* Men classified at the Army Selection Centre as 'redeemables' and 'doubtfuls' were sent to Nos. 1, 2 and 3 Labour Companies, and 'incorrigibles' were posted to No. 10 Company. 'Doubtful' cases could, if necessary, be transferred to No. 10 Company, if it later appeared that they were 'incorrigible', subject to the approval of the Command Psychiatrist and Command Personnel Selection Officer.

It was decided that men serving in these units would continue their military training and be subjected to a high standard of discipline, but that they would at the same time be allowed all normal privileges. The object of Nos. 1, 2 and 3 Labour Companies was the military rehabilitation, by careful individual treatment, of the soldiers sent there, and in this respect they were comparable to the S.T.U.s. The object of No. 10 Company was, by means of firm discipline, regular routine and good administration, to prevent, so far as possible, further deterioration of the 'incorrigibles', and thus to reduce the incidence of their offences.

In April, 1944, a War Office Memorandum was issued, with a view to improving the selection of chronic delinquents for transfer to Labour Companies. As in the case of the S.T.U.s, it was stated that the classification of offenders was not intended to provide rigid criteria, but rather to constitute a working basis for the psychiatrists at Army Selection Centres, and to ensure some degree of uniformity in the types of men sent to the respective Companies.

While the Company for 'incorrigibles' was, at first, run on almost identical lines to the other three units, it came to consist increasingly of the least modifiable criminal element, and it was ultimately decided that either No. 10 Company must be disbanded, or a regime more in accordance with ordinary prison methods introduced. The former course was adopted in September, 1944, and the majority of the men in this unit were discharged from the Army by administrative procedure.†

Apart from the psychiatrists' work in the selection of trainees for the Labour Companies, the Command Psychiatrists visited the Com-

* Nos. 3 and 10 Labour Companies, established near Pembroke, in Wales, and near Halkirk, Caithness, respectively. A.C.I. 134/44 (January, 1944) amplified existing instructions concerning Labour Companies.
† Under *King's Regulations*, 1940, § 390, (xviii) (*a*).

DISCIPLINARY PROBLEMS

panies every six weeks and, in conjunction with the C.O. and Personnel Selection Officer, decided whether men had been effectively rehabilitated and whether they could be posted to a new unit.

By September, 1945, all the Labour Companies had been disbanded.* Reviewing the work and achievements of the Labour Companies, Col. Barbour arrived at the following conclusions. The chronic absentee is frequently a military misfit who is 'redeemable', i.e. able to give efficient service in a non-penal unit, but only if the latter is specially staffed: otherwise, the mistakes of previous units will tend to be repeated. Such Companies can save C.O.s much administrative and training time; they contribute to the morale of normal units by disposing of the impression that the chronic A.W.O.L. obtains his discharge through his offences. In practice, these units earned their keep and rehabilitated at least one-third of the men sent to them.† The experiment of running non-penal Companies had, therefore, been a success and had justified the imaginative outlook of those who planned them.

In a report on the work of Special Training Units and Labour Companies, Major A. J. Hobley, R.A., who had gained considerable experience of these units while commanding No. 10 Labour Company (during the whole of its existence), and Nos. 1 and 3 Labour Companies and No. 2 S.T.U. (during their last few months), attributed much of their success in rehabilitation to the individual attention which was a basic feature of these experiments. The officers in particular, who were available at practically any time, and certain of the better N.C.O.s, were able to deal personally with the men's troubles, and this was, of course, supplemented by frequent visits from Army psychiatrists and Personnel Selection Officers, much welfare work of all kinds, and great efforts to promote educational, athletic and other activites, and to provide entertainments. It was found, in many cases, that misdemeanours were the outcome of uncongenial employment in the Army and consequent demoralization, and great importance was attached to suitable selection and reallocation on discharge from the units. This system of individual attention and rehabilitation involved considerable deviations from ordinary

* No. 2 Company was disbanded in May, 1944. No. 3 Company had never functioned adequately, having twice been moved, and was disbanded in December, 1944. Following V.E.-Day and the consequent reductions in home establishments, No. 1 Company was disbanded in September, 1945.

† From the follow-up reports, it appears that the rehabilitation rate in No. 1 Labour Company was 40%; in No. 3 Company (which, it has been noted, never functioned adequately), 26%; and even in No. 10 Company (for 'incorrigibles'), 28%.

DISCIPLINARY PROBLEMS

military discipline, and the exercise of leniency on many occasions, but these methods were almost invariably justified by results.

Discussing some of the reasons for the limited success of these experiments, Major Hobley referred to the local opposition which was encountered when the units were established.* This was particularly evident in the case of the Labour Companies, and added greatly to their difficulties. The opposition, which in most cases preceded the arrival of the units, went to the length of petitions and questions in Parliament. Stories were circulated and rumours spread that all the men were convicted criminals, that women would not be safe in their vicinity, and so on. Even the permanent staffs and officers were included in the general condemnation, and this 'took a lot of living down'. In fact, however, it was admitted by the local police that there was less crime in the localities concerned, than when other, ordinary units had been stationed there.

Furthermore, there was at times a lack of encouragement from higher authority, and in certain quarters these units were not wanted: this, in turn, may have been partly responsible for another factor militating against greater success, unsuitable staff. In some cases, C.O.s had disposed of 'unwanted' officers and N.C.O.s, when staff was required for the Labour Companies; and it had been laid down that, with the exception of the R.S.M. and provost sergeant, all staff could be of low medical category.†

* This, unfortunately, is a feature well known to those who have had experience of working in the more progressive, 'open' institutions and camps for juvenile and other delinquents, in civil life. Cf., for example, A. Aichhorn.[4]

† It is perhaps relevant to comment on the excessive caution so frequently shown by the authorities concerned, with regard to the more progressive and rational methods of rehabilitating delinquents, in spite of the vast amount of evidence which has accumulated in well over half a century, as to the successful results obtained in many such experiments in different countries. Indeed, the official reaction strikes the psychiatrist or sociologist as one of almost naïve surprise, when it has fortuitously been 'discovered' that delinquents other than the 'safe bets'—i.e. those who are most in need of rehabilitation—can benefit by, and respond to, these methods, as well as the 'star prisoners' who could, in fact, often safely have been placed on probation in the first place. Thus the Commissioners of Prisons: "On the outbreak of war, the bulk of the population of the prison . . . was transferred to Lowdham Grange, which . . . ceased to be a Borstal Institution, and Wakefield received a large number of ordinary prisoners . . . from Leeds, Manchester and Hull. It was impossible for the Governor and staff at Wakefield to alter their whole method of discipline . . . designed to evoke a real sense of responsibility and self-control from first offenders with fairly long sentences, to suit the very different natures and habits of their new charges. . . . The response of the recidivists was a pleasant surprise . . ., and provided much food for thought as to the training of this type of prisoner in the future." Some 250 men were then moved to Lowdham Grange: "Many of these men . . . were at an early stage of a long sentence, but all were now required to pass straight from the restraint of a prison wall to associated life in . . . a perfectly open Borstal. . . . Yet only two absconded . . . and less than 10 per cent. had to be transferred because they failed to maintain the high

DISCIPLINARY PROBLEMS

After the disbandment of S.T.U.s and Labour Companies, it was decided that all men who would previously have been recommended for transfer to such units, and thus first sent to an Army Selection Centre, would be dealt with by units of 45 Division.*

Army psychiatrists had occasion to investigate in some detail the various factors which were liable to lead to absence without leave, and desertion.

In the War of 1914–18, deserters, who not infrequently were suffering from obvious psychiatric disorders, were liable to the death penalty.[60, 97, 124] In the Second World War, desertion was no longer punishable with death as a maximal penalty, but severe sentences of imprisonment were imposed for this offence. Whatever may have been the various considerations which ultimately influenced the authorities in reaching their decision, it can hardly be doubted that the force of public opinion alone would have compelled this alteration in policy.

Army psychiatrists were convinced that the only logical and effective approach to the problem of desertion was a thorough scientific investigation of the causes of such behaviour in each individual case; and, in reply to the repeated, dogmatic assertion on the part of certain senior officers, and others in positions of authority and influence, they pointed out that a considerable number of men had deserted during the First World War even at the risk of facing execution.†

As a result of an investigation, in October, 1941, designed to discover how far misfits and untrainable men were concerned in repeated A.W.O.L., Lt.-Cols. T. F. Main and A. T. M. Wilson came to the conclusion that there was a fundamental relationship between military crime and low morale. Among 300 absentees in detention, it was found that there were twice as many dullards and defectives as in an equivalent random sample of recruits,‡ and that 15% of the

standard of conduct and discipline required. Many with bad records in other prisons worked well and gave no trouble while at Lowdham. Once again the exigencies of war showed that in future a more generous estimate of the trustworthiness of many convicted men may more safely be taken than was commonly supposed." [63]

* The functions of 45 Division, which were taken over (in somewhat modified form) in April, 1946, by the War Office Selection Centre, were the reassessment and reallocation of various groups of men, or their discharge from the Army if it appeared that they could not be usefully employed in any military capacity. Cf. A.C.I.s 389/45 (April, 1945), 164/46 (February, 1946), and 496/46 (May, 1946).

† For comparative statistics of the incidence of desertion in the British Army in the two World Wars, and a discussion of the question of desertion in relation to the death penalty (and its abolition); in fact and fiction, cf. Appendix B.

‡ The high incidence of dullards and defectives among deserters and absentees is discussed in some detail, in the chapter on Mental Defect.

total number were entirely unfit on psychiatric grounds for any form of military service. Furthermore, Cols. Main and Wilson stated that, whereas disciplinary action sufficiently severe to remove the symptom of absenteeism could no doubt be instituted, such action might well prove dangerous, unless accompanied by measures directed towards the improvement of the poor morale which was the basic cause of such behaviour.

The usual sentence imposed for desertion, during the B.L.A. Campaign, was one of three years' penal servitude. During the early part of this campaign, the problem of military delinquency, and particularly of desertion and absence without leave, in 21 Army Group became acute. Prisons and Field Punishment Camps were over-full, and more men were awaiting trial than could be dealt with by the disciplinary organization. The consequent wastage of man-power placed an appreciable strain on combatant units at a time when there was a most urgent need for all available fighting men. The Adviser in Psychiatry, 21 Army Group, therefore decided that a psychiatric examination of as many soldiers under sentence as possible should be carried out.

In November, 1944, over 100 soldiers belonging to units in 21 Army Group, under sentence in Fort Darland Detention Barracks, were examined by psychiatrists in order to ascertain whether they could be regarded, on medical and psychiatric grounds, as potentially 'valid reinforcements', i.e. as medically fit to return at once to duty in a forward area and, in particular, in a combatant unit. It was found that nearly three-quarters of this group of men were physically and mentally fit for immediate front-line duty overseas, and one-fifth were fit for immediate duty overseas in a limited capacity (either with a restricted employment recommendation, or in a lower medical category). Thus, 94% were considered fit for service overseas in some form, and the remaining 6% were fit for home service only. Those who were fit for limited service overseas, or home service only, included a number of neurotics and dullards. Of the neurotics who were fit for service overseas in a reduced medical category, nearly all were still officially in medical category A.1. All the neuroses in this group were mild anxiety states, not requiring hospital treatment and not incompatible with useful service in a lower category. Such men would, however, be very definite liabilities in category A.1. in combatant action, although they were not likely to develop urgent symptoms before they reached a forward area. 13%

DISCIPLINARY PROBLEMS

of the whole group required downgrading for neurosis; and 22% required employment recommendations, or lowering of category.

Among these soldiers under sentence from 21 Army Group, nearly all the offences were A.W.O.L. and desertion. Although a neurosis was often a contributory factor, it was, however, rarely the main cause of absenteeism. The psychiatrists' investigation of these men's histories confirmed the well-established view that good Army welfare, good man management, understanding and leadership, have a direct effect on the incidence of absenteeism.

Lt.-Col. J. C. Penton, with the collaboration of two other psychiatrists, examined over 100 soldiers under sentence in one Military Prison (No. 3) in 21 Army Group, and reached certain basic conclusions which were set out in a report, in November, 1944, to the Adviser in Psychiatry. After careful investigation of each man's personality and ability, of the stress to which he had been subjected at the time of his offence, and the adequacy of his training for the job he was expected to perform, it was considered that the prospect of rehabilitation for further service was fair to excellent in some 90% of cases, if due attention were given to each individual's future allocation. It was concluded that some 90% of all men undergoing long sentences for absence or desertion could be returned to duty with confidence that they would not commit further offences, provided that each man were given a full psychiatric interview which would be taken as the basis for his reallocation. The residual 10% were considered to be anti-social psychopaths and criminals, irredeemable for military service.

After this preliminary survey, an experimental Review of Sentences Board was set up in 2nd Army, consisting of the D.A. and Q.M.G., the A.A.G., and a psychiatrist (Major R. J. Phillips). The Board, which sat twice weekly at No. 8 Field Punishment Camp, interviewed each man personally three months after he had been sentenced, when his case came up for review in accordance with normal military routine. Formerly, review of sentence had always been carried out by the competent military authority, without personal interview, on the evidence of the Prison Commandant's report and documents dealing with the man's military history. At that time, the return of the men to the front line was considered to be the matter of greatest importance, and a man's consciously expressed attitude to further fighting was given great weight in deciding for or against suspension of sentence. No attempt was made to undertake any systematic assessment of personality, and cases were only given a full psychiatric examination if the Board felt some uncertainty concerning them.

The psychiatrist on the experimental Review of Sentences Board confirmed the main conclusions reached by Lt.-Col. Penton in his original investigation. In April, 1945, 159 cases had been followed up: the majority of these men had seen several months' active service since the suspension of their sentences in November and December, 1944. Reports from C.O.s of units showed that, of these 159 men, some 82% had proved 'satisfactory' and some 4% 'unsatisfactory' in their units; the remaining 14% had committed further offences for which they had been returned to the Military Prison. Major Phillips suggested, in his report, the advisability of employing a full-time Board, and of introducing scientific tests of intelligence and aptitude, 'personality pointers', etc., which would be available to the Board. Similarly, Col. Penton observed that, although in the circumstances of the campaign the results achieved might be considered satisfactory, the number of men returned to prison would have been considerably lowered if a more thorough examination of the personality had been possible.

While the original Review Board was working with 2nd Army, Col. Penton devised a questionnaire which was designed to elicit all the factual information necessary for a rough personality assessment of each case, as well as any material suggesting that the man required further psychiatric investigation. This procedure was evolved because of the shortage of psychiatrists, which rendered individual psychiatric interview impossible except in a few special cases. At the suggestion of the Commandant of No. 3 Military Prison, and with the concurrence of the D.A. and Q.M.G., 2nd Army, the report of the Prison Officer and the questionnaire completed by the latter were forwarded, with the Commandant's routine report based entirely on the man's behaviour in prison, to the Reviewing Board. Before the Commandant's final recommendation was made, the soldier was seen by a board at the Prison, consisting of the Commandant, a visiting psychiatrist, and the Prison Officer who had interviewed the man. Cases requiring further investigation or reallocation of employment were then seen individually by the psychiatrist, whose report was also forwarded to the 2nd Army Review Board.

Such was the situation when, on the successful result of the experimental Board, it was decided, in June, 1945, to set up a permanent

DISCIPLINARY PROBLEMS

Review Board for 21 Army Group, to review sentences of a certain type, mainly for desertion and absence. The president of the Board was a line officer (brigadier), empowered by the C.-in-C. to suspend sentences or to order them to remain in execution. The members of the Board included two regimental officers (as vice-president and secretary respectively) and a psychiatrist (Lt.-Col. J. C. Penton). The object of the Board, as stated in a directive issued to the president in June, 1945, was not only to discover men suitable for front line service again, but also to help the soldier under sentence to regain his self-respect and to become a useful member of the Army and of society upon his release from confinement. At the time, application was made for the inclusion on the establishment of the Board of trained personnel necessary for the use of scientific tests of ability and personality, in order that the members might have a full personality assessment before them when the man attended personally for review of his sentence. Unfortunately, this request was not granted. A psychiatrist had been included on the establishment, not merely to interview and report on doubtful cases, but to sit as an executive, expert member. This was decided in acceptance of the principle that, in every case, personality and the psychological aspect of the crime should receive consideration as well as the legal and disciplinary aspects, and that personality assessment was a psychiatric matter.

The procedure of the Board was largely dictated by circumstances, as was the psychiatric technique. All relevant documents having been studied, the soldier whose sentence was under consideration was brought in, and briefly questioned by each member; the president dealt with military matters, the vice-president with domestic affairs and questions concerning the man's background and upbringing, and the psychiatrist with the medical aspects. The great importance of this interview, which was made as informal as such an interview between officers and a private can be, was that the Board had a personal contact with the man and its members were able, after studying the objective documentary evidence, to form an intuitive conclusion concerning him. The psychiatrist was able to give the Board a rough personality assessment on the basis of the Prison Officer's questionnaire (upon which he had, of course, very largely to rely), but it was seldom found necessary to refer a man for further psychiatric examination before a decision could be reached. A thorough psychiatric and psychological examination at a military

DISCIPLINARY PROBLEMS

selection centre invariably took place before the man was posted for duty.

The headquarters of the Board were in Brussels, as this was the most convenient centre and adjacent to the three large Military Prisons situated at Douai, Antwerp and in Brussels itself; three Field Punishment Camps were also in the vicinity of Antwerp. The work of the Board commenced towards the end of June, 1945, with visits to the three Military Prisons, which were then holding a great number of cases long overdue for review. It was found that, with full data available and good organization, the Board could deal with a maximum of 36 cases daily: any larger number per diem caused too great a strain, as it was realized at the outset that anything like irritability through fatigue on the part of the members of the Board during the interviews would be most undesirable and liable to impair the value of the whole procedure. After three months' work, the Board had reviewed 1,300 cases, and were then in a position to deal with cases within a few weeks of the date on which they were actually due for review.

Originally, the Review of Sentences Board was authorized to see only those cases involving so-called 'cowardice' (desertion, absence, etc.), but the powers of the Board were twice extended, and, in April, 1946, came to include the review of all sentences in the B.A.O.R. It was suggested that the powers of the Board be further extended, in order that all men, on admission to Detention Barracks or Military Prisons, should be interviewed, and transferred, on the Board's recommendation, to a Military Prison, Field Punishment Camp, or special rehabilitation unit which would be set up for the purpose, according to the particular case. By this procedure, the adequate selection of delinquents at the outset, and their segregation in the appropriate institution, would be achieved, and this was regarded as an essential measure in their treatment. Such selection would be based entirely on personality, and not on length of sentence, seriousness of the crime, or other (psychiatrically) arbitrary criteria. In particular, those men who were regarded as irredeemable would be segregated from the others, and those who were considered to be easily redeemable would be sent to the proposed Rehabilitation Field Punishment Camp.

As a result of a survey of 2,000 deserters interviewed by the Board in B.A.O.R., Col. Penton was able to confirm previous findings, and, in particular, the relationship between morale and desertion. As he

DISCIPLINARY PROBLEMS

pointed out in his 'Study in the Psychology of Desertion and Absenteeism in Wartime, and its Relation to the Problem of Morale', (July, 1946), experience has shown that when the morale of the unit in war ceases to hold a soldier in his place, one of two reactions is likely: either the soldier will become obviously ill ('battle exhaustion') and will be treated as an invalid; or he will evade action by other means (usually, desertion), whereupon he will be treated as a criminal. It will be appreciated that the dividing line is ill-defined, and in this connection the judge's words, in Samuel Butler's *Erewhon*, come to mind: "You may say that it is your misfortune to be criminal: I answer that it is your crime to be unfortunate."

Some of the important factors in lowering morale and causing desertion and absenteeism in wartime, as clearly indicated by Col. Penton's investigation, must here be summarized. It was found that 57% of the 2,000 deserters showed some form of psychiatric instability (immature and 'inadequate' personalities, dullards, anti-social psychopaths). About one-third of the total number of deserters revealed, even on a relatively brief examination, a history indicative of difficulty in adapting to previous circumstances or of previous instability (e.g. maladjustment at school, unsettled work record, previous neurotic reaction to stress, or frank neurosis, and especially, unsettled home life), and the possible predictive value of these data in selective procedures should not be overlooked. There was a predominance of men in the lower age-groups (35% were under 21 years of age, and 73% were under 26 years, as compared with corresponding figures of 19% and 46% respectively, in the general Army population in B.L.A);* this appears to underline the importance of the factor of emotional immaturity. As already mentioned in the chapter on Mental Defect, a larger proportion of deserters than of the Army population as a whole ranked in the lower half of the intelligence rating scale.

The fact that 25% of deserters had been in previous campaigns, as compared with 6% of the infantry of the B.L.A. as a whole, suggests that previous campaigning and 'campaign stress' are an important factor in desertion: the endurance of a fighting soldier is limited, each man having a specific potentiality dependent on his own basic resistance and the intensity and duration of the stresses to which he

---

* Similarly, of a group of nearly 100 deserters studied in the M.E.F., in March, 1944, 68% were under 26 years of age, as compared with 24% of a control group in an infantry battalion.

DISCIPLINARY PROBLEMS

is subjected. It was found that, proportionately to their total numbers, regular soldiers deserted as readily as conscripts, probably partly because, having served since the beginning of the war, they were more likely to have taken part in several campaigns ('campaign stress'), and partly because of poor selection in peace-time, a number of these men being unstable or 'ne'er-do-well' types. As stated by Col. Penton, this finding points clearly to the need for careful review of the conditions of service and recruitment of men for the fighting arms of the regular Army of the future.

There were more than twice as many young volunteers among the deserters as in the B.L.A. population as a whole. The probable reasons for this striking feature are a high incidence of immaturity in this group, and the fact that voluntary service attracted many individuals with dubious motives and personality structure (e.g. hysterics, psychopaths, 'ne'er-do-well', over-compensating weaklings, etc.). As Col. Penton well observed, in this connection, the rate of desertion amongst young volunteers must cause some misgiving to the protagonists of voluntary recruitment unless they are so wedded to the theory of the survival of the fittest that they are willing to bear the enormous waste that this method of selection has involved during the evolution of species. There was also, among the deserters, a considerable preponderance of infantrymen, who constituted no less than 89% of the total.*

Other causes which, to a varying extent, and directly or indirectly, were shown by this investigation to be operative in a certain number of cases of desertion, were the lack of morale-building factors (lack of training and self-confidence, or identification with the unit, of general adaptation to the Army, etc.), or the presence of morale-destroying factors (inevitable external strains, such as battle or campaign stress; inevitable internal strains, such as changes in, or separation from, the group; poor leadership, grievances, domestic and personal difficulties, etc.). In particular, it may be mentioned that some form of domestic stress appeared to be a significant factor in nearly one-third of cases: and although this was seldom the sole factor, as Col. Penton has pointed out, nor even the most important, it must often have been the deciding one, the one most admissible to con-

---

* The investigation of soldiers from 21 Army Group under sentence in Fort Darland Detention Barracks also showed a preponderance of infantrymen, who constituted more than half the total number. Similarly, the psychiatric examination of nearly 100 deserters in the M.E.F., in March, 1944, revealed that 81% of the group were in the infantry.

DISCIPLINARY PROBLEMS

sciousness, giving the man a feeling that he was justified by the obligations he owed his home and parents in taking to flight.

Col. Penton concluded his careful and detailed study with the comment that, if his thesis concerning the relation of desertion to group morale was correct, the effect of prolonged detention upon a deserter would be to make a second desertion more likely. If personal morale was low, the treatment must be to place the man in a group where morale was high, so that his own might be raised. Removal to an exotic environment, where he would become integrated in an anti-social group and denied the rehabilitative effect of companions and leaders of good morale, would have an effect opposite to that desired. The prison staff just as much as the detainees were the victims of an emotional system designed to satisfy an emotional demand, and erroneously supposed to provide a rational solution to a problem that had not yet been tackled on a rational level.

In September, 1941, the Army medical authorities were asked for their opinion on the general fitness of soldiers undergoing sentences in Detention Barracks, as it was desired to ascertain the potential military usefulness and efficiency of such men if it should prove necessary at any time to release them suddenly in an emergency, e.g. in the event of invasion, when the services of all fighting men would be called upon.

The Consulting Psychiatrist asked for reports from Army psychiatrists in all parts of the United Kingdom, and the information so obtained provided a very useful outline of a number of problems of psychiatric importance concerning military delinquents and penal institutions at that time. There was general agreement that these men were reasonably fit physically, but that it was doubtful how many of them would be mentally fit for useful activity in an emergency, as they included a fairly high proportion of psychopaths and dullards, and it was clear that for this type of man the atmosphere of some at least of the Detention Barracks was not particularly helpful. Brigadier Rees pointed out, in this connection, that more investigation was required, as to the type of man who was placed in detention, and the type of treatment which he received there.

In assessing the reliability and balance of the statements made by Army psychiatrists on the military penal institutions at the time, it should be remembered that all of these specialists were senior medical men of very considerable experience.

DISCIPLINARY PROBLEMS

One psychiatrist, reporting on the Military Prison and Detention Barracks, Aldershot, commented on the fact that 25% of the men in detention had been there before, and that it seemed probable that the somewhat severe treatment which they received produced resentment in the men, and thus lowered their morale. All experienced officers with whom he had discussed the matter, both inside and outside the Detention Barracks, agreed that a vast majority of the soldiers in detention were there because they had been badly handled by inexperienced officers and N.C.O.s in their units.

Another psychiatrist (Major E. A. Clegg), in a memorandum on the 'Effects of Detention on Morale', expressed the view that the military efficiency of soldiers undergoing detention would, on the whole, be impaired. In the case of unstable dullards, sudden release from detention would most probably be regarded as a chance to escape. The psychoneurotic group of prisoners for the most part found themselves in detention because of some impulsive act: in general, detention was not likely to improve the efficiency of these men, and indeed could hardly be expected to do so; their feelings of inferiority were not made any less, by the suffering of indignities which were an essential part of Detention Barracks routine. As to the effect on the individual of military penal institutions at the time, Major Clegg commented that he could not believe that to be shouted at all day long, being made to do everything at the double, or having to stand with one's face to the wall for long periods at a time, could possibly enhance the sense of personal dignity in any man. In his opinion, a period of detention should be synonymous, not with a withdrawal from military training, but rather with an intensification of the latter. He believed that withdrawal of liberty would be perfectly understandable, and even acceptable, to a man under sentence, but the positive suggestion of personal worthlessness or of loss of individuality should be avoided. There would appear to be no good reason why the inmates of Detention Barracks should not be trained as a unit, made up of members of other units.

In January and October, 1941, a group test of intelligence was given to all the soldiers under sentence in the Military Prison and Detention Barracks, Shepton Mallet: on both occasions, it was demonstrated that these men included a greater proportion of dullards than did the population as a whole, and in several such cases it was considered desirable to transfer men to the Pioneer Corps rather than return them to their units. A group intelligence test

DISCIPLINARY PROBLEMS

carried out, in October, 1941, on a small number of men undergoing detention in the Military Prison and Detention Barracks, Aldershot, showed that men in the lower intelligence grades formed a higher proportion of recidivists than of soldiers serving their first sentence, and a higher proportion of first offenders than of the Army population as a whole.*

Investigations by Army psychiatrists, completed in November, 1942, provided evidence confirming much that had already been generally suspected, regarding the incidence of psychiatric disability among soldiers under sentence, and especially among recidivists. Of more than 200 such men examined by psychiatrists, nearly 50% were found to be suffering from psychiatric disorders, of which mental deficiency constituted the largest group (i.e. 25% of the total number examined, or one-half of all those with psychiatric conditions), and anxiety neurosis the second largest group (i.e. 20% of the total number examined). It was also found that absence without leave and desertion together comprised some three-quarters of all the offences for which men were committed at that time. It was noted that much military crime was committed by relatively few men, and that 20% to 25% of soldiers admitted to Detention Barracks were subsequently readmitted for further offences, i.e. were recidivists. In another series of more than 800 soldiers under sentence, the proportion of dull men comprised between one-quarter and one-third of the total number.

Among the various recommendations made as a result of these investigations, and taken up by the Director of Army Psychiatry, were the suggestions that psychiatric (disciplinary) cases be segregated in special detention barracks where they could be dealt with appropriately; that every offender receive individual attention in his unit and assistance after his discharge from detention; and that soldiers under sentence be examined before being posted overseas, in order thus to prevent many psychiatrically unstable men from being sent abroad, and a consequent lowering of the fighting power of their units. These recommendations, so far as can be ascertained, resulted in no significant action at that time on the part of the authorities concerned.

In view of the critical man-power situation, it was the practice,

* Much evidence was subsequently obtained, which fully confirmed the findings of these earlier investigations, concerning the important relationship between military crime and mental backwardness. The later investigations are summarized in the chapter on Mental Defect.

DISCIPLINARY PROBLEMS

in the earlier part of the war, to release certain soldiers on suspended sentence from civil and military prisons, and transfer them immediately to operational theatres. It became clear, however, that, taking the long view, this procedure, unaccompanied as it was by psychiatric screening, was exceedingly uneconomical. A number of dullards, psychopaths, and other unstable and inadequate individuals, who were unfit for front-line duties or, in some cases, for any form of military service, were sent overseas to combatant units, where they not only had an influence deleterious to morale and military efficiency, but also frequently became once more the responsibility of disciplinary or medical authorities and, consequently, consumers of valuable man-power, transport, and other vital resources. Thus, the indiscriminate use of such men proved in fact a false and illusory economy.

Eventually, in December, 1944, it was decided that all soldiers admitted to Group 'C' Military Prisons and Detention Barracks (viz., recidivists and those considered to have an undesirable influence in ordinary Military Prisons) would be examined by Army psychiatrists as soon as possible after admission. The first 500 psychiatric examinations carried out in accordance with this instruction revealed that only 48% of these men were considered mentally fit for overseas service. It was noted that some 30% of the total number were already in the Pioneer Corps, and another 3% were recommended for transfer to that Corps. It was recommended that 27% of the total be discharged on medical grounds or as psychopathic delinquents, and that 2·5% be admitted to a psychiatric hospital. 50% were in the lowest intelligence groups (S.G. 4 and 5), as compared with 30% of a random sample of recruits.

About the same time, the Adjutant-General requested that there should be closer collaboration between the Army medical authorities and the Prison Medical Service, in respect of soldiers under sentence in civil prisons. It was, therefore, arranged that Army psychiatrists would examine all soldiers detained in civil prisons, soon after their admission or immediately prior to review of their sentence by the War Office. Between January and July, 1945, several hundred soldiers were examined in this way, and it was found that 78% of these were fit for some form of service overseas. It was recommended that 14% be discharged on medical or non-medical grounds. The majority of soldiers under sentence in civil prisons were men who had deserted during battle while serving overseas; many of them had

DISCIPLINARY PROBLEMS

deserted only under very severe stress. In July, 1945, following the cessation of hostilities in Europe, there was a change of policy regarding the review of such cases, and it was considered unnecessary for the War Office to have these psychiatric reports. It was then arranged with the Prison Commission that Prison Medical Officers could have direct access to Command Psychiatrists for guidance or advice in any individual case, in accordance with the Adjutant-General's earlier request.

In view of the critical observations which it is presently proposed to make, on such aspects of military disciplinary methods as are the particular concern of the psychiatrists, e.g. selection, morale, and rehabilitation, it is appropriate first to refer to the development of more recent trends towards a reform of the institutional penal system in the Army.

In 1943 and following years, certain incidents, whether fortuitous or of more general significance, aroused much public concern, which found expression in the press and in Parliament, as to the methods of administration and conditions prevailing in Military Prisons and Detention Barracks, and led to various official investigations and subsequent recommendations.

The circumstances in question may briefly be summarized. In March, 1943, the death of a soldier under sentence in Fort Darland Detention Barracks led to the institution of a military court of enquiry;* and to the appointment by the Government of a Committee of Enquiry (Oliver Committee) to investigate and report on all aspects of the treatment of men under sentence in Naval and Military Prisons and Detention Barracks in the United Kingdom and "whether it is in accordance with modern standards and satisfies wartime requirements".[102] In October, 1945, following the suicide of a soldier under sentence at Stakehill Detention Barracks, the Government did not consider that a further public enquiry was necessary, but agreed to requests from Members of Parliament that an Army psychiatrist should be included among the officers forming the military court of enquiry.† In February and March, 1946,

---

* Cf. *Parl. Deb.*, 5th ser., Commons, **395**: 1386–9; 14 Dec., 1943.

† Cf. *Parl. Deb.*, 5th ser., Commons, **416**; 372; 20 Nov., 1945; and 1087; 27 Nov., 1945; **421**: 183–6; 26 March, 1946. In this connection, the Secretary of State for War was also asked "to see that proper . . . arrangements are made from the psychiatric point of view. There are very few psychiatrists attending [detention] camps . . ." (*ibid.*, **416**: 1225–34; 27 Nov., 1945).

DISCIPLINARY PROBLEMS

disturbances or 'mutinies' which received wide publicity occurred, respectively, at Aldershot and Northallerton Detention Barracks,* and the Secretary of State for War informed the House of Commons of his intention to review "the whole system of detention".†

All these enquiries, whether of local military courts of enquiry in particular instances, or the general investigation by the Oliver Committee, agreed in the conclusion that there was, in general, no brutality or gross maltreatment of soldiers under sentence.

Reference will now be made to some of the comments, findings and recommendations of the Oliver Committee as a result of their thorough investigation of all Military Prisons and Detention Barracks in the United Kingdom, where they appear to be particularly relevant to the matters to be discussed below.

The Committee found that the staff, of the Military Provost Staff Corps (M.P.S.C.), were insufficient in number and, to some extent, inadequate in quality and in training; and recommended that a M.P.S.C. training school be established. It was well observed that "The whole problem of securing really efficient and trained staff for these places is beset with the greatest difficulties in these days of shortage of man-power and especially of efficient man-power. The qualities of a capable warder ... are the very qualities of an efficient N.C.O. with a combatant unit." Such men should be volunteers: "It would not be easy to believe that a man who was compelled to take the position of a warder against his wish would make a good one." "In so far as relates to abuse, bad language, and 'chasing', the Committee are satisfied ... that these practices did exist from the earliest days and were worse at the beginning than they are now. In this connection it must be borne in mind that the detention machinery of the Army at the start of the war was just as backward as the rest of the country's military preparation." On the other hand, an important fact noted by the Committee was the adverse effect on the morale (and, presumably, the recruiting) of the staff, of the widespread and unfounded allegations about the general ill-treatment of soldiers under sentence.‡

---

* For statements on the disturbances at Aldershot, cf. *Parl. Deb.*, 5th ser., Commons, **419**: 1572–3; 25 Feb., 1946; **421**: 187–90; 26 March, 1946; and on those at Northallerton, cf. *ibid.*, **420**; 42; 5 March, 1946. In fact, it was at this time officially stated that "three mutinies, one major disturbance and two minor disturbances have taken place recently in Military Prisons and Detention Barracks" (*ibid.*, **420**: 185; 12 March, 1946).

† Cf. *Parl. Deb.*, 5th ser., Commons, **421**: 183–6, 187–90; 26 March, 1946.

‡ "In some places, members of the staff, wearing as they do a prominent red flash with 'M.P.S.C.' on their shoulders, cannot appear in public without the risk of

DISCIPLINARY PROBLEMS

It was recommended that a full-time medical officer should be appointed to each Detention Barracks, although the shortage of medical men at the time was recognized. It was noted that "moreover the most important aspect of these appointments is that the man should have a particular aptitude for this rather specialized and difficult type of work". The Committee "were very much dissatisfied with some of the sanitary arrangements at the majority of the military institutions they visited". It may be mentioned, incidentally, that the old-fashioned 'dietary punishments' were still in use.*

With regard to training and welfare of soldiers under sentence, the Committee made some significant comments: "If the purpose of detention as a method of rehabilitation as well as of punishment is borne in mind, the importance of using the period of a man's sentence as an opportunity for education is obvious." They recommended an extension of facilities for general education as well as for training in technical military subjects. Further, "Welfare Officers are on the strength of all Military Detention Barracks. . . . But while appreciating the value of welfare services in detention the Committee are of opinion that these are frequently rendered too late. They desire to emphasize as strongly as possible the importance of good welfare work in the units from which the men come, as the principal means of saving men from getting into the trouble which leads to detention. They consider that if the admirable Notes for Officers issued by the Adjutant-General under the title 'The Soldiers' Welfare', were fully carried into effect, particularly by Company and Platoon Officers, perhaps as many as fifty per cent. of those who are now soldiers under sentence would never have had to be committed to detention."

The Committee also emphasized the necessity for strictly maintaining the system of segregation of different types of men under sentence (recidivists, first offenders, etc.).[102]

Thus, it cannot be denied that much factual evidence existed that, from the psychiatric point of view, i.e. that of rehabilitation rather than punishment of military offenders, the policy relating to Military Prisons and Detention Barracks, and the conditions prevailing therein,

---

aversion, insult, and assault. Many of the best of them keep within their own precincts. . . . In this way men whose work is hard and thankless enough in the nature of things are deprived of even reasonable recreation and relaxation." [102]

* This senseless, childish, non-reformative type of punishment was still occasionally used, both in the M.C.E., Colchester, and in the M.P. and D.B., Shepton Mallet, at the end of 1948.

DISCIPLINARY PROBLEMS

were in many respects far from satisfactory. It must also be borne in mind that the Oliver Committee carried out their investigations after certain general recommendations made by the military court of enquiry at Fort Darland Detention Barracks had already been accepted. The Committee's Report nevertheless showed that, even at their worst, the general policy and conditions in Military Prisons and Detention Barracks compared very favourably with the very primitive orientation and methods then existing in the majority of the Naval Detention Quarters.

In July, 1946, a "detailed summary of the general post-war policy and plans with regard to Military Prisons and Detention Barracks" was circulated among Members of Parliament by the Secretary of State for War, whose explicit object was, "while there are detention camps, ... to achieve reform rather than punishment". It was proposed to introduce a new type of institution, 'Disciplinary Training Centres' (subsequently known as 'Military Corrective Establishments'), in addition to the Military Prison and Detention Barracks.*

There is reason to believe that the plans for the proposed new system and type of institution for the rehabilitation of military delinquents, were principally the outcome of the successful results obtained by the development of the B.L.A. and B.A.O.R. Review of Sentences Board and of experience in connection with an experimental penal establishment in the C.M.F.

The circumstances which eventually led to the creation of this experimental establishment in the C.M.F. may briefly be mentioned here, although it would appear that little or no use was made of Army psychiatrists in connection with this work. With the invasion of Italy, the incidence of front-line desertion in the newly constituted C.M.F. rose rapidly and necessitated an equally rapid expansion of the number of penal establishments in that theatre. By July, 1944, the situation with regard to prison accommodation had become most acute, and the question of extending the policy of suspension of sentences came once again under consideration. It was left to Prison Commandants to decide, on the basis of a man's expressed desire to 'make good', whether or not to recommend suspension of sentence. Following discussions between the D.A.G. and Inspector of Military Prisons, in August, 1944, it was decided to establish a 'Rehabilita-

* *Parl. Deb.*, 5th ser., Commons, **424**: 1933–5; 2 July, 1946. Legislative provision for the establishment and regulation of M.C.E.s. was eventually introduced by the *Army and Air Force (Annual) Act, 1947*, S. 9, amending S. 132 of the *Army Act.* (Cf. *Parl. Deb., ibid.*, **435**: 1292–9; 26 March, 1947.)

tion Centre', to which men who were considered potentially redeemable as soldiers could be transferred from Military Prisons.

This 'Rehabilitation Centre', which was intended as a development of the Field Punishment Camp system, was opened in December, 1944, and was known as No. 34 Special Training Barracks, C.M.F. Its purpose was to train as 'fighting soldiers' men under sentence, and to act as a transition from a Military Prison to a line unit, and it appears that the intention was that some of these delinquents might be given a chance to 'redeem themselves', following their previous desertion, in front-line action. The Special Training Barracks, therefore, concentrated on military training and strict discipline. The normal period spent at the Barracks was three months, and during this time there was a progressive increase in the 'amenities' of the barrack room, the amount of trust and relative liberty of movement, which a man enjoyed. It was left to the Commandant to decide whether to recommend suspension of a man's sentence or whether he should be sent back to a Military Prison.*

The new scheme for the reorganization of the military institutional penal system was defined (as to object and administration) in a series of instructions issued by the War Office, between August, 1947, and January, 1948.†

Briefly, it was intended that there should be Military Corrective Establishments of two kinds (Types 'A' and 'B'), as well as Military Prisons and Detention Barracks (Type 'C').

The M.C.E.s were intended for soldiers capable of rehabilitation, and, therefore, ultimately suitable to be returned to the Army: military training was to be continued while the soldier was serving his sentence. These men would first be sent to a Type 'A' establishment, where conditions were more rigid, and discipline rigorous, and, after one month or so, would be transferred to a Type 'B' establishment. The latter was to comprise three stages, and normally, two to four weeks would be spent in each stage: these were designed to increase progressively the degree of liberty, until his rehabilitation rendered

* It is regrettable that psychiatric methods played no part in the selection, classification, investigation, and rehabilitation of the men who were sent to this establishment, and it is noteworthy that the reports describing its work make no mention of welfare facilities, although they acknowledge the fact that, in some of these cases at least, domestic and personal factors originally contributed to the poor state of the men's morale.

† Viz., a War Office Letter of August, 1947, on the basic principles of the new policy; A.C.I.s 848/47 and 849/47 (October, 1947), on the object and administration of M.C.E.s and Type 'C' M.P.s and D.B.s, respectively; and a War Office Letter of January, 1948, amplifying these three documents.

DISCIPLINARY PROBLEMS

a soldier suitable for the final (third) stage, which would include a system of parole. Progression to the final stage would not, however, be 'automatic', but (somewhat paradoxically, in this context of rehabilitation) would occur only when it was considered (by the commandant) that a man had been punished for his offence, and was 'well on the road' to military rehabilitation.

Men in both types of M.C.E. would be segregated in four classes: soldiers under 21 years of age of previous good character; soldiers over 21 years of age serving a first sentence and soldiers under 21 years serving a second or subsequent sentence; soldiers over 21 years serving a second or subsequent sentence; and habitual offenders who were considered by their C.O.s to be capable of rehabilitation, and those transferred from Type 'C' M.P.s and D.B.s.

The Type 'C' M.P. and D.B. was intended for soldiers incapable of military rehabilitation: its primary object was, therefore, to rehabilitate as citizens (i.e. for civil life) men of this type who were retained in military custody; its secondary object was the safe custody of habitual offenders or soldiers of bad character who, by reason of their terms of service, would be required to return to the Army. In the Type 'C' institution, there would be no military training, but provision would be made for educational instruction, training in industrial work, and physical training.

The War Office Letter of August, 1947, stated that the principles underlying the new scheme depended for success mainly on three factors: the provision of an adequate and suitable staff for all penal establishments; the organization of military training (at M.C.E.s) on a standard at least as high as that of the Primary Training Centres; and the co-operation of C.O.s in committing an offender to the appropriate establishment, and of superior military authorities in suspending any unexpired portion of the sentence of a soldier who had served a satisfactory period in the final stage of the Type 'B' M.C.E.

The possible function of the Army psychiatrist also received some mention in these various documents. The War Office Letter of August, 1947, stated that the decision as to the type of penal establishment to which a soldier would be sent would be left to his C.O., who would have the most intimate knowledge of his character; Command Psychiatrists might, however, be called upon to advise in regard to this decision. A.C.I. 848/47, on the other hand, did not specifically state that a psychiatrist might be called upon to advise the C.O., who was responsible for making the decision.

DISCIPLINARY PROBLEMS

The War Office Letter of January, 1948, contained instructions concerning psychiatric advice in the case of men committed to Type 'C' M.P.s and D.B.s. The commandants of these establishments were required to review, one month after admission and at two-monthly intervals thereafter, the conduct and character of every soldier admitted. If the commandant had reason to believe that a man would be capable of military rehabilitation, he was to arrange for the soldier's examination by an Army psychiatrist. If the latter agreed with the C.O.'s opinion, the man would be transferred to a M.C.E. and would return to normal duty after successful military rehabilitation. If the psychiatrist did not agree, the soldier would remain in the M.P. and D.B.

In practice, this new scheme of institutional treatment and rehabilitation in the Army, while admittedly still in an early stage of development, left in many respects much to be desired. That this was so, was clear from evidence emanating from various sources, and from two independent reports by Army psychiatrists, in July and December, 1948, which dealt with conditions at the M.C.E., Colchester, and at the M.P. and D.B., Shepton Mallet, Somerset.*

Both reports agreed that, at the Military Corrective Establishment (which, in July, 1948, became a single unit, comprising the previously separate Types 'A' and 'B' units), the quality of the M.P.S.C. staff was poor, and their number inadequate; that the camp provided a most depressing and demoralizing environment, and the conditions of hygiene were very imperfect (a fact which, in itself, must have an important adverse effect on the morale of the men); that there were no provisions for occupational activities, apart from military and physical training and limited educational facilities; that some officers and members of the staff still showed a predominantly 'penal' attitude,† and there was much shouting on the part of the staff. The camp was visited regularly by an Army psychiatrist, who saw cases referred to him but did not see all cases admitted.‡ It

---

* These more recent findings were in many ways similar to those of the Oliver Committee. It is here intended to record facts and not, of course, to imply that the basic principles and organization of the entire military penal system, and the quality of the staff, could be altered overnight by the sole publication of administrative decisions and new policies, however progressive these might be.

† Cf. the Oliver Committee's reference to "the merely punitive conception, traces of which still survive in some places".[102]

‡ The Secretary of State for War had originally stated: "Under this scheme, a soldier sentenced to detention will serve the first period of his sentence in a Military Corrective Establishment, in which there will be psychiatrists who will be able, possibly, to help him, and, certainly, to form an opinion as to his mental attitude. We have found

DISCIPLINARY PROBLEMS

was apparent that there was no adequate selection of the soldiers under sentence sent to the camp, and that redeemable types were mixed with inadequate and psychopathic individuals who were incapable of military rehabilitation; segregation in companies was largely according to age, and not according to individual characteristics and personality. It was concluded that little or no rehabilitation in the true sense, i.e. restoration of individual morale, self-respect and military efficiency, was possible in this environment and under these conditions, unless by a spontaneous process of emotional maturation with the passage of time—what might be called the *vis temporis medicatrix*.*

Similarly, in a report on his visit to penal establishments in M.E.L.F., in November–December, 1947, the Inspector of Military Prisons and Detention Barracks (Col. P. H. Gates) stated that he had formed the impression that in some cases local commanders, under whose command penal establishments were placed, were not fully aware of the new principles. In the Type 'C' Military Prison, work of a constructive or interesting nature had been almost entirely lacking, and the Inspector considered that this would have contributed very appreciably to the unrest, escapes, and low morale of the soldiers under sentence in this establishment. With reference to the selection and segregation of different types of offender, it was observed that, in M.E.L.F., the committal of a soldier was automatically determined by his sentence, and it thus happened that a habitual offender, quite incapable of rehabilitation as a soldier, was sent to a Type 'B' M.C.E. and remained there until his case came before the Review of Sentences Board.

In the Type 'C' Military Prison and Detention Barracks, Shepton Mallet, on the other hand, although the same problems of unsuitable environment and staff existed as in the case of the M.C.E. at Colchester, there was no doubt that in the course of 1948 a very great effort had been made, and much was being done to provide for the vocational training, education and general rehabilitation for civil

---

... that a psychiatrist has been able to help a great deal in eliminating some particular trouble which has affected the soldier or airman, and which might land him into some form of crime or misdemeanour involving him in a sentence of detention" (*Parl. Deb.*, 5th ser., Commons, **435**: 1293–4; 26 March, 1947. Cf. *ibid.*, 1292).

* J. C. Spencer has also pointed out, in connection with the introduction of M.C.E.s, that the failure to develop a probation system is most regrettable: "Administration of such a system would admittedly prove difficult, but the advantages would be considerable in the case of a group of men who need help and advice to enable them to make a success of their Service career." [119]

DISCIPLINARY PROBLEMS

life, of the soldiers under sentence there. In so far as it was possible, the Commandant indoctrinated his staff in the basic principles of the new system, and there was little use of punishment, the emphasis being placed on rehabilitation. There was good co-operation between the Commandant and the visiting Army psychiatrist; the latter saw every man admitted, on the general assumption that almost all soldiers sent to the Type 'C' Detention Barracks would ultimately be discharged from the Army, either on administrative, disciplinary grounds, or as psychopathic delinquents, in accordance with A.C.I. 650/46, and a psychiatric examination and report would consequently be required. Thus it was possible to ensure that special attention would be given to unstable men and dullards, and to the education of illiterate individuals, and a few men were also found, who were considered still suitable for military rehabilitation and were transferred to the M.C.E. Although the forbidding aspect, the thick grey walls and barred gates, of this ancient local prison immediately conjured up for the visitor the vision of Dante,

> Per me si va tra la perduta gente. . . .
> lasciate ogni speranza, voi ch'entrate,

these words were certainly more properly applicable at that time to the M.C.E. at Colchester. Unfortunately, the poor quality of the M.P.S.C. staff and the antiquated prison building, at Shepton Mallet, were without any doubt by far the most important features militating against the attainment of what might well have been a very high degree of success.

From the psychiatric point of view, the official documents relating to the new military penal system, while admittedly stressing the principle of rehabilitation, still appear to place rather too much emphasis on punishment. It would, perhaps, contribute to clarity of thought in planning a rational policy for the 'redeemable' military delinquents, as well as to greater success in its practical application, if the authorities were to decide whether the new system is to be based on the principle of rehabilitation, or on obsolete punitive methods which have been tried and found wanting. It may be doubted that these two divergent points of view can be reconciled with any advantage (either to the individual or to the Army). It is at least questionable whether (as the official documents appear to suggest) a preliminary process of degradation and demoralization by punishment of a potentially useful soldier, in a M.C.E., is likely to constitute a sound or rational foundation for the attempt subsequently to restore his self-respect and self-discipline, i.e., morale, by rehabilitation and military training. Those who hold the opinion expressed in Shakespeare's *King Henry V*,

> Let him be punished . . . lest example
> Breed, by his sufferance, more of such a kind,

should ask themselves *which* example is liable to exert the more potent influence on a man who provides basically good material, whether as soldier or as citizen: that of skilled leadership and informed attention to the factors conducive to a high morale, or that of the first 'old lag' or psychopathic delinquent who happens to come along.

Another tendency to which some exception may be taken, is the persistence of the authorities (as shown by these documents) in their concern that there must be no evasion of compulsory national service by means of misconduct. There is a danger that, if too much stress is placed on this aspect, which has already been discussed with reference to the question of the discharge of psychopaths and habitual offenders from the Army, the result will be the retention in the Service of a large number of unsuitable individuals, incapable of making good soldiers, who will exert a detrimental effect on the morale of their comrades and the military efficiency of their units. Also, it is hard to understand how the military authorities can still adopt the policy (as stated in A.C.I. 849/47) that certain "habitual offenders or soldiers of bad character", who, having been sent to a Type 'C' M.P. and D.B., are presumably considered irredeemable for military purposes, and whom it is necessary to keep in safe custody, must subsequently, because of their original terms of service, be required to return to the Army—and this, after a lengthy term of imprisonment, during which they have received no *military* training, in an institution primarily intended for the rehabilitation of chronic delinquents for useful *civil* life. Is it, then, that such men, who have been clearly acknowledged to be not only useless, but a burden, in the Army, are nevertheless regarded by the authorities concerned as so valuable as to be *worthy* of retention in the Service at all costs, that they may thus continue to undermine morale, destroy efficiency, and commit further offences?

While it was officially recognized at the outset (in the War Office Letter of August, 1947), that the new scheme depended for its success

DISCIPLINARY PROBLEMS

on the provision of an adequate and suitable staff for all penal establishments, and the co-operation of commanding officers in committing an offender to the appropriate establishment, it has already been noted that, in practice, the greatest defects in the new Military Corrective Establishment were the inadequate number and quality of the staff, and the lack of any scientific selection or segregation of the soldiers committed to this institution.*

For, in the absence of such selection and segregation it might well be asked, what shall it profit a man, if he shall advance from stage to stage of this pilgrim's progress of military rehabilitation in the M.C.E., and lose all chance of regaining his morale by being compelled to travel with such dubious companions as delinquent psychopaths and dullards? And for the rest, the futility must assuredly be conceded, of attempting to transmute a base metal into gold.

It is not until the essential basic reforms, i.e. scientific selection and segregation of offenders, and suitably selected and trained staff, have been introduced into the military penal system, that there can be any advantage in employing full-time psychiatrists in the new establishments.† That psychiatrists may make a valuable contribution to the work of rehabilitation of military offenders, in an appropriately organized system of this kind, has been clearly demonstrated by the important work undertaken in the U.S. Army's Rehabilitation Centres which, introduced in November, 1942, were estab-

* For a critical discussion of the important questions of selection and segregation of military offenders, and of the consequences of retaining chronic delinquents in the Army, as also for certain constructive proposals, cf. the relevant excerpts, in Appendix A, from the report by Majors R. H. Ahrenfeldt and P. R. A. May on 'The Disposal of Delinquents in the Army' (September, 1949).

† Concerning the reform of disciplinary procedure in the Army, two additional observations may be made:

(1) The Lewis Committee, appointed in 1946, made a number of recommendations as to necessary reforms of court-martial procedure (and, in particular, the avoidance of delay in bringing the accused to trial, and the right of appeal).[104] The Committee's Report resulted in the acceptance by the Government of some of their recommendations,[32] and notably, in the institution of a Court-Martial Appeal Court—cf. *Courts-Martial (Appeals) Act, 1951*.

Reference may also be made to the recent recommendations of the Select Committees, for the amendment of the Army Act,[105, 106] which resulted in the *Army Act, 1955*.

(2) It is to be hoped that the military authorities concerned will come to deal with sexual offenders in a more enlightened way than has, in general, hitherto been the case. In many such instances, in the Army, the psychiatrist's report as well as his evidence was available to the Court, but was entirely disregarded, and severe non-reformative sentences have all too often been imposed. Careful consideration might well be given to the recommendations made, in this respect, by the Scottish Advisory Council on the Treatment and Rehabilitation of Offenders.[114]

DISCIPLINARY PROBLEMS

lished in each of the nine U.S. Service Commands,[1, 2, 68, 115, 132] as also in the U.S. Disciplinary Barracks at Fort Leavenworth, Kansas.[30] *

* In connection with the matters discussed in this chapter, cf. also J. C. Spencer, *Crime and the Services*,[119] and the paper by J. C. Penton.[90]

VI

TREATMENT AND DISPOSAL OF PSYCHIATRIC CASES

THE IMPORTANCE of psychiatric disabilities in the Army, from the point of view of the Medical Services, will be evident from the fact that they were by far the largest cause of medical discharge among military personnel (other ranks) during the Second World War. In 1943, psychiatric disorders constituted more than one-third of all discharges with respect to disease, and in 1944 their proportion rose to two-fifths. It was also estimated that, of all those men rejected for military service on medical grounds by Ministry of Labour and National Service Boards, between 1939 and 1942, some 12% were so rejected on account of psychiatric disorders (including mental dullness).*

From the end of 1939, questions were from time to time asked in Parliament, which, while revealing a somewhat inordinate degree of complacency in official quarters, nevertheless showed an awakening concern elsewhere, to ensure that the importance of providing adequate treatment for psychiatric cases and an efficient psychiatric service in the Army would not be overlooked, and that the principal recommendations of the Southborough Committee would be implemented.†

It has already been mentioned that, apart from the two Consultants who entered the Army at the beginning of the war, there were in the Service at first only a small number of psychiatrists, and medical

---

* Some of the more important statistical data on the incidence of psychiatric disorders in the Army during the Second World War are summarized in Appendix C.

† Cf. *Parl. Deb.*, 5th ser., Commons, 355: 1217; 13 Dec., 1939; 357: 1137–8; 20 Feb., 1940; 1892–3, 1917; 27 Feb., 1940; 377: 1961; 19 Feb., 1942.

officers with some psychiatric knowledge or experience. By July, 1943, there were 198 psychiatrists serving in the Army.*

In April, 1940, a psychiatrist was attached to the medical headquarters of each command in the United Kingdom. The duties and functions of the Command Psychiatrist, as officially defined, were as follows: to examine all cases referred to him from medical units in the command; to serve as a member of all medical boards held on psychiatric cases, or, where this was not possible, to provide a report for the board; to pay particular attention to the early detection of psychiatric illness or potential mental disorder among soldiers serving in the command; and to be responsible for the selection of cases suitable for transfer to the E.M.S. Neurosis Centres and military mental hospitals.

Military psychiatric out-patient centres were established, which served as a filter for the E.M.S. hospitals, separating out those cases with a good prognosis who appeared suitable for retention in their unit under the supervision of their medical officer.

It soon became impossible for the Command Psychiatrists to deal by themselves with all the clinical work and the numerous advisory duties arising in such large areas. In the latter part of 1940, therefore, it became necessary to appoint more military psychiatrists (specialists and 'graded' specialists) to each command. In July, 1940, the establishment of the 'Command Psychiatric Pool' was increased from one psychiatrist in each command, to three (in Northern Ireland District), four (in Aldershot Command), or five (in all other commands). Further additions to the Command Psychiatric Pool were authorized in April, 1941, and thus, eventually, there came to be in each command from three to ten, or at times fifteen, Area Psychiatrists whose work was co-ordinated by the Command Psychiatrist.

The principal function of the Area Psychiatrists was to provide an out-patient service for every area where there were troops or military hospitals. In addition, they visited units to discuss with regimental officers the military value of men who had been referred to them, and to advise both medical and administrative officers on a great many problems arising in units. Later, they also assisted in the selec-

* Cf. *Parl. Deb.*, 5th ser., Commons, **391**: 7; 13 July, 1943. Nine officers were commissioned in the R.A.M.C. during December, 1939, for psychiatric duties, but of this number all but one were at that time employed on general duties as, it was officially stated, they were not yet required for specialized work (*ibid.*, **357**: 1892-3; 27 Feb., 1940).

TREATMENT OF PSYCHIATRIC CASES

tion procedure. Perhaps more than any other group in Army psychiatry, Area Psychiatrists succeeded in getting 'inside the Army'. They required to understand something of the various jobs, the training, and the intimate lives of the soldiers, and to become thoroughly acquainted with the administrative procedures and methods of disposal in many different types of case.

Although cases of severe psychiatric disorder could, of course, be discharged by a medical board, and specific methods of dealing with dull and backward soldiers were gradually devised as the war proceeded, it was not until January, 1942, that the whole question of the disposal within the Army, and discharge from the Service on medical grounds, of all types of psychiatric case received more careful consideration on the part of the military authorities, and the administrative aspects were clarified and detailed in an Army Council Instruction (A.C.I. 84/42) on the 'Disposal of Soldiers who are Temperamentally or Mentally Unsuited for their Present Employment'. This document may be said to have constituted the 'Army psychiatrists' charter'.*

Simultaneously with the development of an out-patient service, facilities were gradually provided for the care and treatment in the Army of psychiatric patients requiring hospitalization.† The provisions for the treatment of psychotic and psychoneurotic military patients, respectively, are described below.

PSYCHOSES

With the considerable assistance of the Board of Control for England and Wales (and especially, of the late Sir Hubert Bond and Mr. C. F. Penton), and with the help of the General Board of Control for Scotland and the Ministry for Home Affairs of Northern Ireland, military hospitals were opened for psychotic patients.

* This A.C.I. was subsequently amended and replaced by A.C.I.s 904/44 (June, 1944) and 82/49 (January, 1949).

† In a most interesting historical survey of 'The Early Days of Army Psychiatry', Brigadier R. Rosie has drawn attention to the little known fact that among the first mental hospitals to provide rational and humane treatment in this country, was that opened by the British Army in the early part of the nineteenth century: "Military accommodation set aside in 1819 for the insane soldier was reasonably generous and patients were then, though unfortunately the policy was later changed, allowed to receive the benefit of a prolonged stay in a military asylum where the humane care and management could at least compare favourably with any civilian asylum in the country. Those humane methods of management were indeed in advance of what are regarded as the epoch-making innovations of Dr. Gardiner Hill at Lincoln and Dr. Connolly at Hanwell." [110]

TREATMENT OF PSYCHIATRIC CASES

In order to obviate the various disadvantages of the policy adopted in the First World War, of immediately discharging to civil mental hospitals all soldiers suffering from psychosis, and in view of the public protest which such a procedure aroused at the time, it was decided in 1940 to retain such cases in the Service for observation and treatment for a limited period. For this purpose, a number of civilian mental hospitals were, in part or entirely, converted into special military psychiatric hospitals, most of which only admitted psychotic cases. For administrative purposes, the medical superintendents of civil hospitals which were taken over in part, and their deputies, were given an honorary commission in the R.A.M.C., and acted as commanding officer (Lt.-Col.) and second-in-command (major), respectively, of the military hospital, while continuing their duties in respect of the civil institution.

The policy of treating psychotic soldiers in military hospitals had several very definite advantages. In particular, it was possible thus to obviate the necessity for certification, and to ensure the careful consideration, in each individual case, of the question of attributability of the illness to military service. Patients suffering from acute psychotic episodes of short duration could remain under treatment in the Army until recovery. Furthermore, such policy greatly facilitated the inevitably complex administrative procedures connected with the holding of periodical military medical boards, the invaliding of men from the Army, the disposal of such disciplinary difficulties as might have arisen prior to a patient's admission to hospital, and various other matters.

That the civil mental hospitals, already overcrowded and understaffed during the recent war, were thereby saved an additional burden will be evident when it is realized that not more than some 7·5% of psychotic patients admitted to military psychiatric hospitals were subsequently discharged to civil mental hospitals.[97] It has also been stated by the Ministry of Pensions that, as a result of dealing with military cases in this way, pensions were awarded to approximately 20% of men discharged with psychosis, as compared with some 90% of men so discharged during the First World War.

Before the war, it was the official policy that all soldiers suffering from mental disease should be discharged by a medical board, with the exception of those suffering from certain transient psychiatric disorders of traumatic or toxic aetiology, and those with psycho-

TREATMENT OF PSYCHIATRIC CASES

neuroses.* In May, 1940, the War Office directed that psychotic patients whose condition was such that, after a reasonable period of observation, there appeared no likelihood of recovery to a degree compatible with fitness for military duty, should be brought before a medical board without delay, with a view to their discharge from the Army.†

The peace-time policy of normally discharging from the Service *all* recovered psychotics was modified, in November, 1940, to enable medical boards to recommend, in appropriate cases, for retention in the Army men whose illness, though psychotic in nature, was of short duration and associated with a good basic constitution, severe precipitating causes, and an apparently perfect recovery.

The work of centres for the prompt treatment of psychiatric cases overseas was greatly facilitated by the adoption of this scheme. Thus, in areas such as the Middle East, where the provision of transport and the evacuation of cases to the U.K. constituted an extremely difficult problem, a number of psychotics who recovered after receiving treatment overseas returned to duty and made a satisfactory adjustment.

During the war, it was possible to provide all forms of modern therapy for psychotics in military hospitals: there was, for the most part, an adequate number of medical officers and trained Mental Nursing Orderlies with previous civil experience, and sufficient hospital beds were available for psychotic cases. After the cessation of hostilities, however, many difficulties were encountered: a number of military psychiatric hospitals were closed down, some of them being once more required as civil mental hospitals, and, with the demobilization of many of the trained Mental Nursing Orderlies, there was a considerable shortage of adequately trained mental nursing staff in the remaining military hospitals.‡

---

* Cf. *Regulations Med. Services Army*, 1938, § 546. For the procedure at that time for discharge of 'soldiers of unsound mind', cf. *Army Act*, S. 91, and *King's Regulations*, 1935, §§ 399 and 403–6.

† In November, 1940, the War Office directed that cases retained in the Army for observation and treatment would be reviewed at the end of 3 months. In practice, psychotics were usually retained in military mental hospitals for 3–6 months (exceptionally, 9 months). In December, 1945, it was decided that a patient whose psychosis had been accepted by the authorities as attributable to military service could be retained in a military hospital up to a period of 2½ years (Long-Term Treatment Scheme). Other cases were entitled to such treatment for a period of 8 months, as originally authorized in February, 1945.

‡ Some of the military psychiatric hospitals were staffed, in addition to the Mental Nursing Orderlies, with nursing sisters of the Q.A.I.M.N.S., but it was difficult to obtain the services of a sufficient number of sisters with a double qualification (i.e. in both general and mental nursing). Between March, 1945, and May, 1946, 508 Mental Nursing Orderlies, out of a total of 1,161 (nearly 50%), had been released

TREATMENT OF PSYCHIATRIC CASES

These conditions made it difficult to carry out forms of treatment such as insulin therapy and continuous narcosis as adequately or intensively as would have been desirable, and the diminishing hospital accommodation made it increasingly impracticable to retain the more chronic psychotics for long periods. The situation was a difficult one for the military psychiatric hospitals, which were confronted with the paradoxical position of having to admit for treatment an appreciable number of cases of psychosis occurring among the younger section of the population, subsequent to enlistment, which cases would normally have been absorbed by the civil mental hospitals; whereas, at the same time, an increasing number of trained Mental Nursing Orderlies were returning, on demobilization, to the civil mental hospitals, so that the latter no longer suffered from the acute shortage of staff—at least, in the case of male nurses—which had so greatly limited their activities during the war.

In view of these circumstances, the War Office decided, in October, 1946, to modify the existing procedure. At that time, psychotic soldiers undergoing in-patient treatment in a military hospital could not be transferred under certificate to civil mental hospitals, until the period of treatment to which they were entitled under the 8 months' rule or the Long-Term Treatment Scheme had elapsed. The object of the new regulations was to limit the entitlement of such patients to treatment in military hospitals, without depriving them of the benefits to which they were entitled under the previous procedure. It was laid down that the normal maximum duration of treatment in military psychiatric hospitals of soldiers suffering from psychoses, whether or not these had been accepted by the Ministry of Pensions as attributable to military service, would, in future, be 9 months. In any particular case, as soon as it became apparent to the psychiatrist that a patient was unlikely to recover sufficiently within the period of 9 months to enable him to be discharged to his home, arrangements could be made to transfer him under certificate to a civil mental hospital. Provision was also made for the transfer of soldiers to civil mental hospitals as voluntary patients in suitable cases.

from the Service, and the establishments in the Army, in 1946, were 40% below strength. The difficulties experienced in the post-war period, in spite of every effort on the part of the authorities concerned, in recruiting and selecting men suitable for training in this physically and mentally most exacting of duties, were, of course, in many respects similar to those encountered in attempting to obtain a sufficient number of suitable trainees for mental nursing in civil mental hospitals. Cf. *Parl. Deb.*, 5th ser., Commons, **423**: 290–6; 21 May, 1946. Also, *ibid.*, **420**: 181–2; 12 March, 1946.

TREATMENT OF PSYCHIATRIC CASES

PSYCHONEUROSES

A Conference was convened by the Ministry of Pensions in July, 1939, to advise the Government as to the general principles to be followed in dealing with cases of neurotic breakdown which might become manifest in time of war. The Conference, whose members included Lord Horder (chairman), Sir Hubert Bond (Board of Control), the Directors-General of the Medical Services of the Royal Navy, Army and Royal Air Force, and others, made a number of recommendations, intended to combat, so far as possible, any potential 'epidemic' of so-called 'war neurosis'.[96] The policy which they advocated formed the basis of further recommendations made, in November, 1939, by a Conference of Representatives of the Service Departments, Ministry of Health and Ministry of Pensions, as follows: first, so far as practicable, no man should be discharged from any of the Fighting Services in consequence of developing a neurosis, and treatment should be carried out while the man remained in the Service; and, secondly, no man should be given a pension on account of neurosis, during the war, except in special circumstances. The Conference recommended, therefore, that consideration be given to the provision by the Army of rehabilitation centres for cases of neurosis.

In September, 1939, Brigadier Rees had also put forward 'A Brief Outline of Suggestions for the Psychiatric Service of the Army', which included a statement of the general principles of treatment of the war neuroses, and stressed the desirability of establishing separate hospitals for these cases and avoiding their being scattered among general hospitals. He similarly pointed out that the provision of special rehabilitation centres for neurotic patients would be of the greatest importance.

From the outbreak of the war until April, 1942, the majority of soldiers suffering from psychoneurosis were treated in Emergency Medical Service (E.M.S.) Neurosis Centres. Cases of psychoneurosis evacuated from Dunkirk were treated in these E.M.S. Centres, and in No. 41 General ('Neuropathic') Hospital, which had been mobilized in January, 1940, for service with the B.E.F., but did not have the opportunity of proceeding to France before the Dunkirk evacuation.

In a report reviewing the problem of psychoneurosis in the Army from September, 1939, to June, 1940, Brigadier Rees noted that there

TREATMENT OF PSYCHIATRIC CASES

were available at that time for the treatment of military neurotic patients, eight special E.M.S. units. Those at Mill Hill and Sutton, which had been functioning from the beginning of the war, were run by the L.C.C. with the staff of the Maudsley Hospital, and, therefore, provided excellent facilities for treatment. These two units had returned approximately 50% of their military patients to duty of some kind. In the early months of the war, they served as a filter for Army cases, and consequently, they received defectives, psychotics, and many equally hopeless cases of neurosis. Since the Command Psychiatrists began work in April, the patients referred to E.M.S. units had been of a far more suitable type: these hospitals still continued, however, to receive from Army medical specialists (i.e. specialist physicians), from E.M.S. specialists, and from other hospitals and Army units, cases which were quite unsuitable for treatment. They were, in this way, nevertheless carrying out a diagnostic function for the Army, and, through their out-patient and in-patient services, greatly assisting in the disposal of these military cases.

The provincial E.M.S. units, on the other hand, although they had not been so burdened with unsuitable cases and their patients had, in general, a better prognosis, were inadequately organized and staffed. The D.G.A.M.S. had, in fact, been notified of the 'availability' of these units some two months before they were functioning, and many cases were subsequently refused because of a lack of accommodation.

The E.M.S. Centres had, in any case, the inevitable and obvious disadvantage, from the point of view of the rehabilitation of neurotic patients for further military service, of not being military hospitals and therefore, as Brigadier Rees observed, of allowing the patient to drift away from everything that his Army training had given him. It was also pointed out that, in the E.M.S. units, the standard of treatment might perhaps be rather higher for certain cases, were it not for the principle, very much emphasized by the Consultant Adviser in Neurology of the Ministry of Health Emergency Hospital Scheme, of 'rushing everybody out in a few days', which could not, if it were followed, produce satisfactory results.

Brigadier Rees concluded that, with the proposed addition to the number of Army psychiatrists, it should be possible to improve the diagnostic and selection procedure, and to provide early, rapid out-patient treatment at military hospitals for cases of psychoneurosis

TREATMENT OF PSYCHIATRIC CASES

(including those induced by the stress of war). Moreover, the establishment of a 'general' military psychiatric hospital would ensure that every type of psychiatric disability could be dealt with effectively by the Army, that standards of treatment would be based on, and adapted to, the specific conditions and requirements of the military organization, and that there would be more adequate provision for the unpredictable emergencies of the near future.

Although a number of specialized military psychiatric hospitals were opened after the outbreak of war, it was felt that there might yet be definite advantages in being able to admit certain military psychiatric cases, for observation and treatment, to a psychiatric unit attached to an ordinary (non-psychiatric) military hospital. It was, therefore, decided to establish, in association with the Military Hospital, Bath, an experimental 'Psychological Centre', which might also provide an opportunity for evolving methods of treating and rehabilitating military psychoneurotics. This Centre (35 beds), which constituted a 'Psychoneurotic Department' of the general military hospital, was accordingly opened in September, 1940, and was located in a separate building at some distance from the main hospital. As an experimental unit, it served a very useful purpose in the early part of the war, before the development, on a large scale, of methods of treatment and rehabilitation of psychoneurotics at Northfield Military Hospital.

Northfield Military Hospital, Birmingham, was taken over for military patients in April, 1942, and was originally divided into a 'Hospital Wing' (200 beds), and a 'Training Wing' (600 beds) where psychoneurotic soldiers could be rehabilitated before their return to duty. From the Hospital Wing, where patients received active psychiatric treatment, and wore 'hospital blue' clothing, convalescent soldiers were transferred to the Training Wing. Here they wore khaki, and were given modified military training under combatant officers and N.C.O. instructors, while remaining under medical supervision, and receiving further 'out-patient' treatment where this was considered necessary by the psychiatrists of the Hospital Wing. This approach to the rehabilitation of soldiers suffering from neurosis was merely a logical application to the military sphere, of the concepts of occupational therapy and rehabilitation which had long been incorporated in the treatment of similar cases in civil life. It should be noted that patients were, at first, admitted to Northfield Military Hospital only where it appeared probable that, following

TREATMENT OF PSYCHIATRIC CASES

treatment, they would be fit for further military service in some capacity. The cases for admission to this hospital were either selected directly by the Area Psychiatrists, or else transferred from E.M.S. Neurosis Centres on the recommendation of E.M.S. psychiatrists.

In December, 1943, it became necessary to review the existing policy, determining the disposal of soldiers suffering from long-standing neurotic disabilities. Experience had shown that chronic neurotics with a poor constitutional background, even after treatment in hospital and, in some cases, with the aid of restricted posting to special employment, did not, as a general rule, give effective service in the Army, and subsequently required to be discharged on medical grounds. There was evidence that the maximal number of such men who could at that time economically and usefully be employed in the Army had been reached, especially with regard to those soldiers who were capable of performing full regimental duties. It was also necessary to take into consideration the shortage of medical man-power and the need to utilize available military medical resources in those directions most helpful to the war effort. It was, therefore, decided that admissions to military hospitals for neurosis would be restricted to cases in which there was a high probability of return, after treatment, to high grade military duties (i.e. not merely simple administrative and domestic duties, or service in the Pioneer Corps). All other cases were to be admitted to E.M.S. Neurosis Centres, with a view to their rehabilitation for civil life.

The gradual development of administrative and therapeutic methods at Northfield Military Hospital, to deal with the difficult problem of psychoneurotic soldiers, was a matter of experiment and of trial and error, but was also necessarily determined to some extent by the changing man-power requirements of the Army and by the military situation at any given time. Thus it was, that in this early stage, which lasted until the middle of 1944, in which the hospital was divided into two distinct units, there were several features which proved to be unsatisfactory. There was little or no co-ordination between the various therapeutic, occupational and other activities in the hospital, and no really continuous, consistent plan for the treatment, rehabilitation and disposal of various types of patient admitted there. The general state of morale was not very satisfactory. Many of the patients were unwilling soldiers with long-standing difficulties, and not infrequently their chief preoccupation was discharge from the Service. The dichotomy of the Hospital emphasized

TREATMENT OF PSYCHIATRIC CASES

to many the contrast between Army life and hospitalization, health and disability: as Major S. H. Foulkes has well observed, "the contrast posed for all the problem of the future and showed the unwilling soldier his first target, namely, to remain sufficiently ill and unserviceable to the Army to avoid his transfer to khaki and the Training Wing".[47]

The two units were sharply delimited, and there were no nursing sisters or medical officers in the Training Wing, but military training officers who regarded the psychiatrists with some degree of suspicion: "For the medical staff seemed to the military men to be . . . inexperienced in the 'old soldier' tricks which were practised upon them. They saw the men running to their psychiatrists like children, and often blamed the psychiatrists' attitude for the patients' condition. The administrative attitude towards this schism in the staff was that the psychiatrists must be left alone to do their job in the Hospital Wing, and when they had 'cured' their patients they must send them to be made back into soldiers in the Training Wing, but each wing must leave the other alone to do its job." [47]

Nevertheless, during this phase of the Hospital's history, some valuable preliminary experiments were being carried out in devising methods of treating and rehabilitating these neurotic patients as a group, and not only as individuals. Problems of administration, discipline and morale, as well as therapeutic considerations, suggested the desirability of such experiments, which were carried out notably by Major W. R. Bion, in the Training Wing, and Major J. Rickman, in the Hospital Wing;[20] and Major S. H. Foulkes introduced analytic group therapy amongst his own patients in the Hospital.[47] In November, 1943, Majors Bion and Rickman concluded an account of their work with the following observation: "These experiments . . . suggest the need for further examination of the structure of groups and the interplay of forces within the groups. Psychology and psychopathology have focused attention on the individual often to the exclusion of the social field of which he is a part. There is a useful future in the study of the interplay of individual and social psychology (viewed as equally important interacting elements), and wartime makes this study an urgent issue." [20]

With the opening of the Second Front, in June, 1944, there was a marked change in the type of patient admitted to the Hospital, the majority being young, active soldiers who had broken down in battle. At the same time, the exigencies of the situation, and the urgent need for active therapy, resulted to an appreciable extent in the attenuation of the clear-cut division of the Hospital into two parts. There was better co-operation between the staff of the two units, who came more frequently into contact, and the psychiatrists were now encouraged to visit their patients in the Training Wing. There were also greater facilities for the occupation of patients in the Hospital Wing.

In November, 1944, a new phase—the so-called 'Northfield Experiment' proper—was initiated. A military staff was selected, who had acquired positive understanding of the psychiatric point of view, and, in particular, of group-psychological orientation, through experience with the War Office Selection Boards.

The Training Wing was abolished and replaced by an organization for the promotion of activities of all kinds, and the military staff, psychiatrists and patients were able to regard the tasks of the now unified Hospital as a common concern. The Hospital was gradually allowed to develop into a self-responsible community, with some degree of self-government in so far as the organization and activities of the community were concerned. Occupational, recreational, social and educational activities underwent a very considerable expansion, with the full support and co-operation of the new staff. The function of the former Training Wing was taken over by a Convalescent Depot through which most patients passed who were returning to the Army.[23, 47, 74]

It need hardly be stated, however, that certain difficulties arose in the attempt to reconcile strictly military concepts with the organization of a community along these lines. Major Foulkes has judiciously described the situation as follows: "The ordinary Army claims for discipline and procedure were forcefully represented by the commanding officer, a regular soldier. This prevented the experiment from assuming an artificial note unrelated to military and other reality.... An essential test of the success or failure in treatment was that the patients ... should satisfy the claims he represented, and he for his part never failed to give us what support he could reconcile with the claims he had to maintain. However, it is not astonishing that a hospital which was ostensibly run in a manner so contrary to the usual military code would find only his reluctant approval. Nevertheless the impression grew that he himself was more easily in sympathy with the methods adopted, and he was at a later stage even seen to apply them himself, and very competently at that!" [47]

TREATMENT OF PSYCHIATRIC CASES

After V.E.-Day, the atmosphere and conditions within the Hospital changed again, and tended to resemble those obtaining in the first phase of the Hospital's development. Lack of enthusiasm for the Japanese war and hope of early demobilization were a general problem of morale in the Army, and this was reflected in the attitude of patients and staff alike. The patients, afraid of further service overseas, were unwilling soldiers anxious for discharge. The staff, both medical and general, were concerned with their civilian future. Experienced members of the staff were gradually withdrawn or demobilized, and were replaced by less experienced and constantly changing personnel. "The spontaneity of the activities diminished. What had developed out of the current needs of the Hospital ... now was in danger of being out of tune and of becoming institutionalized. To the soldier coming new to the Hospital these institutions now again appeared to be more of an imposition from above than a way of meeting their own wishes and expressing ... their needs." [47]

Subsequently, also, all types of neurotic patient were admitted to Northfield Military Hospital, without much consideration being given to the question of their potential fitness for further service; and, in contrast to the fairly large number of cases of acute 'battle neurosis' admitted during the actual war, of whom a majority responded rapidly to treatment and made a good readjustment to military life, after the cessation of hostilities a far greater number of chronic neurotics were admitted, who could be of little further use to the Army in the post-war period. The man-power situation no longer required that so great a number of men be returned to military duty, whereas, during the acute stages of the war, medical considerations had frequently to be subordinated to the exigencies of the military situation. Thus, particularly after the cancellation of the 'Annexure' Scheme in August, 1945, the very great majority of cases of psychoneurosis admitted to hospital, having received treatment, were discharged from the Army by medical boards as permanently unfit for military service, and emphasis was therefore placed rather on the civil resettlement and civilian occupational training of the patients, than on their military rehabilitation. Where the latter was required, it was carried out at a Convalescent Depot.

The military hospitals for psychoneuroses were staffed with Mental Nursing Orderlies, and also, in some cases, with nursing sisters (Q.A.I.M.N.S.). The problems arising from the shortage of Mental Nursing Orderlies were, of course, similar to those already

TREATMENT OF PSYCHIATRIC CASES

mentioned in connection with the hospitals for psychoses. Although the treatment of psychoneurotics in the Army included all forms of individual psychotherapy short enough to be applicable to military cases, as well as occupational therapy and experiments in group psychotherapy, considerable difficulties necessarily resulted from the shortage of trained nursing staff, as also from that of Army psychiatrists, each specialist having to treat an unduly large number of cases. A further, unfortunately inevitable, disadvantage in the treatment of neurotics in military hospitals derived from the continual changes of specialist personnel, necessitated by the frequent posting of psychiatrists to theatres overseas, or to other hospitals or areas in the U.K., where their services were urgently required.

In view of the fact that psychoneurotic soldiers were treated, during the recent war, in civilian Emergency Medical Service hospitals as well as in military hospitals, it is perhaps relevant to compare the two different types of hospital in so far as the treatment of service cases is concerned. The general conclusions which may be drawn from wartime experience have been summarized by Brigadier Rees: "So far as one can judge after five years' experience, the E.M.S. hospitals have one great advantage in a stable and adequately arranged staff. Their personnel does not shift like the military personnel.... The civilian psychiatrists can give their whole time to professional work. In an Army hospital there are certain inevitable military duties which take some time. These civilian hospitals quickly found that they needed certain help from the Army to deal with these cases, and physical-training instructors, non-commissioned officers for disciplinary purposes, educational sergeants and others were introduced. The best of these hospitals, where they have made real efforts to understand the Army's point of view and to work with and for the Army, minimizing the civilian influence, have produced extremely good results, slightly better in fact than the military psychiatric hospitals. But that is not true of all of them, and probably over all it would be better to have any man whom it was hoped to send back to the Army under care in a military hospital all the time, and only use civilian hospitals for the necessary rehabilitation of those who are going back to their civil occupations." [97]

An important factor in the successful military rehabilitation of psychoneurotic patients was their suitable disposal and employment after discharge from hospital. It was found that many such patients, who had responded well to treatment, subsequently relapsed after they had returned to their original units and duties. In an attempt to obviate such occurrences while meeting the urgent need for economy in man-power, and reducing to a minimum the number of men who had to be invalided from the Army on account of neurosis, a special scheme was introduced in May, 1941, largely at the suggestion of Professor Aubrey Lewis who was working in the E.M.S. at Mill Hill Emergency Hospital. By this procedure, which came to be generally known as the 'Annexure' Scheme,* soldiers could be discharged from military or E.M.S. neurosis hospitals to restricted employment of a suitable type, if necessary in a selected environment.[140]

At the beginning of February, 1941, in a letter to Brigadier Rees, Dr. Aubrey Lewis indicated the principal considerations which he had in mind. He pointed out that soldiers who failed to adjust to Army conditions and developed neurotic symptoms, fell into two main groups (although these, of course, overlapped): "(i) Men who are too timid, immature, or otherwise psychopathic to endure any danger and discomfort, camp or campaign life, discipline, and separation from their home; (ii) Men who have been put on jobs for which they are unsuited and which they therefore dislike." Those neurotic soldiers who belonged predominantly to the second group might cease to be misfits, and consequently cease to show neurotic symptoms, if they were placed in a suitable job. A provisional review of military cases at Mill Hill Hospital showed that in about one-sixth of these, provisions for their placement in suitable jobs might either permit men who were at that time being invalided from the Service by medical boards to be returned to duty, or permit men sent back to duty to remain fit whereas, at that time, they soon broke down again and had to be discharged from the Army as permanently unfit for military service.

Dr. Lewis gave a general outline of the problem and of various possibilities for its solution, and concluded: "I should make it clear that it is not suggested that men, having once broken down, should be recommended for exactly the work that they had been doing in civilian life. . . ; but only that they should if possible be given the type of military work, within broad limits, that they are fitted for. It is not a question of being kind and grandmotherly to the man, but of making him a useful soldier of a particular kind, instead of letting

* This name was derived from the forms for recommendations and information which were forwarded in such cases to the War Office, and were originally issued as 'Annexure A' (for training or employment other than in agriculture) and 'Annexure B' (for employment in agricultural work) of the War Office Letter introducing the scheme.

him remain a useless soldier of another kind—and eventually discarding him. I recognize that the causes of neurosis are also the causes of discontent; and that they are all well known difficulties, which would be remedied, or are being remedied, if possible: also that plenty of men allege they are in an unsuitable job, whatever job they are in. I have only been referring to men in whom the facts indicated that they had been in quite unsuitable jobs: more stable men might have adapted themselves, but these men, with their neurotic tendencies, could not."

Under the 'Annexure' Scheme, each man's capabilities were carefully assessed, and more or less specific suggestions were made as to the particular jobs they could best perform. Such postings as were recommended, whether to specified units or to individual extra-regimental employment, could only be varied on the authority of the War Office and after further psychiatric examination. The employment recommendations were made by psychiatrists until October, 1943, when selection testing and the services of Personnel Selection Officers became more generally available and were introduced into the Scheme with a view to improving its efficiency.

A follow-up investigation in 1943 indicated that some 60% of men who had been treated for neurotic complaints and who would otherwise have been considered suitable only for discharge, were retained in the Army by the 'Annexure' scheme; about five-sixths of these had continued to give satisfactory service in their new work, were contented and had made an adequate adjustment.

Brigadier Rees, reviewing the situation in 1945, stated: "This experiment is not only of considerable importance in that it has helped to maintain the man-power of the Army and to ensure that certain jobs are well done by men whose employability is limited, so releasing other fitter men, but also it should be of some value to us in planning for the treatment and disposal of the chronically neurotic men and women in civilian life." [97] When it is realized that some 10,000 cases were dealt with under the Scheme, and that it would otherwise have been necessary to discharge these men from the Army on medical grounds at a time when the man-power situation was acute, it will be seen that this experiment was fully justified. In August, 1945, the altered man-power requirements made it possible to cancel the 'Annexure' Scheme, and the great majority of psychoneurotics subsequently discharged from hospital were invalided from the Army, as unfit for further military service.

TREATMENT OF PSYCHIATRIC CASES

Early in the war, and before the introduction of the 'Annexure' Scheme, an attempt was made to rehabilitate men who had been discharged from hospital following treatment for neurosis but were not considered sufficiently stable for immediate return to their units, while retaining their services within the Army, by drafting them into special 'N' Companies of the Pioneer Corps which were employed solely on agricultural work. At that time, the farmers throughout the U.K. and the agricultural committees responsible for increasing the output of the land were very short of labour, so that the services of these soldiers, consisting for the most part of unskilled work, were welcomed, and were regarded by the men themselves as well as by the public as an important contribution to the war effort. These agricultural companies were run on a basis of military discipline less strict than the normal. So far as possible, men were allowed to visit their homes at week-ends, and excellent welfare was provided for them. It was found that those men who had been reasonably well selected for this job did good work, made very few complaints regarding their health, and had good morale.

With the introduction of the 'Annexure' Scheme in May, 1941, the transfer of neurotic patients to agricultural companies became known as the 'Annexure B' Scheme. However, a War Office Letter issued in February, 1942, stated that, although it had been hoped that a period of duty in an agricultural company under this scheme would facilitate the rehabilitation of some cases of neurosis, the results of subsequent psychiatric examination showed that few if any of the men concerned were ever likely to be sufficiently fit to return to full military duty, and it had therefore been decided to discontinue such transfers.*

In May, 1942, a psychiatrist (Major J. Wishart) who had been associated for some eight months with the 'N' Companies of the Pioneer Corps, in a report on the 'Annexure B' Scheme, stated that the Scheme had suffered from its inception from a lack of settled policy, and it seemed that there had not been in the past a true realization of its possibilities and limitations. While the companies contained a majority of men who were never intended by the hospitals for anything other than permanent agricultural work, the original policy, which provided for either permanent or temporary allocation

---

* For various reasons, but principally because from the Army's point of view the nature of their work was necessarily very restricted, these 'N' Companies were disbanded in the autumn of 1942.

to such work, had apparently undergone reconsideration in November, 1941, after which date incorporation of neurotic cases in a permanent agricultural company was no longer officially contemplated.

Referring to the results achieved, Major Wishart commented that a large proportion of the men were doing excellent work in agriculture, but for one reason or another would never be suitable for normal military service. It was not reasonable to expect six months in agricultural work to increase the mental capacity of a defective, or to rehabilitate a chronic neurotic, or so change a psychopath that he would become an efficient soldier, although it was the case that in sheltered agricultural work the symptoms of many of these men were minimal. On the other hand, it was noticeable that those men whose neurosis was either attributable to, or aggravated by, their war experiences derived great benefit, and it was in this group that the agricultural companies were doing by far the best work. These men were usually suffering from acute neurotic symptoms when first admitted to hospital; under treatment in hospital, the acute symptoms subsided, but convalescence was a prolonged matter, and there came a time when further retention in hospital, even with occupational therapy or other rehabilitatory methods available there, became deleterious to the individual. Moreover, hospital accommodation was precious and limited. It was at this point that transfer to agricultural work proved most beneficial. Although it might not be possible to return more than a few of these men to military service —which in itself was the ultimate test of recovery—they could nevertheless be discharged from the Army with every likelihood of being useful citizens instead of nervous invalids, incidentally with a consequent saving in the matter of pensions.

It is relevant here to quote the critical comments of Brigadier Rees on the limitations of such experiments as this, from the purely psychiatric point of view, in so far as their actual curative value is concerned: "It did not produce cures, as some optimists had hoped it might, but it did provide work and an environment that allowed the neurotic men to contribute without coming under greater stress. It is perhaps worth noting for our post-war problems that here is further evidence that the return to beautiful surroundings and to mother earth does not produce cure of war neurosis.* It will be

---

* "O fortunatos nimium, sua si bona norint,
   agricolas! quibus ipsa, procul discordibus armis,
   fundit humo facilem victum iustissima tellus."
   VIRGIL, *Georgics*

TREATMENT OF PSYCHIATRIC CASES

tried again and will be said to work, for it is a very popular piece of homoeopathic magic. Nevertheless its therapeutic dividend is negligible."[97] Psychiatrists are, of course, well aware that neuroses and other mental illnesses cannot be cured merely by environmental changes, but it was generally considered that, at a time when considerable demands were being made on Britain's resources and manpower, such an experiment, even if it effected only partial rehabilitation, was fully justified by the contribution which it made to the general war effort.

It may also be mentioned that, in January, 1942, an Army Council Instruction (A.C.I. 84/42) authorized psychiatrists to recommend employment of a special nature for men who were employed on jobs for which they were temperamentally unsuitable. This procedure resulted in an appreciable decrease in the number of men who broke down and had to be admitted to a neurosis hospital, and was a notable achievement in vocational selection and psychiatric prophylaxis.

The important question of the rehabilitation of psychoneurotic soldiers, after treatment in hospital, with a view to their return to civil life as efficient members of the community, had already been the subject of a memorandum by Brigadier Rees as early as July, 1940, in which he had advocated the institution of special rehabilitation centres for this purpose.

In a valuable survey of the civil resettlement of a number of soldiers discharged from the Army after treatment in an E.M.S. Neurosis Centre, Dr. Aubrey Lewis stated (at the beginning of 1943): "The present arrangements sponsored by the Ministry of Labour, the Ministry of Pensions and the Ministry of Health provide for co-operation between doctor and employment exchange officer in arranging training for the handicapped when they wish it, and in helping their return to suitable work. These arrangements are a remarkable advance, but they apply too exclusively to the phase just after departure from hospital. There is much less possibility of collaboration between psychiatrist and employment exchange officer once the patient has been put into his first civilian job after discharge; there may then be no psychiatrist at hand to consult.... Sometimes the general practitioner may be in a position to give valuable guidance, but in the series of cases here reported the doctor had not, as far as could be ascertained, usually taken an active part in advising on the industrial and social problems involved in the man's treatment. The improved medical and industrial arrangements for rehabilitation, and the readiness with which a man can now get employment of some sort, however handicapped he may be, probably account for an improvement in the state of affairs disclosed by the follow-up at different periods since it was begun." [70]

In August, 1941, when half of the series had been followed up, the survey showed that 22% were unemployed, and only 35% could be classed as socially satisfactory in respect of work and general adjustment; whereas, by June, 1942, when the whole series had been visited, the corresponding figures were 12% and 50% respectively. Dr. Lewis commented: "What has been found is not a salutary state of affairs. If the investigation had been limited to postal enquiry, a fairly reassuring picture would have been disclosed, but postal enquiries are often specious and deceptive when used for a psychiatric follow-up. The far more reliable home enquiry by psychiatric social workers showed a disturbing situation. The men had gone downhill as a group; they were less usefully employed than before, earning less, less contented, less tolerable to live with, less healthy." The social condition of discharged neurotic soldiers, as revealed by this survey, was still far from satisfactory, but "further development of the arrangements for co-operation between psychiatric and social, especially industrial, agencies would be likely to bring about further improvement".[70]

A subsequent investigation was carried out at the beginning of 1943 by Dr. Eric Guttman, assisted by a psychiatric social worker, Miss E. L. Thomas, into the readjustment in civil life of soldiers discharged from the Army on account of neurosis. This survey showed that 6% of the men investigated were unemployed, i.e. only half of the incidence found in the earlier investigation by Dr. Lewis. Dr. Guttman's general conclusions were as follows: "... The men discharged from the Army on grounds of neurosis have not entirely recovered and readjusted themseves. They form a population with a high incidence of neurotic complaints and neurotic illness 15 months after their discharge. A large proportion of them find it difficult to return to civilian occupation, as shown both in delay in taking up work and in the frequency of job changes. There is a high rate of absenteeism due to sickness requiring a considerable amount of medical attention. Moreover the men feel unhappy in their private lives; they feel self-conscious, and they are liable to social frictions. There is enough evidence to show that they differ in all these respects from an average working population in wartime, and their handicap is clearly indicated by their failure to participate in the increase of earnings, which must lower their living standards as compared with their equals. The group investigated was not a normal one before enlistment. It showed a high incidence of neurotic heredity; of earlier neurotic symptoms; of earlier breakdowns; of poor adjustment to work. Though it is impossible to assess the exact degree of their deterioration, it is certain that a considerable proportion of men now show more marked symptoms, and a poorer adjustment than before they served in the Army." [55]

It is perhaps relevant to refer here to another important investigation by an Army psychiatrist (Major E. D. Wittkower), related to the problem of the rehabilitation of servicemen with severe physical disabilities. It was realized that, although such disablement was commonly regarded as merely a surgical and financial matter, in fact the social readaptation and working capacity of disabled men depended to a large extent on their state of mind. Thus, a psychological study of the emotional reactions to severe disablement was considered to be of the greatest importance. In the course of his investigation, begun in 1944, Major Wittkower studied three large groups of disabled men, suffering from loss of a limb (200 cases), loss of vision in one eye and blindness (some 100 cases each), respectively.[42, 135, 136, 137, 139]

Although it appeared that there were certain specific differences, both quantitative and qualitative, in the emotional reaction of men in the several groups, it was also found that these showed certain common psychological characteristics. The following excerpts from an article by Major Wittkower on the rehabilitation of amputees, may therefore be taken as a summary of some of his general findings: "An able-bodied man who goes out to fight and comes back badly maimed encounters a variety of problems arising from his disability which according to his temperament and character he is either able or not able to solve. If he fails, he creates a good deal of unhappiness for himself and those around him, and eventually he becomes a liability to the community. While great strides have been made in many aspects of the after-care of the disabled, it is felt that the psychologic aspects have received insufficient attention.... The disabled man struggles against a fair number of difficulties both in the outer world and in his own inner world. About 50 per cent. of the patients studied were in a state of emotional maladjustment.

TREATMENT OF PSYCHIATRIC CASES

Mourning is the normal emotional reaction to bereavement, and just as the mourner either gives way to his feelings or conceals them in front of others, so the disabled man, inevitably mourning his losses, is either frankly depressed or hides his grief behind a wall of psychologic defences. However good the substitute limb may be, it never replaces the loss he has incurred. Hence the psychologic approach to disabled men requires skilful handling of depression based on understanding of its fundamental nature, and not pity, praise or a 'cheer up ol' man' approach.

"Main factors determining the type of reaction to disablement are the personality previous to the injury, the site of the disability, the probable functional efficiency of the artificial limb for the particular case, and the social, occupational and financial situation. The previous personality determines the mode of reaction, and the other factors determine how far the pendulum swings. Prominent among the disabled soldier's difficulties are his attachment to and detachment from the Army, his reciprocal relationship with women and his present and future employment. Faulty placement of disabled men may be the result of physical unfitness for the job, of emotionally conditioned overestimation or underestimation of the disabling effect of the injury, of low intelligence inadequate for the job, of acceptance of second rate jobs for want of better ones, and of erroneous vocational guidance. Satisfactory employment of disabled men could be ensured only by a joint effort of . . . surgeons, psychiatrists and psychologists." [136] *

---

* Similarly, in a survey of a group of 50 unemployed disabled men in Manchester, it was noted: "The most important single medical factor was a mental one, in the main that of personal attitude towards disability. . . . The striking feature of the group was the pathological attitude of resentment, aggression, depression, and, in many, severe anxiety. . . . In 6 cases periods in the regular Armed Forces had never been recovered from so far as resettlement was concerned. . . . Personality and mental factors, excessive subsidy, physical disability, and age, in that order, were of importance in hindering return to work." [58]

VII

FORWARD PSYCHIATRY

> Busy the preachers, the politicians weaving
> Voluble charms around
> This ordeal, conjuring a harvest that shall spring from
> Our hearts' all-harrowed ground.
> I, who chose to be caged with the devouring
> Present, must hold its eye
> Where blaze ten thousand farms and fields unharvested,
> And hearts, steel-broken, die.
> C. Day Lewis

IT IS PROPOSED HERE to consider some general aspects and principles of military psychiatry in forward areas and theatres of operations overseas, which were applied with certain appropriate modifications, or proved relevant, to developments in relation to specific campaigns and local requirements; and, very briefly, to summarize a few data on the incidence, treatment and disposal of psychiatric casualties under varying conditions of environment and warfare, in the several theatres at different periods of the war.

Such matters as the relationship between morale, mental stability, and desertion during fighting, and the importance of adequate selection and allocation in drafts proceeding overseas, in preventing psychiatric breakdown and ensuring the maintenance of high morale among soldiers under conditions of stress in battle or after prolonged service abroad, are highly relevant to the subject of forward psychiatry, and are discussed elsewhere in the present work.

It is an undeniable, if regrettable, fact that the attitude is not infrequently encountered, even in this allegedly enlightened age, among laymen and medical men alike, that no man should break down, or indeed be 'allowed' to break down in battle: "Behind this belief is the idea that somehow courage and cowardice are alternative free choices that come to every man, overriding all emotional stress, that a man can choose which he prefers and that he can be courageous if he is told he must be." [97] *

It is, however, both interesting and significant that in the Second World War men were—in the words of Brigadier Rees—"less scared of being afraid", and, when they did break down under stress, tended to develop straightforward anxiety states rather than hysterical conversion symptoms (as was so frequently the case in the previous war).† "All of us are nicely balanced between courage and cowardice, and we find ourselves with anxiety controlled, expressing itself only through the autonomic nervous system;‡ yet there must for many come a time when courage, however well cultivated and maintained, fails to operate. . . . Broadly speaking, it is true that any man *may* break down, granted that there are sufficient predisposing causes. . . . The man who has a high personal morale, and . . . is well trained and happy in a well-disciplined group, will manage his fear better than the man who has not got those qualities or circumstances. Many men with well-marked neurotic predispositions stand up for a long time to the most trying front-line fighting, but on the whole, the inadequate man and the dullard crack very quickly and are better excluded." [97]

---

* In this connection, the late General G. S. Patton's own account of the notorious incident in a U.S. field hospital in Sicily, involving a soldier who was suffering from battle neurosis, is revealing: "I said, 'You mean that you are malingering here?' He burst into tears and I immediately saw that he was an hysterical case. I, therefore, slapped him across the face . . . and told him to get up, join his unit, and make a man of himself, which he did. . . . I am convinced . . . that, had other officers had the courage to do likewise, the shameful use of 'battle fatigue' as an excuse for cowardice would have been infinitely reduced." [89] In the British Army, notices were posted, on instructions from the C.R.A., in all gun units in Malta, when the bombing was at its height in March, 1942: these stated that anxiety neurosis was the term employed by the medical profession to commercialize fear, that if a soldier was a man he would not permit his self-respect to admit an anxiety neurosis or to show fear, *ceteraque similia*.

† Cf. W. Sargant, *Battle for the Mind*;[112] also, W. Sargant and E. Slater,[113] and A. E. Moll on 'Psychosomatic Disease due to Battle Stress'.[82]

‡ " Fear has so many symptoms— , . .
The bones, the stalwart spine,
The legs like bastions,
The nerves, the heart's natural combustions,
The head that hives our active thoughts—all pine,
Are quenched or paralysed
When Fear puts unexpected questions
And makes the heroic body freeze like a beast surprised."
C. DAY LEWIS.

FORWARD PSYCHIATRY

Evidence is not wanting, to demonstrate all too clearly the consequences of the absence of any scientific selection procedure in the British Army at the outbreak of war, as indeed of the considerable and serious delay in its subsequent introduction, and in its effective application in the face of obstacles which might have been avoided, in addition to those inevitably inherent in conditions of war. Certain formations, where the commander had insisted upon very careful sorting of his men, proved highly efficient in battle and showed an outstandingly low rate of psychiatric casualties. On the other hand, in those units that were far below the requisite standard with respect to the selection of personnel, and contained, in consequence, a large proportion of men of low intelligence and too many dull N.C.O.s, there was a very high incidence of psychiatric disorders.

The basic problems of forward psychiatry have been so clearly and pertinently stated by Lt.-Col. T. F. Main, that to attempt either paraphrase or summary would be both futile and presumptuous:

"The mental health of a fighting force is not the same thing as the mental health of a nation at war. With the differing functions, different standards are needed. If a sergeant can recover his poise for one month, it can be regarded as a satisfactory therapeutic result in an Army fighting for its very life, though such a result would not be worth having in civilian life. Then the stresses which such a man must be capable of withstanding are very different from those which would operate upon him in civilian life—and they must be fully understood by the psychiatrist. Lastly, the positive factors which will support the mental health of such a man are different in the forward area from those in the rear areas. The job of the psychiatrist, in fact, demands a grasp of the social as well as the medical variants which influence treatment and disposal.

"One campaign does not seem to train a psychiatrist automatically for another. In the Middle East the great separation from home, the flat barren wilderness in which the men lived, the poor food and water supply, the rarity of action, the occasional big battles dominated by the spandau, the 88 mm. and the mortar, lasting only a few days, contrast with the battles of the Normandy Bridgehead which went on without remission for over two months in familiar green fields and copses, with scarcity of sleep, the multi-barrelled mortar, and the continued carnage, as the great stresses. In Burma, I am told, it was not the noise of explosions nor the power of enemy weapons that were the stresses, but silence in jungle patrols, the fear of being seen without seeing, the difficulty of sleeping with a calm mind, and the long separation from home.

"Yet these stresses can be classified. The sense of separation from home, from its security and its comforting permanence and its familiar reassurance of one's personal status, is a permanent stress. A camaraderie is the only human recompense for a threatening sense of impotence in the face of death and the waywardness of elemental forces and the decisions of the mighty who use soldiers like pawns.

"The lonely homesick man, overwhelmed by insecurity, showing anxiety and hysterical illness, is met sometimes before he has even been in battle, together with the men who have carried out their social obligations in the face of fantastic dangers until their sense of security too has gone. There are others who have contained their anxiety, supported by comradeship and affection until the death of their friends has left them bereaved, to face further dangers alone. The man who has killed too much, the officer who has lost his men through an error of judgement, the tank commander who escaped alone from a burning tank—present pictures of guilt and depression that may be psychotic in depth. Fleeting schizophrenic screens may be drawn for a few days over anguish too gross to be borne.

"These acute clinical pictures arise very often in conjunction with loss of sleep. While this can be a symptom, it is often a necessary condition of some battles, and gross fatigue alone leads some men to the psychiatrist.

"Acute cases repay simple forward treatment of rest and sedation, and justify the existence of forward psychiatric centres. The bonds which tie men to their fellows have not yet been broken, and some 30% to 60% can be returned fit to carry on. The numbers correlate indirectly with the surgical casualties—following about 3 days behind the curve of daily incidence. But it is not a parallel curve; as the surgical casualties rise, the psychiatric casualties rise out of all proportion. Depending on the type of battle, 2% to 30% of all casualties may be psychiatric.

"When the numbers are high during a big battle, you may imagine the alarm in high places, the increase in diagnosis of 'cowardice' by administrative staffs, and the reluctance to recognize the problem as a psychiatric one. At these times all the slack in senior super-egos is taken in, and some of the wrath falls of course on the patients and occasionally even on their therapist. That is in the day's work.

FORWARD PSYCHIATRY

One popular view at such times—popular in rear areas at least—is that access to the psychiatrist will discourage the fighting men who are sticking it out. This may be so, but I have yet to meet a regimental medical officer who knows of a single instance of a good man being discouraged by the knowledge that if he became a casualty of any sort he would get looked after.

"The 'chronic' cases seen in quiet periods are a mixed bag. Some of them are chronic neurotics, but many are men with persistent symptoms from earlier battles, particularly of guilt and depression about comrade-loss or with anxiety which has not resolved spontaneously after rest. The home worries, too, mount as a campaign goes on and become increasingly a source of military inefficiency. The prognosis with the cases that appear during quiet periods is not as good as with the acute cases, and hospital treatment and reallocation are needed.

"The forward psychiatrist has made himself a familiar figure in the war, and has proved his value in every theatre since 1940. He cannot work miracles, but by persistently plying his craft, keeping his head amid the shifting moral attitudes towards his patients, and remaining, in so far as his own situation allows, objective and unsentimental, honest about his failures and modest about his successes, he can serve the men of his formation in a way granted to few medical men. Such a result, however, is achieved not by heroics, but by good psychiatry." [73]

The local organization of psychiatric services in forward areas necessarily varied to some extent with the requirements specific to a given theatre of war, and was also gradually evolved as a result of experience in dealing, under existing local conditions, with psychiatric battle casualties.

The problem of the military psychiatric casualty was reviewed by Lt.-Col. H. A. Palmer in 1944, on the basis of experience derived from a study of over 12,000 cases in three theatres of war during $4\frac{1}{2}$ years with British armies at home and overseas. Col. Palmer pointed out that the procedure at first evolved, during the recent war, to deal with this problem, tended to rely on a hospital organization based in principle solely on experience of neurosis in civilian life and on the doctor-patient relationship. Treatment was, by implication, 'medical' (in a narrow sense), and was based on a conception of the problem solely in terms of individual psychoneurotic conflict.

The patient was treated in hospital for his illness and he was then passed on for routine convalescence, and finally disposed of in his correct medical category. Col. Palmer observed that such an approach, "in so far as it fails to take cognizance of what appear to be factors more immediately involved in the causation of the casualty, has tended to neglect ways and means whereby such factors, viz. those concerned with morale, can be restored", and stated that, in his opinion, it had wrongly placed its emphasis, "by selecting for therapeutic attack the more personal and less socially orientative trends of the patient's personality make-up".[88]

Realizing that this situation had arisen, the Army commenced, in the summer of 1943, to set up an organization in the Middle East—which at that time was the main theatre of war—whereby this 'faulty emphasis' might be corrected. Specially designed military psychiatric Rehabilitation Centres resulted from the experimental centres developed in relation to the 8th Army and, subsequently, in the C.M.F. in Italy (February, 1944). The experiments were so successful that it was recognized that psychiatric Rehabilitation Centres should be provided for all cases of battle neurosis who could not be returned to duty within a few days of their withdrawal from the front line. Such Centres were ultimately established in all theatres of war. The rehabilitation of psychiatric cases was possible within the general framework of an ordinary military Convalescent Depot, provided that there was a special psychiatric wing under the care of a psychiatrist. The four-week scheme of rehabilitation of an ordinary Convalescent Depot had, of course, to be modified to meet the special requirements of psychiatric cases as compared with the usual physical cases.

Col. Palmer considered that a psychiatric service for a task force required five subsidiary organizations:

(i) and (ii) *The Filtration Units:* (i) the Forward Filtration, or Corps Exhaustion Centre, attached to a C.C.S.; (ii) the Main Filtration Centre, or Advanced Psychiatric Wing of a forward general hospital.
(iii) *The Rehabilitation Centre.*
(iv) and (v) *The Base Psychiatric Units:* (iv) the Base Psychiatric Wing of a base general hospital; (v) an Evacuation Unit, which should ideally be attached to the main evacuation hospital for the command.

The first four of these constituent units were to be regarded as

FORWARD PSYCHIATRY

providing the means of restoring the psychiatric casualty by a process of rehabilitation (which included an immediate phase of psychiatric first-aid). The fifth unit was for the ultimate disposal of the residual casualties, who were permanently unfit for further military service with the force.[88]

The aim of psychiatrists with the armies overseas was, wherever possible, to provide a psychiatric organization on these or similar lines.

As summarized by Major C. Kenton, the military problem arising from psychiatric battle casualties resolved itself, in practice, into the following several objects: first, to prevent psychiatric casualties from impeding actual fighting operations, or the evacuation and treatment of the wounded; secondly, the selection and treatment of those casualties who would be capable of early return to further effective combatant duties; thirdly, the prevention of deterioration in those unable to return early, or at all, to further combatant duty; and finally, due consideration of the factor of long-term conservation of man-power.[67]

With adequate triage at R.A.P. and M.D.S., and an adequately constituted 'Exhaustion Centre' at C.C.S. level or its equivalent— (e.g. one F.D.S. might be taken over as a Corps Exhaustion Centre) —it was possible to return the majority of cases to fighting within a week (figures varied from 70% to 56%), and only some 5% of these broke down again in the course of the same battle. The contribution of even these 5% outweighed any possible deleterious effect on their comrades of their subsequent incipient breakdown.

The essentials of treatment were adequate sedation by the regimental medical officer immediately after the breakdown, and continuance of this sedation at the M.D.S. and Corps Exhaustion Centre.

All those cases for whom there appeared to be a reasonable probability of early return to fighting duty, were retained for treatment at the Corps Exhaustion Centre, where treatment was based on the following principles: continuation of sedation, where required; maintenance of military, rather than 'hospital', discipline; continued contact with comrades of the same or neighbouring fighting units; some reinforcement of a man's individual and group morale; and the maintenance of a 'curative' atmosphere, such as would lead each soldier under treatment to anticipate an early return to duty.[67]

Of the cases retained at the Exhaustion Centre, only a certain

FORWARD PSYCHIATRY

proportion became fit to return to their unit, varying from corps to corps in the same and different theatres of war, and in the same corps in changing conditions of warfare. On the average, rather less than 30% of cases could be returned to duty from the Exhaustion Centre. The remaining 70% were evacuated to an Advanced Psychiatric Centre, where the majority of those admitted could be sufficiently rehabilitated within a month, to return to duty in lines of communication or 'B' Echelon work. Cases of poorer prognosis were evacuated to a Base Psychiatric Hospital or to the equivalent ward of a base hospital. One of the major difficulties, however, in the triage and treatment at the Corps Exhaustion Centre, was that, at a time of great operational activity, cases arrived at such a rate that the staff were more than fully occupied, and it was consequently impossible, on many occasions, to give the requisite time for adequate treatment, with the inevitable result that it was necessary to evacuate some cases, where this would normally have been considered unnecessary and unwise.[67]

The whole success of forward psychiatry depended on early treatment, and the results were as good as those mentioned above only when treatment could first be given within a matter of hours.

In the last phase of the war, a Divisional Psychiatrist was attached to each actively fighting division whenever this was practicable.* If there were insufficient specialists, the Corps Psychiatrist always attempted to set up Divisional Exhaustion Centres under specially trained General Duty medical officers. It was, of course, not possible for the Corps Psychiatrist himself to run an advanced Exhaustion Centre, because he had to be available for his many specific duties, and particularly to advise his D.D.M.S. as to the total morale situation in the corps, and to plan new administrative procedures for the disposal and treatment of psychiatric casualties.

Experience proved beyond any doubt the importance of ensuring that patients from psychiatric Rehabilitation Units should proceed direct to their future unit, without an intermediate period of waiting in R.H.U.s, etc., as a very marked deterioration invariably occurred in cases remaining in such holding stations for a few weeks. It is well

---

* "In January, 1918, on the recommendation of the division of neurology and psychiatry, the U.S. War Department created the position of division psychiatrist, with the rank of major, one for each tactical division. The creation of this position, which was the first recognition of the Army of the utility of specialists for troops in the field, proved of the utmost importance." [124] In the Second World War, Divisional Psychiatrists proved to be of fundamental importance in the Burma campaigns.

recognized that it requires high morale and firm internal discipline to withstand boredom and inaction, and soldiers who have recently had a psychiatric breakdown are obviously not fit to endure this kind of strain. In the opinion of Army psychiatrists, it is essential that the whole progress from breakdown to final return to active, effective duty shall be continuous if the results of the treatment are to be good.

Corps Psychiatrists were used for the first time, in the recent war, in North Africa and Italy. Their functions, as officially defined in February, 1944, were as follows: to advise in all matters pertaining to mental health; to eliminate (by 'screening') men who were mentally unfit for duty with the corps; to undertake the early treatment of men with minor maladjustments to military service; to advise on the psychiatric aspects of discipline, morale, and training, and assist, by lectures and informal discussions with staff, regimental, and medical officers, in the promotion of mental health and in preventive psychiatry; to attend medical boards, and assist in the reclassification and suitable reallocation of men, as required; to visit medical units and Regimental Aid Posts, and advise on the management of psychiatric and psychosomatic problems; to keep themselves informed of changing psychiatric problems during training and fighting periods, with a view to the development of 'mental toughness' essential to fighting troops; and, finally, to supervise the management of psychiatric casualties during action—in particular, the avoidance of indiscriminate evacuation, and adequate selection of cases for treatment on the spot, in the interests of the conservation of man-power.

Reference must also be made to the development of 'campaign stress', or 'campaign exhaustion', in men who have been subjected to the strain of active warfare for a relatively prolonged period of time. An important and significant psychiatric study of this condition, and of the average 'psychiatric life' of the infantryman in active combat, based on experience in the 5th Army in Italy, in the middle of 1944, was made by two American investigators, Lt.-Col. J. W. Appel and Captain G. W. Beebe.*[13] In view of the importance of this work, for British as well as for American Army psychiatry, and the light which it throws on such problems as the incidence of psychiatric breakdown, desertion and the various indices of low morale,

* Cf. also the detailed report on 'Combat Exhaustion', by L. H. Bartemeier, L. S. Kubie, et al.[16]

at different stages of a campaign or after successive campaigns, it is relevant to quote this valuable report at some length:

"There is no such thing as 'getting used to combat'. . . . Each moment of combat imposes a strain so great that men will break down in direct relation to the intensity and duration of their exposure. Thus, psychiatric casualties are as inevitable as gunshot and shrapnel wounds in warfare. Prevention can be thought of only in terms of preventing needless waste of man-power. . . .

"Precisely because the infantry is exposed to the greatest danger it also suffers the greatest loss of man-power from psychiatric disorders. . . . In the North African Theatre practically all men in rifle battalions who were not otherwise disabled ultimately became psychiatric casualties. Although only 1 to 3 per cent. of the combat strength was lost from this cause during any single offensive, apparently the intensity and duration of the continued campaigns surpassed the limit of endurance of the average soldier. Just as an average truck wears out after a certain number of miles, it appears that the doughboy wore out, either developing an acute incapacitating neurosis or else becoming hypersensitive to shell fire, so overly cautious and jittery that he was ineffective and demoralizing to the newer men. The average point at which this occurred appears to have been in the region of 200 to 240 aggregate combat days.* The number of men still on duty with this amount of combat experience is small and their value to their units is negligible. . . . From the Sicilian Campaign onward it was noted that an increasing number of the psychiatric patients being sent back from the lines were not 'weaklings' who had merely broken down after a short exposure to combat but experienced veterans, strong men with excellent combat records, often including decorations. Most of them were non-commissioned officers, either squad, section or platoon leaders. By the spring of 1944, following the Volturno, Rapido and Cassino actions, there were more of these old men than new men coming in as psychiatric patients. . . .

". . . . A survey was made of battalion and regimental surgeons, of division psychiatrists and experienced combat unit commanders. Particular emphasis was placed on obtaining the opinion of company-grade commanders, since they had the most direct contact with troops. It was found that both the medical and the line officers were

* In this article, 10 combat days were taken as equivalent to 17 calendar days.

in unanimous agreement that by the time a man had served 200 to 240 aggregate days of combat in a rifle battalion he was non-effective. He was worn out. . . . Actually, many of the line officers were emphatic in stating that the limit of the average soldier was considerably less than 200 to 240 aggregate combat days. Most men, they stated, were ineffective after 180 or even 140 days. The general consensus was that a man reached his peak of effectiveness in the first 90 days of combat, that after this his efficiency began to fall off, and that he became steadily less valuable thereafter until finally he was useless. They agreed that actions such as those at Rapido and Cassino accelerated this process, that men who had survived these actions were never the same again. They indicated, however, that even relatively light, successful actions such as were experienced by certain units in the Rome push, could not be considered light in their effect on the infantryman.

"Individuals developing psychiatric disorders after less than 200 combat days can and have been successfully returned to full combat duty by the excellent front line treatment developed in the North African Theatre. The man who is 'worn out', on the other hand, is through as a combat soldier. At least six months would be required to make him effective again for combat, although he still might be very useful in a noncombat assignment.

"The effective combat life of the average infantryman appears to depend largely on how continuously he is used in combat. The British, for example, estimate that their riflemen in Italy will last about 400 regimental combat days, about twice as long as U.S. riflemen in the heavily used U.S. divisions in Italy. They attribute this difference to their policy of pulling infantrymen out of the line at the end of twelve days or less for a rest of four days. The American soldier in Italy, on the other hand, was usually kept in the line without relief for twenty to thirty days, frequently for thirty to forty and occasionally for eighty days. Although tactical requirements may have required this policy, the fact that a man wears out in combat has apparently been insufficiently recognized by command." [13]

It is not possible, in a work of this size, to undertake a detailed account of the organization of the psychiatric services in the various theatres of operations overseas, as they were developed, during the Second World War, to meet the general medical needs of the Army as well as the specific requirements of forward areas. Indeed, the

FORWARD PSYCHIATRY

extensive and detailed (and, for the most part, unpublished) records of these important aspects of British military psychiatry, which were compiled throughout and following the recent war—and, it may be added, subjected to a very thorough analysis by the author—would require a substantial volume to themselves. The brief summary which follows is intended merely to provide in outline a few facts of possible interest and significance for comparative purposes.

BRITISH EXPEDITIONARY FORCE

The main problem during this initial phase of the war (September, 1939, to June, 1940), in France as elsewhere, was to sort out and deal with the psychiatrically unstable and backward men who had been passed as fit for service by the Recruiting Boards. The large number of psychoneurotics constituted a particular difficulty. Of the total number of cases dealt with at a B.E.F. general hospital before fighting started, although these were trained men who had already been considerably 'filtered', 8% were suffering from pure neurosis. Some 8% of the convoys from Norway were stated to be cases of neurosis, but according to the medical specialist of the 22nd General Hospital at Narvik, neurotic disorders were one of the principal problems at that time, although it was possible to return most of the men to duty after a few days in hospital.

Of the cases admitted to the psychiatric wards at Dieppe, during a period of six months in the 'passive phase' of the war, some 50% were psychoneurotics, 30% psychotics, 10% mental defectives, 7% alcoholics, and 3% epileptics: approximately 60% (including slightly less than half of the neurotics) were evacuated to the U.K., and 40% were returned to duty. During the 'active phase', on the other hand, the great majority of cases admitted were acute psychiatric disorders precipitated by experiences of bombing and shelling: many of them had no ascertainable previous history of psychiatric trouble, and their prognosis was consequently far better than that of the cases seen during the 'passive phase'. Psychiatric disorders constituted some 10–15% of all casualties, during the 'active phase'.

Major R. J. Phillips, a psychiatrist working as a R.M.O. during the Dunkirk evacuation, found that, in his battalion, about 10% of the cases which passed through the R.A.P. were psychiatric casualties. Except for morphine and hyoscine which were required exclusively for the wounded, sedative drugs were non-existent; he reported

FORWARD PSYCHIATRY

that "there was, however, an ample supply of alcohol, an excellent sedative, which proved most effective", and that, by its aid, together with strong reassurance and encouragement, about 75% of these cases were persuaded to remain with the battalion and eventually returned to England. The acute war neuroses which occurred at Dunkirk have been well described from the clinical point of view by Drs. W. Sargant and E. Slater, who noted that, in general, they showed the physical signs of exhaustion and mixed anxiety and hysterical symptoms.[113]

BRITISH LIBERATION ARMY

Within 10 days of D-Day, the psychiatric problem in 21 Army Group had become evident: 10–20% of battle casualties were psychiatric cases of 'exhaustion'.

The medical unit principally used in the forward treatment of psychiatric casualties was the Field Dressing Station. Within four weeks, the need for Divisional, as well as Corps, Exhaustion Centres became clear, and by mid-July, Exhaustion Centres were functioning at Divisional, Corps, and Army levels. The lack of accommodation and of personnel on the bridgehead, during June, unfortunately made it impossible to retain patients for more than 48 hours: only some 10% of cases recovered during so short a period and could be returned to their units; the remainder were evacuated to England. In July, patients could be retained for 7 days' treatment, and the number of men returned to duty rose to 50–70%.

The Advanced Section of No. 32 General (Psychiatric) Hospital arrived in Normandy at an early date, and opened exactly 30 days after D-Day. As Lt.-Col. J. F. Wilde observed, the one and only novel feature was that, in this invasion Force, for the first time in British military history the possibility of psychiatric casualties in large numbers had been envisaged, and at least some provision made to meet it: for the first time, an adequately equipped general hospital had been sent to within ten miles of the front line to deal with the problem.

The Hospital (now comprising its combined Advanced and Rear Sections) moved from Normandy to Belgium at the end of October; during the intervening period, when it was closed, psychiatric casualties from the fighting in the neighbourhood of Arnhem and the Scheldt Estuary were evacuated to England. After the Hospital had reopened near Malines, with 600 beds, not more than an average of 10–20% of cases admitted there required evacuation to the U.K., and these represented a very small fraction of the total number of psychiatric casualties occurring in the forward areas. In the middle of the battle between the Meuse and the Rhine, it became necessary to move the Hospital to a new site near Louvain, and as a result of reduced accommodation and the large number of acute cases requiring treatment, it was necessary to reduce drastically the length of time for which patients could be retained (even to 2 or 3 days, in the milder cases). Although a considerable number of men consequently received at that time insufficient individual treatment, it was nevertheless possible to avoid large-scale evacuation.

In the early months of the Campaign, L. of C. psychiatrists in the U.K. were engaged in the 'screening' of reinforcements to 21 Army Group: many unstable men were thus found in the stream of reinforcements. On examination of the surgical and psychiatric cases returned to 21 Army Group from military and E.M.S. hospitals, in June and July, it was found that more than 90% of the 'exhaustion' cases were in the wrong medical category and had to be reclassified, and 50% of the same group had not previously seen a psychiatrist; and that, of the surgical cases referred to the psychiatrists, 6–10% were unfit for further duty because of psychiatric disability.

Statistics concerning the incidence and disposal of psychiatric casualties in 2nd Army, for the entire North-West European Campaign, from its commencement on 6th June, 1944, to its termination on 9th May, 1945, show that the total number of 'exhaustion' cases was 13,255, and that these constituted some 16% of all battle casualties. The incidence of psychiatric casualties in 2nd Army rose from about 10% of *battle* casualties (9% of *all* casualties) in June, 1944, to a maximum of 20% (10%)* in July–September, 1944, and thereafter gradually decreased, to 14% (5%) in October–December, 1944; 10% (3%) in January–March, 1945; and 8% (3%) in April–May, 1945.

During the first month of the Campaign, the average rate of return to full duties of some kind, from Corps Exhaustion Centres, was 30–40%. When Divisional Exhaustion Centres were set up in July, 1944, the average rate of return to full duties approximated 60%; thus, the Corps Centres received cases with a poor prognosis, and

*.The figures in brackets represent percentages of *all* casualties, and the other figures, percentages of *battle* casualties, in 2nd Army.

FORWARD PSYCHIATRY

comparatively few of their patients, at that time, could be returned to full duties. In spite of an appreciable relapse rate, it can, however, be stated that, over the entire Campaign, about one-third of all psychiatric casualties treated in the North-West European theatre eventually returned to full duties, and remained so employed: this represents just over 4,400 men saved for combatant duties, at a time when our man-power situation was critical.

MIDDLE EAST FORCE

One of the inherent and fundamental problems, in organizing the psychiatric services in the Middle East, was the extent of the area concerned, and the consequent difficulties in travel and communication: this area included Egypt, Palestine, Syria, the Sudan, Eritrea and Abyssinia, Libya, Cyprus, and originally, also Iraq and Iran. These difficulties were of obvious importance in attempting to establish a co-ordinated service itself, and also in arranging for the evacuation of psychiatric cases: thus, the evacuation time between the forward areas in the Libyan Campaign and a suitable base hospital or centre was rarely less than seven days, and the process usually involved a considerable degree of mental and physical strain. A second problem, of very great practical importance, was the wide diversity of races and nationalities encountered—(in one centre alone, during a period of 12 months, patients of some two dozen or more nationalities and races—European, African and Asiatic—were admitted for treatment, in addition to British and Dominion troops, and German and Italian prisoners of war).[35]

Although the policy originally formulated for this theatre envisaged such an extensive psychiatric organization that very few casualties would require to be evacuated from the Middle East Force, problems presented themselves, which by 1942 seemed likely to overwhelm the psychiatric services then in existence, and it is certain that there were many cases of breakdown among men who should never have been accepted for military service: for the latter (including schizophrenics, epileptic or post-traumatic personality disorders, unstable defectives and psychopaths), the only possible method of disposal was evacuation. On the other hand, at first, a number of psychiatric casualties were evacuated, who would at a later date have been retained in the Command. Hospital ships were in short supply, and psychiatric cases had a very low priority and consequently tended to accumulate: towards the end of the Libyan Campaign, in late 1942 and early 1943, this became a very serious matter, as accommodation at No. 41 General Hospital was heavily compromised by the necessity for retaining for long periods large numbers of psychotics of many nationalities.

During 1941-2, the average duration of stay in hospital for psychiatric cases was 25 days; the proportion of patients returned to duty varied from 70% to 90% (of which some two-thirds to full duty of some kind, and one-third to base duties). It would appear that not more than 5-6% of these patients subsequently broke down and required to be readmitted to hospital.[35]

It was estimated that at least 40% of psychiatric casualties in the Middle East Campaigns could have been foreseen by a careful psychiatric survey, or even by obtaining, in the case of men to be sent overseas, a reasonably detailed medical history. The Consultant in Psychiatry (Brigadier G. W. B. James), referring to this situation, stated that an important lesson could be learnt from the fact that, taking as a sample over 6,000 psychiatric cases in the M.E.F., in less than 40% was the illness related in any way to war stress, and over 60% were men with no experience of battle conditions.*

Summarizing the work accomplished by Army psychiatrists during the first two years in the Middle East, Lt.-Col. H. B. Craigie stated that, although the results obtained had been reassuring, as demonstrated by the high proportion of patients returned to duty, the indifferent quality of many of the drafts sent overseas was often only too obvious: not only were many of these men unfit for service overseas, but in a number of cases, they were "candidates for hospital treatment on enlistment".† [35]

Practical experience during the actual Campaign in 1941-2 demon-

---

* The author is greatly indebted to Dr. James for kindly placing at his disposal a most detailed (unpublished) history of Army psychiatry in the M.E.F. from September, 1940, to July, 1943: much of the information on the M.E.F. included here was derived or completed from Dr. James' manuscript. Cf. also G. W. B. James, 'Psychiatry in the Middle East Force 1940-1943', in the official British medical history of the Second World War.[61]

† Brigadier James, who drew the attention of the War Office to these conditions resulting from the lack of adequate selection of recruits and drafts for service overseas, as early as February, 1941, recorded the following instances: In 1941, there were 27 mental defectives in a draft of 80 men for a searchlight unit; in 1942, a draft of 200 men contained 4% of illiterates, some of whom were untrained and untrainable for infantry; and, in spite of a great improvement in the situation at the end of 1942, even in 1943 four illiterates arrived in a small draft of Guardsmen—"Externally they appeared admirable soldiers, but were discovered after leaving the Depot to be emotionally too unstable for battle."

FORWARD PSYCHIATRY

strated that the most important features of desert warfare, in relation to psychiatric casualties, were its extreme mobility, the vast extent of the areas over which actions took place and the remarkable speed of the latter, and the long and arduous lines of evacuation. The constant movements of medical units and the long distances between medical posts made static treatment even for a few days a matter of difficulty. The policy, therefore, in the early days, was to get the men back to general hospitals (and special centres, when these became available) in the Delta Area or Palestine for treatment, followed by a period of rehabilitation at a Convalescent Depot. The great importance of early and adequate treatment of these cases, where it was practicable, was, of course, realized. As the responsibility for providing such immediate treatment in forward areas necessarily lay with the regimental medical officers, it was essential to ensure that the latter should have a sufficient knowledge of the principles of early psychiatric treatment, as well as an adequate supply of the appropriate sedative drugs.[33, 34]

In 1941, there was a very forward psychiatric unit, 'Z' Ward of the 4th Australian General Hospital, at Tobruk. With the advice of the Consulting Psychiatrist, the Australian Army Medical Corps was thus able to provide accommodation and treatment for psychiatric casualties, and consequently very few of these required to be evacuated during the eight months' siege of Tobruk (April–December, 1941). At the Consultant's suggestion, the Australian Army medical authorities also started another centre, on the open beach, which provided accommodation and treatment for various cases, including 30 beds for psychiatric patients.* At the time of the siege, it was vital to retain for some form of duty every possible soldier, and therefore to evacuate psychiatric casualties sparingly. One of the Field Ambulances acted as a filter for all psychiatric cases evacuated from the front, and through prompt treatment was able to return 56% of such casualties—some of them admittedly still in a somewhat unstable condition—to their units after a few days. The remaining 44% were sent on to 'Z' Ward, a deep concrete dug-out in a hillside on the summit of which was a heavy A.A. gun post; this dug-out shelter was nevertheless reasonably quiet and quite safe, and it was thus possible, after more lengthy treatment, to return to their units 50% of the patients admitted.

* In October, 1941, No. 62 British General Hospital proceeded from Jerusalem to Tobruk, and took over these units from No. 4 Australian General Hospital.

FORWARD PSYCHIATRY

In the middle of 1942, psychiatric cases constituted 7-10% of the total (sick and battle) casualties of the 8th Army: the majority, however, were cases of simple exhaustion who recovered rapidly and completely with rest and sedation, and the proportion of true psychiatric casualties requiring further treatment was found to be approximately 2% of all casualties of the 8th Army. An Army Rest Centre was set up by the 200th Field Ambulance, for cases of physical and mental exhaustion, and worked from the end of July to the beginning of November, 1942. During the opening phases of the battle of El Alamein, there was a high proportion of cases of severe neurosis requiring to be evacuated, but, as the battle continued, the cases of simple exhaustion became relatively more numerous. Some 60% of all admissions to the Rest Centre made a full recovery within a week.[65]

Following the exacting retreat to the Alamein line over hundreds of miles of desert, when the problem of 'exhaustion' had shown itself to be one of the most urgent psychiatric emergencies in war, experience proved the value of rest and rehabilitation. It became the practice that a number of beds in Convalescent Depots should be allotted to psychiatric casualties. Results showed that about 90% of men breaking down in battle could be restored to a good standard of stability; in practice, a fairly constant 30% returned satisfactorily to combatant duty, the remainder requiring work, temporarily or permanently, at bases or on lines of communication.[65]

Brigadier James has summarized the psychiatrically significant aspects of this part of the Campaign as follows: "The worst period of the Campaign for fatigue was undoubtedly May, June and July, 1942. . . . The state of exhaustion of the 8th Army after the summer fighting in 1942 was partly due to the fact that so little organised rest and change was possible for units engaged in the Western Desert. The men got tired of fighting, became somewhat apprehensive of the German power and leadership and were 'fed up' with the desert, the rough conditions of living, the flies, the sand storms, the disappointing movement in the wrong direction, and the chronic shortage of effective arms and equipment." The brief periods of rest in the Desert during continuous operations, while successful in relieving physical fatigue, did very little to alleviate the cumulative effects of constant mental strain. "Men went back to the battle willingly enough, but unless arrangements are made in theatres of war for whole battalions or large formations to get away from fighting for a generous period of rest and training in fresh surroundings, the incidence of war worn soldiers is bound to rise to a high level."

The incidence of psychiatric casualties in the M.E.F. rose from about 8 per thousand troops in 1940, to 24 per thousand in 1941, after which it gradually decreased to about 21 per thousand in 1942, and 15 per thousand in 1943.

After the fall of Tripoli, during the period from March, 1943, to the end of the Tunisian Campaign in the middle of May, the psychiatrist with the forward unit (No. 1 Mobile General Hospital) was able, by immediate treatment, to retain some 18% of cases in the field, and 82% were evacuated to the Advanced Psychiatric Unit at Tripoli. Of the total number of psychiatric cases seen by this psychiatrist, an appreciable proportion gave a history of previous neurotic breakdown, whether in civil life (23%), as a result of earlier operations prior to arrival in the Middle East (5%), or in the Middle East (23% having received in-patient, and 6% out-patient, treatment); and 40% of the total number gave evidence of significant demoralization before breakdown. Thus, there was a previous history of psychiatric instability or demoralization in no less than 97% of these psychiatric casualties. During this latter part of the Western Desert Campaign, psychiatric cases constituted some 9% of battle casualties, and 4% of total casualties.

Of those psychiatric cases admitted during this period to the Advanced Psychiatric Unit (Filtration Centre), 33% were sufficiently restored to be disposed of direct to the Reinforcement Unit, either for redistribution on lines of communication or for return to their units; 65% proceeded to the Convalescent Depot (Rehabilitation Centre); and only 2% required evacuation to the base hospital in Egypt.* From the Rehabilitation Centre, 60% (of the total admissions to the Filtration Centre) were then disposed of direct through the Reinforcement Unit, and 5% were sent to the Special Rehabilitation Unit (Farm Depot) for prolonged rehabilitation before they were finally dealt with by the Reinforcement Unit. From the Reinforcement Unit, 68% (of the original total) were given special postings on L. of C., and 30% were returned to their units. The importance of the results achieved is sufficiently demonstrated by the fact that 93% of cases admitted to the Filtration Centre were returned to some form of duty within 28 days of evacuation from forward units.

* Fortunately so: cases had to be evacuated by sea, and No. 41 General Hospital, at El Qantara (Canal Zone), was some 1,100 miles from Tripoli.

FORWARD PSYCHIATRY

Certain observations by Brigadier James, on the varying incidence of psychiatric casualties during the Tunisian Campaign, may be mentioned. In the first part of the Campaign, the incidence of such casualties remained low: however, some of the most severe cases of acute anxiety reaction resulting from battle conditions in the entire operations in North Africa, were seen at this time, especially among men of very high morale, of the Royal Engineers, whose dangerous and arduous task was to clear a passage for the infantry and tanks through enemy minefields, while being subjected to barrage and mortar fire. As the Campaign progressed, and particularly after the capture of Tripoli, when the troops reached the rocky, wooded and more built-over areas of Tunisia, the neurosis rate rose considerably. This was partly due to 'campaign exhaustion' after the long series of battles—to which were added the exacting battle of the Mareth Line and operations around Enfidaville, and partly to environmental physical conditions. Brigadier James stated, in this connection, that it had been noted before that the occurrence of psychiatric breakdown was least in desert fighting, and increased as soon as a change of terrain was experienced. "Thus psychiatric cases tended to rise every time the troops went through Cyrenaica, with the appearance of hidden danger in the hills, buildings and trees."

As a result of his extensive experience of the M.E.F. campaigns, Brigadier James reached certain conclusions, of which the following may be quoted: "Uninterrupted and unhindered dive-bombing by Stukas was only too often the fate of the infantryman in the early days of the M.E.F., and it left its mark on men, which hastened the onset of nervous bankruptcy which evidences the 'burnt out' soldier. . . . Once a 'campaign neurosis' is established, neither officer nor man is ever quite the same. . . . Continuous fighting will exact its price, and . . . an officer should not be more than a year in unrelieved operational work, for the sake of his men. The same is true of N.C.O.s. Men can probably do two years, after which there is an increasing risk of nervous breakdown, or of loss of interest, and . . . of delinquency, with consequent failure in morale and fighting efficiency."

The whole situation in the Middle East underwent a marked change in the course of 1943. As Brigadier R. F. Barbour has well expressed it, during the twelve months from Midsummer, 1943, to Midsummer, 1944, the Middle East Command sank quietly into oblivion: instead of the 'Victorious 8th Army' one heard of 'Men England Forgot' (M.E.F.); from being the main base for the Western Desert Campaign, Egypt became a staging camp on the route to the Far East. He pointed out, however, that the conversion of a command from a primarily fighting role to that of supply did not necessarily diminish psychiatric problems, and in fact might increase them.*

BRITISH NORTH AFRICA FORCE AND CENTRAL MEDITERRANEAN FORCE

Because of intense hostility and opposition on the part of both medical and non-medical military administrative authorities with the 1st Army in North Africa, it was impossible to arrange for an adequate and efficient psychiatric organization in the B.N.A.F. during the Tunisian Campaign. The medical authorities had made no arrangements, and sent out no hospital, for the treatment of psychiatric casualties when the Force landed early in November, 1942. In spite of representations by the Director of Army Psychiatry, not only some months before, but subsequent to, the Allied landing in North Africa, there was no Psychiatric Adviser at Medical Headquarters throughout the Campaign, and the specialist resources of the Force amounted to two psychiatrists who were not sent out until December, 1942, and two General Duty medical officers whose help they had enlisted.† [71]

In spite of considerable difficulties and administrative obstruction, one psychiatrist (Major J. W. Wishart) worked for a time in the forward area, where he obtained the co-operation of the unit medical officers, and did everything possible in the circumstances to provide immediate treatment for psychiatric casualties and prevent unnecessary evacuation.

Major Wishart investigated the causes of a generalized panic which occurred in January, 1943, in one brigade. The principal factors which combined to produce this mass reaction were found to be the following: fatigue following three days' mortar fire, with very little

* Official statistics relating to the M.E.F. are recorded for the period, October, 1943—March, 1945; as are figures showing the relative morbidity and wastage in the M.E.F. during 1943, with respect to psychiatric and various other illnesses.[130]

† In contrast, as Brigadier Rees observed, the American psychiatric organization in the same theatre clearly demonstrated "how proper forward treatment, coupled with a good sane military attitude to the soldier, can operate".[54] Belatedly, and through experience of the inevitable consequences of their opposition, there was a change of attitude on the part of the British medical authorities.[28] Finally, in March, 1943, the D.D.M.S., 1st Army, became so worried about the situation which had developed, that he flew to Cairo to consult the D.M.S., M.E.F., and was given advice by the Consulting Psychiatrist, M.E.F.

sleep; inadequate food supplies; poor selection (with a relatively high proportion of dull and backward men, and neurotics); heavy losses of officers and N.C.O.s; and the fact that the men had not been long in this theatre, and were inexperienced in this type of warfare.

At the base at Algiers, at No. 95 General Hospital, Major C. Kenton, at first working single-handed, "with opportunism, skill and immense industry, built up an unofficial rear psychiatric centre . . ., where he did his best under difficult conditions to get the psychotics handled suitably, and, in the treatment of the enormous numbers of neurosis cases, brilliantly employed narcotic, abreactive and psychotherapeutic techniques".[71] In this work he had the support of the C.O., and the Officer i/c Medical Division, of the Hospital. He also obtained the generous assistance, for part of the time, of the Consultant to the U.S. Army Air Forces (Lt.-Col. Roy R. Grinker), and of two other American psychiatrists who helped in the treatment of British cases as well as caring for their own.[54]

In February, 1943, partly owing to pressure of work at the base, but principally because of the administrative opposition, Major Wishart was transferred to Algiers, where he assisted Major Kenton in the treatment and disposal of the more severe psychiatric casualties recently evacuated from the forward areas, as well as of the patients who had accumulated in large numbers before the psychiatrists' arrival in North Africa. At one time, this base psychiatric unit accommodated 500 patients.

Treatment in the Hospital was inevitably commenced at a relatively late stage of the illness because, before they reached the base, the men had to undergo a long and tiring journey, and had usually been in other hospitals in the course of their evacuation. "They travelled, without sedation, by slow stages along the winding valley routes from the front. In turn they were bullied, ignored, and mollycoddled. . . . Many of the cases, therefore, had become much more complicated, with emotional deterioration, fixation of their original symptoms, formation of new symptoms, and the development of much 'secondary gain'. Some of them regressed to states of hysterical stupor very difficult to distinguish from psychosis." [71] It is not surprising, therefore, that only a small number of men were returned to full duty with combatant units, but some 75% of cases were returned to full duties of some kind, with special postings in North Africa. The number of psychotics was somewhat less than 5% of the total cases admitted.

FORWARD PSYCHIATRY

The result of the absence of trained staff to deal with these patients and with the rush of cases—many of whom should never have been evacuated to the base at all—was that treatment, in some cases, was less thorough than it should have been, and this accounted for the large numbers of unstable, 'bomb-shy' men who were constantly awaiting disposal at the Base Depots. The difficulty of giving these men extra treatment was due to the fact that, as late as June, 1943, there were in North Africa still no additional psychiatrists and, in fact, by then the assistance of the American psychiatrists was no longer available as the latter had moved to a psychiatric hospital of their own on the L. of C. Another obstacle to effective rehabilitation of these cases was the fact that, owing to ignorance at Headquarters and the lack of personnel selection facilities, most of the psychiatrists' well-considered recommendations for changes of employment were never carried out.[71]

It should also be mentioned that the Consulting Physician (Brigadier Boland)—who, in the absence of an Adviser in Psychiatry, did everything in his power to instigate action with regard to the management and treatment of psychiatric casualties—made arrangements, during the fighting, for the establishment of a Rest Centre for cases of physical and mental exhaustion.

One psychiatrist, supplied by the M.E.F., worked with the British troops in Sicily, after the Allied landing in July, 1943, but only for a few weeks. Lt.-Col. S. A. MacKeith, who had eventually been allowed to proceed to B.N.A.F. towards the end of May, 1943, as Adviser in Psychiatry, also served in this capacity in the C.M.F., and was able to outline the fundamental principles of a policy for dealing with psychiatric casualties during the impending Italian Campaign, on the basis of the experience of Army psychiatrists in North Africa (principally, in the 8th Army in M.E.F.). Psychiatrists were attached to two of the three British corps invading Italy in September, 1943 (viz., Major Wishart, from B.N.A.F., to 5th Corps, and Major H. D. Hunter, from M.E.F., to 10th Corps), although at this time "no one was quite sure what their functions would ultimately be. Not altogether unwisely, they were sent into the field to build up the job for themselves."[64] At a later date, a Corps Psychiatrist was also attached to 13th Corps.*

---

* The psychiatrist of 10th Corps was subsequently attached to H.Q., 8th Army (at Pesaro). Another Corps Psychiatrist was appointed to 3rd Corps during the invasion of Greece, and was attached to No. 97 General Hospital, Athens.

FORWARD PSYCHIATRY

During the fighting in Sicily and in the early part of the Italian Campaign, there were no facilities for retaining for treatment the more severe psychiatric casualties, and these consequently had to be evacuated to North Africa and Malta—(the majority of cases from Sicily being evacuated to Tripoli). Statistics available in respect of the cases evacuated from Sicily and Italy to Tripoli, in July–September, 1943, indicate that the psychiatric casualties constituted some 11% of battle casualties, and some 4·5% of the total casualties (as compared with 10% and 4%, respectively, in the latter part of the Western Desert Campaign).

Thus, when Major Hunter landed with 10th Corps at Salerno, his first task was to check the evacuation to North Africa of minor psychiatric casualties, with the purpose of avoiding secondary deterioration and wastage of man-power: "Necessity gave birth to improvisation and, in face of many obstacles, a Forward Psychiatric Centre accommodating 50 patients was opened at C.C.S. level, precariously staffed by one or two borrowed Nursing Orderlies and a number of enthusiastic convalescents." During this period, patients could not be retained for longer than an average of four days, because of the large number of casualties in the intense fighting in the neighbourhood of the Volturno. Nevertheless, it was possible to reduce the proportion of psychiatric casualties evacuated from Italy to less than 10%.[64]

During 1944, the technique of the Corps Exhaustion Centres was gradually evolved. At the same time, the Advanced Psychiatric Centre, initiated in December, 1943, developed from two inadequate 100-bed 'expansions' of general hospitals in forward areas (one on each side of the peninsula), into a single unit with 200 beds (later increased to 400 beds), situated immediately behind Army H.Q., in the L. of C. Area, at Assisi (some 300 miles from the base). Very few of the patients received by this unit from the Corps Exhaustion Centres, were returned to combatant duty: most of them were allocated to employment in the L. of C. Area.[71]

The organization for the rehabilitation of psychiatric patients in the C.M.F. originated in the formation by Lt.-Col. Palmer, in February, 1944, of a unit at the base—eventually known as the Reallocation Centre (All Arms), C.M.F.—intended to deal with the large number of psychoneurotic cases evacuated from operational areas in the Command, which would otherwise occupy much valuable hospital accommodation required for urgent surgical and medical casualties. It was also felt that this Centre could fulfil an important function in dealing with the considerable number of un-rehabilitated psychiatric casualties and chronic psychoneurotics who were, at that time, deteriorating in Convalescent Depots, Transit Camps, Training Depots, and other units, where they were mixing with future reinforcements, to the inevitable detriment of the morale of the latter.[88]

In the C.M.F., in 1944, as a result of these various developments, regimental medical officers in forward areas had been taught when to evacuate psychiatric cases, how to effect adequate sedation for their journey, and how to 'label' them so as to ensure that they reached the Corps Psychiatrist. At the Corps Exhaustion Centre, one-third of the cases, i.e. those with a good prognosis, were retained for simple treatment, for three to five days, and then returned to their units; the remaining two-thirds were evacuated to the Advanced Psychiatric Centre. Of these cases, a small number (including all psychotics, gross psychopaths, and those neurotics requiring prolonged treatment or evacuation to the U.K.) were sent on almost immediately to a Rear Psychiatric Centre in the Base Area. The remainder of those admitted to the Advanced Centre were retained for an average period of ten days and received specialized hospital treatment, followed by some weeks of rehabilitation at the Reallocation Centre. Most of the cases admitted to the latter unit, having been placed in a lower medical category, were tested and interviewed by Personnel Selection staff, and reallocated to non-combatant duties in the L. of C. Area. On an average 90% of cases admitted to the Advanced Centre, and 38% (about two-fifths) of those dealt with in units at the base, were returned to full duty of some kind in the C.M.F.

As a result of this organization, the clinical findings and results in the C.M.F. were in very marked contrast to those existing in the B.N.A.F.: "Thanks to earlier evacuation, sedation for their journey, and contact with a psychiatrist (in the Corps Exhaustion Centre) at an early stage, practically none of the patients severely 'regressed'. The psychiatric syndromes they displayed were much milder...; there was less fixation of symptoms, no new symptom formation, and amazingly little 'secondary gain'. Continuous narcosis was less frequently needed, and abreaction much less often employed. Treatment was, in general, much less specialized." [71]

In the early, administratively stable, stage in the C.M.F., a forward organization based on Corps Psychiatrists and their teams was found

FORWARD PSYCHIATRY

to work well in practice, and the corps remained as compact entities. At a later stage, the methods of conducting the Campaign altered to such an extent, that divisions changed their corps frequently and at relatively short notice, thereby very considerably reducing the efficacy of forward psychiatry based on a corps structure, and the undoubted advantages, in these circumstances, of a system involving the use of Divisional Psychiatrists very soon became apparent.

MALTA

Although a psychiatric specialist had been requested by Malta Command, and was sent out from the U.K. in June, 1942, he was subsequently retained in the Middle East, as the D.D.M.S., Malta, at that time, stated that he did not want a psychiatrist. Indeed, the Army medical authorities in Malta had by then appointed one acting 'Command Psychiatrist' and three acting 'Area Psychiatrists', who were all medical specialists (i.e. specialist general physicians). It thus happened that, during the period of the siege (June–November, 1942), there was no actual psychiatric specialist on the Island.*

Needless to say, this regrettable state of affairs resulted from an intense hostility towards psychiatry, on the part of medical and non-medical military administrative authorities in Malta. It was fortunate, therefore, that through the efforts of the medical specialist (Lt.-Col. R. E. Tunbridge) who had to act as Command Psychiatrist on the Island, the psychiatric cases which occurred during this period received as much care and treatment as it was possible to give them in the circumstances.†

Col. Tunbridge, reviewing the experiences of medical specialists in Malta from September, 1941, to June, 1943, recorded a number of

* It was not until July, 1943, that a psychiatrist was eventually admitted to the Island's medical establishment, subsequent to certain administrative changes which occurred (in May, 1943) shortly after a visit by the Adjutant-General (Gen. Sir Ronald Adam).

† It is relevant here to record an unfounded and irresponsible statement which was originally made at a meeting of the Royal Society of Medicine, and was subsequently widely quoted, e.g. by the late Col. E. C. Cutler, Chief Consultant in Surgery, U.S. Army, European Theatre of Operations, who declared: "There are statistical data to support the fact that where there is no escape route, these psychological casualties do not arise, or arise but rarely. Thus . . . few on the island of Malta were afflicted once escape was found impossible. If it is quite as unsafe to run away as to stay, perhaps the unconscious processes that lead to such desertions will not arise and such casualties will diminish." [38] Col. Cutler's departure from the, no doubt, more familiar and concrete realms of surgery, into somewhat unorthodox and speculative theory in psychopathology, and the similar assertions of others, have but one disadvantage, that of not being founded on fact.

factors which affected the morale and mental stability of the men stationed there, and certain widespread and significant symptoms which occurred among them.* The following observations are of particular importance, in the present context: "At first, dullness and mental backwardness were not much in evidence, which was all the more surprising as the units had left the U.K. before the introduction on any large scale of the newer methods of selection and testing.... As the strain of the siege conditions increased and the necessary equipment for the more technical training of the modern infantryman became available, mental backwardness became increasingly important. Dullards who had in the past been tolerated as the platoon or company comic began to be despised, for they delayed the training programme and brought the platoon into disfavour, and they sought refuge in sickness or crime." [123]

Rest, sedation, and reassurance were the only treatment available for psychiatric cases. "The smallness of the Island meant that no area was immune from enemy action or from anti-aircraft or aerial activity. The Convalescent Depots and hospitals were all within a mile of military objectives; hence the value of these institutions as rest centres was limited. The patients with severe symptoms had to be admitted to hospital, as they could not be retained in their units, but once in hospital they created many administrative and medical difficulties, chief of which was the inability to transfer them to the mainland. The men were employed wherever possible, but their continued presence about the hospital for months, their behaviour during air-raids, and their apparent physical well-being... had a bad influence on the other patients.... Many of the patients with a reasonably good background, after rest, sedation, and repeated interviews, returned to their units and performed useful work, if sheltered from exposure by arrangement with the Company Officer and unit medical officer. Had an invasion occurred, they would have proved a serious liability." [123]

It was noted by the medical specialists that, soon after the bombing began in 1941, some 50–60% of all the out-patients seen by them at the three hospitals were primarily psychiatric cases. Col. Tunbridge stated: "The limited investigation of the possible effects of bombing suggested that at least 25% of the garrison showed a pathological

* The conditions and reactions observed by Col. Tunbridge and others in Malta, are in many respects similar to those which occurred in other isolated areas overseas— e.g. Gibraltar, and East and West Africa—and which are described in the chapter on Morale.

FORWARD PSYCHIATRY

degree of response to aerial attack in March, 1942, a percentage which in my opinion had increased by the end of April, 1942." [123]

Brigadier Rees, who had previously been able to discuss the situation with several medical and surgical specialists who had left the Island, visited Malta in June, 1943, and had occasion, at that time, to meet a number of medical, and senior non-medical, officers: thus, the D.D.S.T. had informed him that all the officers suffered from "ineffectiveness and loss of grip, great sleepiness and jumpiness", and that "there was much neurosis all through the Island". Brigadier Rees further ascertained that when, in February, 1942, conditions were becoming worse, there was a gradual, steady increase of fear states, and drinking was heavy; one officer stated that they "were very near to a crack in April, 1942".

Col. Tunbridge had suggested, early in 1942, that an adequate survey should be made to assess the state of the troops, and that a rest camp for the Gunners should be established. Although at that time there were three or four raids daily, with an average of 100 bombers on each occasion, these suggestions were rejected. As Brigadier Rees pointed out, if the medical advice in these matters had been followed, a good deal could have been done to avoid the potentially serious situation which arose.

INDIA AND SOUTH-EAST ASIA COMMAND

It is only possible here to refer briefly to the general psychiatric organization in India, and to mention a few aspects of forward psychiatry in relation to the campaigns in South-East Asia.

The general situation has been well summarized by Brigadier E. A. Bennet, who was the Consultant in Psychiatry to India Command: "The development of the medical services was at first gradual, and it was not till 1942 that it became evident that the psychiatric needs of the Army were not being met. At that time there were six psychiatrists in the Army in India, and some of them were doing general duty as well as psychiatry. By 1945 the number of whole-time psychiatrists had risen to almost one hundred. This rapid development was accompanied by the provision of over three thousand beds for psychiatric patients. The policy was to link the treatment of these patients with that of the general hospitals. A 'standard psychiatric ward' of twenty-five beds was designed and one or more of these units was added to the smaller general hospitals according to local needs. In addition,

FORWARD PSYCHIATRY

large psychiatric centres were formed in base areas, with accommodation for several hundred patients. These proved insufficient and in 1945 a psychiatric hospital of 1,200 beds was opened. Towards the end of the war there were between forty and fifty psychiatric centres in India, Burma and Ceylon." [18] *

Forward psychiatry was gradually developed, in this theatre, during the fighting in Burma and on the India-Burma front, from 1942 onwards. The psychiatric requirements in these campaigns obviously presented a problem very different from those which were encountered in M.E.F., B.N.A.F., C.M.F., and North-Western Europe. In Burma, the psychiatrists worked in a combat zone which lay in hilly and thickly wooded (bamboo and scrub) jungle country, where communications were difficult to maintain. Units in the same corps or division frequently fought far apart. The lines of communication within the Corps Area were long, and evacuation was slow and hazardous.

The geographical features of the country on the borders of India, Assam and Burma made it necessary for divisions to operate alone, and this led to the need for Divisional Psychiatrists. Each Corps Psychiatrist formed a Centre with 50–100 beds in a convenient medical unit, usually a C.C.S. or a forward hospital; and each Divisional Psychiatrist established, as far forward as practicable, an Exhaustion Centre to which were sent all patients considered by the regimental medical officer to be suffering from psychiatric disorders.

The difficulties in selecting a suitable site for the Divisional Centres were considerable: rest and quiet were obviously desirable, but were, of course, only obtainable at some distance from the line, and consequently some of the Centres were located a few miles to the rear. In certain engagements, 'boxes' (defended perimeter sites) were occupied by fighting units; and at least two Divisional Psychiatrists treated their patients in these 'boxes', i.e. virtually in the front line. The Divisional Centres were set up in a variety of structures, ranging from a mere dug-out with tarpaulin head cover, to tents or, in one instance, a corrugated iron shed capable of holding 30–40 'charpoys' (string beds). The Divisional Psychiatrist retained some cases for

---

* The inadequate and out-of-date features of the majority of civil mental hospitals in India were described in the Report, published in 1946, of the Health Survey and Development Committee (Bhore Committee) which was set up by the Government of India.[103] (The author is greatly indebted to Lt.-Gen. Sir Bennett Hance, late D.G.I.M.S., now Medical Adviser, Commonwealth Relations Office, for kindly placing at his disposal a copy of this almost unobtainable Report.) Cf. also the comments by Brigadier E. A. Bennet.[17, 18]

FORWARD PSYCHIATRY

treatment and the remainder, requiring more complete investigation, were sent to the Corps Centre where they could be retained for two weeks or longer, depending on the operational situation. Each Divisional Psychiatrist had been provided with two panniers (which could be carried on mule or jeep) containing a supply of sedatives and suitable equipment, so that he could work, if necessary, apart from a parent medical unit.[17, 39, 40]

It is important to note that the Adviser in Psychiatry to 14th Army (Lt.-Col. A. A. White), as a result of very extensive experience of psychiatric organization in this type of warfare, expressed the opinion that it would be a mistake to make any firm pronouncement as to where the Divisional Psychiatrist should be located, especially when operating in territory so wild as that of the Assam-Burma border. He should, according to Col. White, be sufficiently mobile, and his organization sufficiently elastic, to enable him to undertake his work wherever the opportunity allowed in any circumstances. It would, therefore, certainly be a mistake to have a conception of a linear evacuation route, with A.D.S., M.D.S., and C.C.S. all located at succeeding points along it. With aerial evacuation from the actual battlefield, it might be that the M.D.S. and C.C.S. would cease to exist in their traditional form, and that the psychiatric unit would be one of several specialist units which would continue to work at the point of battle itself.

The majority of the casualties referred to the Exhaustion Centres, although presenting psychological rather than physical symptoms, were not psychiatric cases in the usual sense, but were suffering from the effects of a combination of factors of which, as a rule, the most prominent was physical and mental exhaustion. This was to be expected, for the conditions under which the men fought on the India-Burma front, quite apart from enemy action itself, were severe. Although these conditions naturally varied to some extent at different periods, the more important stresses to which the men were subjected were common to all the Burma Campaigns: "The climate (particularly in monsoon conditions), the nature of the ground, shortage of food and water, fatigue and the lowered resistance following malaria and other illness, acted adversely even on the most stable. The fighting was intermittent in character. In quiet periods, particularly from sunset to dawn, the presence of Jap patrols made sleep difficult. During attacks on defended positions there was added the emotional strain of battle—danger, loss of comrades, incessant noise of gun and mortar fire, and the unrelenting demand on physical endurance." [17]

Particularly following the introduction of Divisional Psychiatrists in November, 1943, there was a very marked improvement in the efficiency of the forward psychiatric organization, and it became possible to effect a considerable saving of man-power by avoiding the unnecessary evacuation of casualties. Divisional Psychiatrists were eventually appointed to no less than ten divisions engaged in the Burma Campaigns. Behind them, at Corps level, were three Corps Psychiatrists (of 4th, 33rd and 15th Corps).

A problem specific to the Burma Campaigns was that arising in the forward areas during the semi-resting phase enforced by the rainy season. "During the monsoon period, positions were relatively static in certain sectors, and patrol activity became the main military task. The true battle casualty was rare as the stress of active fighting lessened, but more resistant disabilities were seen. There was, for example, an increase in toxic confusional conditions, in which the precipitating factors were multiple. Thus, malaria and amoebiasis, or malaria, hookworm infection, and anaemia, were frequently found in conjunction with severe psychiatric symptoms. Symptoms which developed as the outcome of active fighting were recognized and treated before they became assimilated in the personality, and recovery was rapid. But the recovery rate fell during the relatively quiet phases of the campaign, both in Indian and British troops. The majority suffered from chronic rather than acute psychoneurotic conditions, complicated by organic disorders." [17]

It was fortunately possible, as a result of the diminished intensity of battle at such periods, to undertake the treatment of these more chronic cases at a really forward level. The therapeutic results were most satisfactory and showed how much could be done to retain for further military duties men who, untreated, would have been added to the number of chronic military patients in hospitals at the base, unlikely ever to return to the field. For example, of the British cases treated at the 33rd Corps Psychiatric Centre during a period of three months in the semi-resting (monsoon) phase on the India-Burma border, preceding the second Campaign, in 1944, less than 8% were evacuated to India, some 65% were returned to their units in their original medical categories, and the remainder in a lower category.

The frequent occurrence of organic conditions in association with psychiatric disorders was, in fact, a matter of considerable importance in this theatre, and especially in regions such as Assam and Burma. For example, no less than 50% of a group of Indian 'mental cases', examined by Lt.-Col. A. A. White in June, 1943, were found to be suffering from infective conditions to which their psychiatric symptoms were secondary. In consequence, a hospital order was issued, and subsequently circulated widely in the Eastern Army Area, pointing out that the following organic causes might give rise, as a presenting symptom, to mental disorder: malaria, typhus and heat exhaustion—the most common causes; and typhoid, meningitis, pneumonia, alcohol (native spirit), and drugs such as opium and hashish ('ganja').

The results of forward psychiatric treatment were good, and on an average, approximately 60% of cases were returned to their units, and of these only a small number broke down again. In the stringency of the general military and man-power situation, it was considered that if a man, returned to duty, fought even for three or four days, his return was justified.[17]

A few available figures relating to psychiatric casualties in the Burma Campaigns may be quoted. Psychiatric cases in the second Arakan Campaign constituted less than 10% of the total casualties. The incidence of psychiatric casualties among British troops (1·5%) was higher than among Indian troops (0·6%), but amongst the latter, on the other hand, there were a fair number of self-inflicted wounds and cases of desertion. The cases seen by the Corps Psychiatrist, 15th Indian Corps (Lt.-Col. J. Matas, R.C.A.M.C., attached R.A.M.C.), in this same Campaign, during the monsoon period (June–October, 1944), were distributed as follows: Of the British cases, three-fifths were psychoneuroses, and one-fifth dull and backward; of the Indian cases, two-fifths were psychoses (one-eighth of all cases being toxic psychoses), and more than one-third were cases of hysteria (with or without associated organic illness). Of the British cases, one-fifth were returned to their units, one-quarter evacuated, and the remainder downgraded at Corps level; of the Indian cases, rather less than one-quarter were returned to their units, and about three-quarters were evacuated.

During the first Assam-Burma Campaign (Kohima to Imphal), in March, 1944, one of the Divisional Psychiatrists recorded that, at a time when Japanese infiltration was taking place and operations were, in consequence, 'fluid', the forward unit was located in a defensive ('box') position, to which casualties made their way: treatment was carried out at the M.D.S.; cover from shelling was secured by digging in, but there was no head cover—("a splinter-proof room would have been a great asset"). Nevertheless, more than 50% of the cases were returned to duty in less than three days.[40]

During the whole of the second Assam-Burma Campaign (Imphal to Rangoon), there was uninterrupted evacuation from the Divisional Psychiatric Centres direct to the Corps Centre, by light aircraft. Of the total number of psychiatric casualties in this Campaign, some 50% of British cases, and some 36% of Indian cases, were returned to full duty from Divisional level. The Corps Psychiatrist, 33rd Indian Corps (Major A. Milne), expressed the opinion that this rate of 50% was "about the best that can be achieved by a Divisional Psychiatrist, especially when the men have been, as ours had been, in the field a long time and the effects of cumulation of stress become obvious." From *all* levels, in this same Campaign, 72% of the total number of British, and over 60% of the total number of Indian, psychiatric casualties were returned to full duty in their units.

VIII
PROBLEMS OF TRAINING AND MORALE

> To give moderate liberty for griefs and discontentments to evaporate (so it be without too great insolency or bravery), is a safe way: for he that turneth the humours back, and maketh the wound bleed inwards, endangereth malign ulcers and pernicious imposthumations.   FRANCIS BACON

DURING AND FOLLOWING the Second World War, Army psychiatrists were called upon to investigate, and to advise on, a large number of problems of morale, which arose in very various circumstances, and in widely separated and diverse theatres of operations. On many occasions also, the Consulting Psychiatrist was personally asked for advice by 'A' and 'G' Staffs on many different questions relating to morale. It is noteworthy that it was the medical authorities who, throughout the war period, frequently showed by their decisions and attitudes that they had failed to appreciate the immense potential contributions of psychiatry to the understanding and management of the manifold problems involving morale, whereas, on the other hand, senior officers on both 'A' and 'G' Staffs, through the pressure of circumstance, very soon became keenly aware of the value and importance of these potentialities of applied psychiatry.

A substantial amount of evidence is recorded elsewhere in the present work of the considerable 'indirect' contributions of Army psychiatry to the maintenance of good morale: in particular, by the detection, treatment, or disposal of those men who exerted a deleterious effect on group morale, by reason of their mental instability, low intelligence, immaturity or inherent inadequacy (whether manifested by psychiatric breakdown, delinquency, desertion, alcoholism, frequent minor illness, a high incidence of V.D., or other symptoms of their maladjustment, e.g. abysmal inefficiency or obstructiveness);* and by attention to the problem of the 'misfit', through adequate selection and allocation of personnel, thereby eliminating such important causes of low (individual and group) morale as employment of men on unsuitable jobs, and the presence in ordinary units of large numbers of dullards (whose morale improved as surely as did that of the unit, as soon as they were segregated in specially organized companies).

With a view to lowering the incidence of psychiatric breakdown, and promoting mental health, Army psychiatrists also contributed directly to the maintenance of good morale principally by giving advice on the psychiatric aspects of leadership and 'man-management', propaganda, training, and welfare.

Since the first introduction of psychiatrists into the Army, at the beginning of the war, lectures were given by Consultants and specialists to regimental officers, staff courses and O.C.T.U.s, on 'man-management', i.e. on the psychology of morale and leadership. One psychiatrist in particular (Lt.-Col. T. F. Main) was, from February to July, 1942, primarily concerned with questions of morale, and gave a series of lectures to officer students and commanders of infantry battalions attending Battle Schools, on such subjects as the following: methods of maintaining the mental health of the soldier, weeding out unsuitable men before battle, and handling incipient breakdowns during a campaign; the principles of group feeling (esprit de corps); the place of discipline in mental health; the foundations of morale; the effect on morale of various enemy weapons; the proper place and use of 'battle inoculation'; factors militating against individual and group morale; methods of maintaining mental stability under stress; and the function of leadership in relation to morale. The School of Infantry subsequently continued to include lectures on these subjects in its courses.

In June, 1942, Lt.-Col. A. T. M. Wilson compiled some notes for Army psychiatrists who might be called upon to discuss questions of morale. A few of the points emphasized by Col. Wilson may be mentioned: In modern war, victory depended not so much on the

* These symptoms of poor individual adjustment and morale, if they became widespread, were of course undoubted evidence of a serious state of low group morale.

PROBLEMS OF TRAINING AND MORALE

number killed as on the number demoralized. Weapons, no matter how good or how abundant, could not bring victory if units had poor morale: and morale was 'forged by the officer'. The building up of good morale was an active process: there was no really effective passive defence against either air attack or bad morale. For twenty years, the enemy had given as much thought to the importance of morale as to the preparation of physical weapons. "Officers and men cannot be attached and removed like articles of equipment. A unit is a living organism in which grafting is as difficult as in trees." A summary was also given of the factors which could damage trust in leaders, group morale, and individual morale, respectively.*

Early in 1942, the Army formed its first Battle School. The principal aims of the Battle Schools were, first, to establish a battle drill which would replace older methods of training in tactics, and secondly, to condition men to the noise and turmoil of war, by using the maximal amount of live ammunition and high explosives throughout the course. At the request of G.H.Q., Home Forces, a psychiatrist (Lt.-Col. T. F. Main) was attached to the newly formed G.H.Q. Battle School, in February, 1942. He was asked to give advice to the Chief Instructor of the School on the psychological aspects of the investigation and development of new forms of battle training.

It was realized by Army psychiatrists that adequate preparation of this kind, if conducted along correct lines, might help to prevent breakdown under actual battle conditions.† For this reason, such

---

* "When the Captaine electeth his Caporals, he ought to do it with such consideration, that amongst his souldiers, one, chosen to this office, none should excell him in valour, vertue, experience and diligence; yea and in age also, to the end he might be respected with more loue and reuerence: so that he deport himselfe among them, as a father with his children, his conditions being a patterne vnto them, asswaging and ending their debates and quarrels, reducing them vnto amitie, . . . in such sort that they may all be of one will, desire, and ligue.

"Let him learne . . . to know the qualitie & valour of euery one in particular, & be earnest with them to keepe their armor neat, cleane and bright, and often to practise the weapon they carrie, he himselfe ensigning and teaching the . . . rawe men. . . .

"He shall reprehend them for swearing and lewd speeches: and shall not permit them any prohibited games, the which he must doe with such sagacitie and warie meanes, that they result not against him, and so reiect and contemne his reputation, thereby loosing their loue and his former respect. . . ."—Robert Barret, *The Theorike and Practike of Moderne Warres* (London, 1598).

† Cf. the following statements by the Southborough Committee, in 1922: "As the production of good morale is the most important object in military training, . . . the best possible training should be given to every man intended to serve as a soldier, and . . . by such means, . . . he will be protected against the occurrence of 'shell-shock'. . . . It is recommended also . . . that troops should, when possible, be entered into battle gradually and not precipitated into the thick of war." [128] In 1881, General Sir George Balfour had asked the Secretary of State for War to take such necessary

measures, based on correct psychological principles, became known as 'battle inoculation'. The psychiatrist, in his advisory capacity, exerted considerable influence on the development of techniques towards this end.

It was the intention of the School, at its inception, not only to use maximal amounts of live ammunition, but to combine this with a training in 'Hate', to be induced by the excitement of students by instructors' cries, atrocity photographs, and special lectures. Plans had also been made for attempts to 'condition' students to the sight of blood, by visits to slaughterhouses and the throwing of blood about the training areas during active exercises. The psychiatrist was asked to devise further measures of this kind. The opinion given by the psychiatrist was that the training in 'Hate' and this kind of 'conditioning' to bloodshed were not only socially undesirable but liable to increase rather than decrease the incidence of breakdown in the Army; on the other hand, it was considered that 'inoculation' with live ammunition and explosive noises held promise, but that more facts were needed before it could be regarded as ideal in its existing form of maximal intensity in the early stages of training. Col. Main reported that there was a reluctance to accept this advice, as what had been hoped for was the intensification of both of these kinds of training, with the uncritical aid of psychiatry. Certain subsequent events, however, suggested that the advice given was sound.

'Hate' training was, therefore, discouraged at the outset by the psychiatrist. Indeed, as Col. Main well observed, the analogy of the battlefield to a slaughterhouse did not seem to be relevant or inspiring, and the emphasis on the less skilled and more sadistic aspects of war appeared to upset many students. Incidents of fainting and vomiting among students gave point to the psychiatrist's emphatic advice, and the attempt to teach 'Hate' was abandoned by the G.H.Q. Battle School in March, 1942, after the first course.

It subsequently appeared, however, that among some of the newly formed Battle Schools further attempts were being made to create a

---

action "as will . . . enable commanding officers to enforce and carry on military discipline without the aid of flogging", including the introduction of "stringent rules, requiring all recruits to be thoroughly trained, and before being passed into the ranks, reported on by a responsible officer of rank, as to their fitness by age, bodily powers, and military instruction to perform all the duties of a soldier in the field as well as in garrison" (*Parl. Deb.*, 3rd ser., 260: 375-6, 562; 31 March, 4 April, 1881). Thus, thorough training (and hence good morale), rather than fear and coercion, was seen to constitute the basis of good discipline.

PROBLEMS OF TRAINING AND MORALE

sadistic atmosphere. The strange and primitive—and from the standpoint of psychopathology, highly revealing—methods of the new Battle Schools, which purported, by the process of 'blooding' and by instilling hatred, to create a desirable and efficient type of military leader, were described in vivid and lurid detail in a talk broadcast by the B.B.C. Home Service, immediately after the 1 p.m. news, on 27 April, 1942. According to this account of one particular School, the aim was "to teach men from different units in the Command how to hate the enemy and how to use that hate".

This talk, and the methods it described, aroused widespread criticism, and protests were made by informed and educated members of the public, in the press, in Parliament, and by religious leaders (on psychological as well as ethical grounds).*

At the beginning of May, 1942, further representations on this matter were made by the Directorate of Army Psychiatry to the military authorities concerned. It was pointed out that, from the beginning, the psychiatric view regarding attempts to work up hate, and the use of blood, had been clear, definite and antagonistic; and that this opinion was supported by that of a large number of extremely competent soldiers of all ranks: the main body of contrary opinion was to be found among the Nazis and among those who had a deep fear of them. From the psychiatric point of view, Brigadier Rees has recorded that "Some of the men who had been the best and keenest students going through these Battle School courses had afterwards lost interest and become rather ineffective; in fact, they had gone into depression." [97]

The whole position with regard to this type of 'training' was stated with admirable clarity, in a Memorandum on Battle Drill, in May, 1942, by the Army Commander, South-Eastern Command (Lt.-Gen. B. L. Montgomery), who observed that any attempt to create an artificial blood-lust or hate during training was worse than futile. Such an attitude was foreign to the British temperament and attempts to produce it by artificial stimulus during training were bound to fail in battle, as was the case in the previous war. Officers and N.C.O.s must be made to realize the difference between this artificial hate, and the building of a true offensive spirit combined with the

---

* Cf., for example, an article by the military correspondent of *Time and Tide*[8]; *Parl. Deb.*, 5th ser., Commons, 379: 1715; 13 May, 1942; a letter by the Moderator of the General Assembly of the Church of Scotland, *Glasgow Herald*, 5 May, 1942; and a statement by the Archbishop of Canterbury, Dr. William Temple, to the full Synod of Convocation, in May, 1942.

will-power which would not recognize defeat. Men stood up to the wear and tear, and the stress of war, just in proportion to their character and will-power, and it was these qualities we must seek to develop. There were no synthetic ways of doing so, and no short cuts. The methods we adopted must be suited to our national character, which did not include blood-lust.

In the middle of May, 1942, the Commander-in-Chief, Home Forces, issued definite instructions that this kind of training should cease, and at the same time, the psychiatrist attached to G.H.Q. Battle School made a tour of these schools and gave advice to the commandants and instructors on the potential harm of such methods.

During 1941, certain experiments were carried out at No. 41 General Hospital (Bishop's Lydeard, Somerset), in the use of special gramophone records of air-raid noises in an attempt to accustom or 'condition' to such stimuli neurotic patients who had been seriously upset psychologically by air-raids. Referring to these experiments, in August, 1941, Brigadier Rees expressed the opinion that, although this was a superficial method of treatment it was of some value in these cases; and he added: "What I have always visualized, however, is that it might be of some small value as an adjunct to training."

In the same months, Majors F. L. McLaughlin and W. M. Millar reported on these clinical experiments as follows: "A large proportion of patients admitted to a neuropathic military hospital revealed that their neurotic breakdown was either determined or in part precipitated by the unaccustomed stress of noises, such as gun-fire, shell-bursts, exploding bombs, sirens, planes, and dive-bombing. Some of these soldiers were Dunkirk casualties, but the majority were men who had not served outside England. Experience showed that treatment along orthodox psychotherapeutic lines ... was impeded in these cases by too quiet an environment in hospital. While other symptoms had been resolved, there remained a certain hypersensitiveness to air-raid noises. ... An attempt was made to 'decondition' the state of hypersensitiveness to warfare sounds by reproducing the disturbing noises till the patients gradually became more normal in their reactions. At first the apparatus used for reproducing these noises was rather crude.... Later, with the helpful co-operation of the B.B.C., it was possible to make use of gramophone records of actual warfare. Technicians made to our specification records of sirens, the firing of A.A. and machine guns, sounds of planes, dive-bombing, and explosions. Individual sounds or a composite effect could be reproduced when required." [72]

These psychiatrists concluded that "Fear, which is simply a normal protective instinct, can be countered by enlightenment, and aerial bombardment is unlikely to achieve its demoralizing object if the experience is not a complete surprise. Apprehension and anxiety concerning air-raids are more likely to affect those who are inactive and have not been accustomed to warfare noises. Repetition of bombardment noises would appear to assist in raising the power of endurance and in enabling the individual to stand up to this new form of attack." [72]

At the end of 1941, a proposal was put forward that, "during the present conditions of comparative peace", far more should be done to train the Army to face the noise and conditions of the battlefield. It was pointed out that, in the First World War, with the trench warfare, it had been possible to introduce the men to these conditions gradually, whereas, in the current war, the men might suddenly find themselves involved in a battle of the first magnitude. The conditions, and particularly the noises, of warfare would have an adverse effect on the efficiency of many men, because they would come as a surprise. Certain arms, such as the Artillery and R.A.C., carried out some of their training under conditions of noise, but the infantry did not do so. These noises could be reproduced by amplifying from records sounds of guns firing, bombs bursting, and so on, and by the explosion of charges; but the Director of Military Training realized that psychology was very closely connected with this form of training, and that if it was not considered, harm might be done.

The Director of Military Training invited a psychiatrist (Lt.-Col. Main) to attend an experimental demonstration of 'noise training' at Ripon, Yorks., in March, 1942, and, at the psychiatrist's suggestion, the War Office arranged a further experiment at Warley, Essex, in May. As a result of his observations, Col. Main concluded that the important condition for the use of explosives during training was that small 'doses' should be used first so that the men might become adjusted to the experience, and that the intensity should then gradually be increased, so that finally the men should not react unduly to dangerous maximal explosions. Psychological experience in clinical work and elsewhere supplied abundant evidence that attempts to 'condition' men, say to noise or danger, might, unless great care were taken, actually produce the opposite result to that intended, i.e.

in the case of noise, make men more afraid of it than they had previously been.

Thus, the working hypothesis was laid down that, by beginning slowly with battle-like experiences, it was possible to assist the growth of military judgement and to reduce the over-estimation of the 'noise and fog of war' as such, during training. It was also clear that training of this kind would have little value unless the conditions reproduced approximated as nearly as possible to those of actual battle. It was found possible to design useful measures to combat exaggerated fears about being overrun by tanks, or exposed to bombardment at close range by mortar bombs and artillery, or to near-hits by small-arms weapons, and to counteract the effects of noise, blast, earth-shake and smoke, so caused. It was not, of course, possible to reproduce the actual dangers of war, but occasional accidents made it plain that the students were not free from all risk. The C.-in-C., Home Forces, who had welcomed and encouraged this development in battle training, accepted the implicit risks.

The G.H.Q. Battle School had, in two months, trained the commandants and instructors of the Divisional Battle Schools which were about to be formed, and by June, 1942, these were carrying out 'battle inoculation' as part of their training programme. One inherent danger of encouraging the use of live ammunition was that officers were liable to use it as a test of nerves rather than a training expedient, i.e. to begin it suddenly and with too violent effects. This fact had already been recognized in March, 1942, and the psychiatrist had issued verbal and written warnings in this connection to all the Battle Schools which were being newly formed. In order to ensure the proper use of such training methods, he also made a tour of over twenty Battle Schools in June and July, 1942, to advise on this subject, and at the same time to give lectures to the officer students on the maintenance of mental health and high morale among men under changing conditions of war.

In November and December, 1942, while with the 8th Army in the Middle East, Col. Main was able to obtain confirmation of the value of some of the methods used in training in England. The opinion was strongly held by fighting men and officers, that 'battle inoculation' was a most important part of the training of battle reinforcements, and should be given to all troops before their first action. The psychiatrist was able to meet, after the Battle of Alamein, a number of officers who had received this training: they were emphatic that

PROBLEMS OF TRAINING AND MORALE

their first experience of a set battle at Alamein had been well prepared for in Britain, and that they had been the steadier for it.

The investigation by Lt.-Col. J. C. Penton of deserters in B.A.O.R. showed that desertion and absenteeism could be regarded very largely as an index of morale. Thus, a specific cause of desertion was found to be the lack of morale-building factors, such as training (and, therefore, self-confidence), general adaptation to Army life and discipline, and identification with a given group (e.g. through transfer from one unit to another, inertia due to sudden change, or the adverse effect of waiting in Reinforcement Holding Units or Transit Camps). Other specific causes of desertion were morale-destroying factors, such as inevitable external strains ('battle or campaign stress', etc.), inevitable internal strains causing individual emotional trauma (e.g. changes in, or separation from, the group; death of a comrade or officer; personal guilt or injury, etc.), or domestic stress and personal worries.

While this investigation was, of course, only concerned with facts which it was possible to elicit directly from the subjects, and, therefore, could not provide evidence on the important influence of the quality of the leadership on the morale of a unit, it nevertheless confirmed the fact that the strength of morale of the group depends very largely on the morale-building and morale-destroying factors mentioned above. Col. Penton pointed out that, as this strength altered with respect to any particular man, so did his personal morale and reliability as a fighting man. There were two natural reactions to danger: fight was the response of the man well integrated in a fighting group; flight, that of the unintegrated. Thus, desertion would take place when group morale disappeared and individual morale sank to 'flight level' or 'desertion point'.

With particular reference to the adverse effect on morale of lack of training, Col. Penton observed that technical mastery of a weapon was only half of training, and was worth little unless accompanied by confidence in the ability to use it under battle conditions. Though the cynics might say that all that was required of an infantryman was that he should walk, run or crawl where he was told to, and fire when the order was given, and that his marksmanship was of little importance, the private soldier going into battle would not be comforted by such an exegesis of his duties. If he felt that his training had been skimped or hurried, or that he was being given a job for which he had not been trained, he would lack confidence; his morale

PROBLEMS OF TRAINING AND MORALE

would be low, and if he should succumb to the temptation to run he would feel resentful and hard done by if classed as a convict. Inadequacy of training was stressed sufficiently often by the men interviewed to justify its designation as a factor in the causation of desertion, and to establish the inadvisability of quick conversions and changing of men's duties during a campaign.

Reference has already been made, elsewhere in the present work, to the relatively very high incidence of desertion in the infantry, and the significance of this fact, from the point of view of morale and training, will be obvious. In this connection, Col. Penton considered, in the light of his careful investigation, that the most important factor accounting for the considerable preponderance of infantrymen among deserters was undoubtedly the dangerous, arduous, unspectacular and unrewarding nature of their job—(aptly summarized, already in the First World War, by the popular term, 'P.B.I.'). It was, however, necessary to take into consideration other factors: it would, for example, be important to ascertain whether the standard of training demanded of the infantry was as high as in technical arms; whether their esprit de corps was as strong as that of the Paratroops, Commandos or Recce Corps; and whether the selection for the infantry, at Primary Training Centres, was as good as that for other arms. Indeed, as Col. Penton observed, the results of his investigation showed that the infantry required a better standard of man than the technical arms: the stress they meet with in battle is greater, the conditions are worse; the tasks that fall to their lot—night patrols and work in extended order—call for a higher standard of individual morale than is needed by those arms that always fight in compact groups, and no other soldier is called upon so frequently to endure prolonged and unrelieved stress under the worst physical conditions.

Similarly, in a report on the state of morale in the C.M.F., in September, 1944, the Adviser in Psychiatry (Lt.-Col. S. A. MacKeith) expressed the opinion that, in this theatre as elsewhere, of all the matters relating to morale the question of the status of the infantry was by far the most important. He stated that it already affected the morale of the Army in every theatre of operations, and that, in the future, this influence was likely to increase progressively. The subject was also highly relevant to the question of desertion. Infantrymen felt that they were subjected to greater degrees of danger and discomfort than were soldiers in other arms. They were aware that their modern role demanded of them considerable intelligence and initiative, and a very high standard of training. Yet they found themselves regarded with 'semi-affectionate contempt' by civilians and others, they received the lowest pay in the Army—with no 'hard-lying money' or 'combat pay'—and they were provided with no badge or flash indicative of their combatant role and their efficiency therein. Col. MacKeith observed that it was difficult to imagine a situation more destructive to morale.

An interesting corollary, in the post-war period, to the foregoing information is provided by an opinion-survey carried out among other ranks in A.L.F.S.E.A. in April, 1946, in order to obtain facts likely to be of use in reinforcing Army morale, and to throw light on some shortcomings in welfare, information, education, and other facilities. Especially noteworthy was the marked tendency, revealed by this survey, of the infantry, as compared with other arms of the Service, to depreciate themselves and their chances in civil life. As stated in this report, the work of the infantryman in war had, fortunately, little similarity to his civilian occupation, while a man in a technical arm might often be doing work more closely akin to his peace-time job; but the boredom and monotony of the repetitive training, together with the comparative suppression of initiative, must, no doubt, also colour the infantryman's outlook; and the poorer pay and lower general estimation from which he still suffered were an additional cause of his appreciably lower morale.*

The practical importance and interdependence of the various factors which have been mentioned above, in relation to the state of morale in a force overseas, are well illustrated by the following statement by Lt.-Col. S. A MacKeith, based on his experience with the C.M.F.: "If it were not for the 'immunizing effect' in the psychiatric field of this well-braced morale structure, half the expeditionary force would become psychiatric casualties, or desert, however harsh

> * " Yes, makin' mock o' uniforms that guard you while you sleep
> Is cheaper than them uniforms, an' they're starvation cheap;
> An' hustlin' drunken soldiers when they're goin' large a bit
> Is five times better business than paradin' in full kit. . .
> For it's Tommy this, an' Tommy that, an'
> 'Chuck him out, the brute!'
> But it's 'Saviour of 'is country' when the
> guns begin to shoot;
> An' it's Tommy this, an' Tommy that, an'
> anything you please;
> An' Tommy ain't a bloomin' fool—you bet
> that Tommy sees!"
> RUDYARD KIPLING, *Barrack-Room Ballads*

the disciplinary regime might be; and the psychiatrist's job would be impossible.... Different front-line battalions, made up, apparently, of similar human material, and fighting under similar conditions, produced startling differences in their numbers of psychiatric breakdowns, and parallel differences in the frequency among their soldiers of petty disciplinary troubles—and of venereal disease. In almost every case of a contrast of this sort between two similar units we found, not a striking difference in the standard of physical fitness between the two lots of men, and not an obviously higher average degree of psychiatric instability among the men in the more troublesome unit, but some, or all, of the following—poor leadership, poor team-spirit, and poor training in the past, with consequently a much less strong feeling of professional soldierly competence. To these were sometimes added a protracted experience of the passive role in warfare, or perhaps the recent memory of a sudden military disaster involving a large element of surprise. As in the pathology, so in the prophylaxis of breakdown in all its forms, the positive factors of morale were of predominant importance. The negative use of discipline in the narrow sense could exert only a limited, and very short-term, effect. When, in rare instances, individual officers tried to inculcate hate and blood-lust into their men, the attempts recoiled upon them,* and the last state of morale was worse than the first." [71]

An interesting example of some of the factors influencing the morale of combatant troops overseas, under exceptionally difficult and unfamiliar conditions, is provided by a comparison between two consecutive campaigns on the India-Burma front, in 1942–3 and 1943–4, respectively.

Referring to the first Arakan Campaign, Lt.-Col. A. A. White, who was then Command Psychiatrist to Eastern Command, India, stated that no purpose would be served by counting psychiatric cases on this occasion; in particular, the whole of 14th Indian Division was for practical purposes a psychiatric casualty. The survivors of the Wingate Expedition of 1943—who were interviewed in June, 1943, when returning to India through Kohima—came out as bands of disorganized stragglers, each man attributing his survival entirely to his own efforts plus an element of luck: as Col. White has graphically

* As stated by the Moderator of the Church of Scotland, "... if it is persisted in, it will end in the perversion of human nature and will have results which its authors little dream of" (*Glasgow Herald*, 5 May, 1942).

PROBLEMS OF TRAINING AND MORALE

observed, in their eyes the hand of authority, normally expected to guide and support them, seemed to have lost its grip. In such circumstances, the level of unit morale was at zero. Individually, many of the men were good soldiers but their attitude to authority at the time of coming out was one of hostility. Some of the causes of low morale in the force were: inadequate selection of the original force, and lack of training in this specific type of warfare (map reading, river-crossings, etc.)—as shown, for example, by instances of men balking at river crossings, and of others panicking and bolting into the jungle at the threat of ambush; lack of a sense of purpose, when it became apparent that the force was not to be the spear-head—as had been widely believed—of a general advance by 4th Corps into Burma; irregular supplies of food and clothing, and, consequently, poor conditions of health and hygiene; defective leadership, and lack of information given to the men as to their approximate location, etc.; and the absence of any means of evacuating the seriously ill and wounded, who were left in the care of villagers—this was an important factor not only in lowering morale, but also in arousing a certain amount of hostility towards the expedition on the part of those men who were still fit.

The basic difference between the first and second campaigns, as noted by Col. White in July, 1944, was in the degree of organization shown by the forces concerned, at the end of the respective campaigns, at the time of their arrival in India from Burma. In the second Arakan Campaign, the men arrived as part of a prearranged evacuation and in an orderly fashion, while operations were actually in progress, with the result that they retained confidence in the ability of their leaders to maintain control of the situation and to look after their interests. With better training, the men looked on the jungle with less fear; the better enforcement of anti-malarial precautions and improved hygiene considerably reduced the incidence of illness;* more publicity was given to the fighting in this theatre; and, with

---

* It was held by the late General Wingate that, if a man was sufficiently 'tough' physically as well as morally, he was immune to all disease. The disastrous losses in effective man-power, through illness alone (particularly malaria and dysentery), which resulted from this attitude, and the officers' consequent failure to enforce adequate prophylactic measures, all but wrecked completely the first campaign. Subsequently, it was possible for the Army medical authorities to bring sufficient pressure to bear, and the physical health of the troops in Burma promptly showed a very great improvement, which was not without its effect on their morale. The General's theory was finally disproved, when he himself became ill with typhoid. It will thus be seen that medical branches of the Army other than the psychiatric services also had their difficulties.

the increasing Allied military successes on other fronts, there was a change of attitude in the Indian civilian.

The foregoing observations on the contrasting state of morale in these two campaigns under similar conditions of jungle warfare, provide an adequate illustration of the truth of the statement by Lt.-Col. F. Spencer Chapman: "It is the attitude of mind that determines whether you go under or survive.... The jungle itself is neutral." 29

Psychiatric reports on certain isolated areas overseas—in particular, Gibraltar, and East and West Africa—during the war, provided evidence of widespread mental instability and an exceedingly low state of morale among officers and men who were stationed there for relatively long periods.*

One of the most important predisposing causes, in this respect, was the lack of any selection procedure in the early years of the war, with the inevitable result that a high percentage of men who were sent to such areas were basically unstable and inadequate, and many of them had a long history of social maladjustment or mental disorder. In addition to this, however, there was also a 'negative selection', in so far as a number of men who had been considered unsatisfactory or ineffective in their units at home, were posted to these localities. It is not surprising that the influence of these 'misfits' on the morale of their new units was deleterious, and particularly so, in view of the trying conditions and mental stress under which the men stationed in such areas were required to live and work; and that their presence and inefficiency placed an additional strain on even the most stable of their comrades.

Precipitating and aggravating factors were also not wanting: unfavourable climate, primitive and monotonous living conditions, an

* Only after much effort and persistence on the part of the Directorate of Army Psychiatry, was it possible to obtain official agreement to the appointment of one psychiatrist to each of these areas: Command Psychiatrists were appointed to Gibraltar (Major G. de M. Rudolf) and East Africa Command (Major P. B. De Maré) at the beginning of 1943, and to West Africa Command (Lt.-Col. D. L. Mackenzie) at the end of the same year. In spite of considerable physical contrasts, these several areas provided strikingly similar problems from the points of view of psychiatry and morale: Gibraltar ('the Rock'), which accommodated a large number of personnel from the three Services, is an area about 3 miles in length and ¾ mile wide. East Africa Command included British Somaliland, Kenya, the Uganda Protectorate, and Tanganyika Territory, with a total area of over 741,000 square miles. West Africa Command comprised the Gambia, the Gold Coast, Sierra Leone, and Nigeria, with a total area of over 498,000 square miles. (Yet, East and West Africa Commands had only *one* Army psychiatrist each! It is, of course, true that troops were to *some* extent localized—but distances had to be covered.)

almost complete lack of any welfare or recreational facilities, the absence or scarcity of women, infrequent and irregular home leave, long separation from home without news, infrequent mail, domestic problems, and physical illness (in tropical areas) or the fear of it. Thus, it was inevitable that there should develop, among the men in these isolated areas, a widespread and increasing feeling that they had been forgotten, that they were unwanted elsewhere and had therefore been exiled, relegated indefinitely to remote and undesirable parts of the world (and, in Gibraltar, 'shut in')—a conviction that was reinforced by lack of active work, and of participation (even in a combatant capacity) in the war, and intense and unrelieved boredom.

The considerable strain to which these men were subjected was shown, not so much by overt mental disorders, as by such prevalent symptoms as insomnia, irritability, apathy, depression, inability to concentrate and impairment of memory, mild paranoid reactions, and alcoholism: in fact, their psychiatric condition was in many respects similar to the 'prisoner-of-war mentality'.*

A Special Research Section (No. 1 Biological Research Section, R.A.M.C.) was formed by the Director of Biological Research in the early part of 1944, and was first sent to the C.M.F.; as the war proceeded, it became clear that the greatest need for such a unit was in South-East Asia, and the Research Section was accordingly sent to A.L.F.S.E.A. in 1945. Both in the C.M.F. and in A.L.F.S.E.A., this unit, working under the direction of the Adviser in Psychiatry to the Force concerned, carried out opinion-surveys and other investigations amongst the troops, and much important information was

* The following data are available, concerning the incidence of overt psychiatric illness in these areas:
Gibraltar: in 1942, more than half of the Service medical out-patients were suffering from minor functional disorders or neuroses. In 1943, the number of psychiatric out-patients was greater than that of all other medical out-patients. The majority of psychoses were depressive.
E. Africa: In 1944, of the neurotic cases attending out-patient clinics, one-sixth had to be evacuated (invalided), and one-sixth were placed in a lower medical category. In Somaliland, the suicidal rate was disturbingly high (at least 10 cases in 4 years).
W. Africa: In 1940–2, psychiatric cases (excluding the large number of psychosomatic cases) were the third most frequent group (15%) requiring to be evacuated and invalided—(the first two groups being malaria and respiratory diseases, respectively). In 1943, psychiatric disorders were the second most important cause (19%) of evacuation (after chronic malaria); and in 1944, they were the first most important cause (18%) of evacuation (and malaria, the second)—this reversal was not due to any increase in psychiatric cases, but to the reduction of the incidence of chronic malaria.[130] 25% of psychiatric cases were on, at least, their second tour of duty (of 18 months). Conditions were aggravated, in all these areas, by considerable delay in evacuation of medical cases to the U.K.

PROBLEMS OF TRAINING AND MORALE

thus obtained on various matters relating to morale—e.g. the soldier's attitude to Army life; leave; recreational facilities; sexual promiscuity and V.D.; prophylaxis against diseases; etc.

The attitudes of the men serving in South-East Asia, which both contributed to, and reflected, their low morale after the cessation of hostilities, when there was no longer the incentive of 'war aims' and the 'stimulus of battle', are clearly shown by the results of an opinion-survey undertaken by the Research Section in 1946, at the suggestion of the Adviser in Psychiatry, A.L.F.S.E.A.*

It was thus demonstrated beyond doubt that many soldiers in A.L.F.S.E.A. felt, with more or less justification, that they were required to waste their time, while losing their skills and abilities— as it were, through 'disuse atrophy'—with 'red tape' and 'bullshit'. The latter term (of most current usage in the Army), as so admirably interpreted by the authors of the survey, "may be defined pedantically as 'excessive insistence, in military administration, on the specious and showy, rather than on things really contributing to military efficiency'". Opinions might differ as to whether an order was 'bullshit' or conducive to essential smartness, 'red tape' or a necessary formality; and although these were matters upon which other ranks were in many cases not the best qualified to pass judgement, their attitude could not therefore be entirely ignored, nor indeed should it be underestimated. "Useless 'messing around' is antipathetic to the spirit of contemporary men, so largely dependent on job-efficiency. Here the situation ... arises out of the essentially unstable and improvised nature of military life and organization, at any rate in a theatre of active operations; it is this which gives the Army, in the mind of the other rank, its character of being all feet, no head, and vaguely malignant, like one of the more incoherent tropical insects magnified ten million times. Everything is fluid; rapidly changing situations lead to rapidly changing orders; armies move, units move from command to command, from shanties to canvas and back again, take men on strength, strike men off strength, and disband; in consequence, drafts of men roam about the country like droves of armed sheep, but more articulate—the Transit Camp, that slaughterhouse of hope, looming menacingly before them. All this fluidity gives an impression of administrative inefficiency, so different

* The report, by E. W. Browne, W. B. Coates, and A. F. Wells, was entitled, 'The Soldier and the Army—Opinions on Some Aspects of Army Life, expressed by Troops in S.E.A.C.'

from the stable, peaceful and well-oiled bureaucracy of Great Britain. This cannot be helped; but some minor, though not unimportant, remedies may be suggested. In particular, some further effort might be made to explain to men the purpose of orders and regulations: such purpose is by no means always apparent. . . . Such a procedure would . . . have a marked effect on morale."

The conclusions reached by the authors of this opinion-survey are, it is felt, so highly relevant to a true understanding of the state of morale, not only of the men serving in A.L.F.S.E.A. during the postwar period, but also of those subsequently stationed in many theatres overseas, that it is important here to quote them: "In the future it will have to be constantly borne in mind that the outlook of the conscript—present in body but so often absent in spirit—is totally different from that of the professional soldier, and that in consequence discipline and morale, in conditions of peace-time conscription, will be more difficult to maintain than they were, not only during, but before the recent war. This need not be so; the opportunities it provides of seeing the world and of meeting men could give the Army a unique place in the training of good citizens. The danger would be avoided by making the Army a sphere in which a youth may be formed, not only into a well-equipped soldier, but into a well-equipped man. This must be done positively, by increasing the place of education, both general and vocational, and the volume and quality of information about contemporary events with which he is provided. This would offset to a considerable degree his missed opportunities of training at university, evening-school or job. But it must also be done negatively, by reducing those feelings of frustration and discontent which the Army's present air of all-pervading witlessness so often inspires in the other rank. To be physically hardened is very different from being mentally stunted, but there is reason to think that, in practice, this distinction is overlooked. If it were not, to the ordinary soldier, his Army service would seem much less of a Rip Van Winkle's nightmare and more of a period of his life to be lived and enjoyed."

Investigations were undertaken to ascertain the principal causes of the high incidence of venereal disease among troops serving in various areas overseas. It was found that, where selection had been poor, a large proportion of the men who contracted V.D. were of low intelligence, or mentally unstable or immature. It also became obvious that the lowering of morale, in particular due to prolonged service overseas and separation from home, showed itself in the increase of the V.D. rate.[24, 93, 137, 138]

Thus, in the course of 1947, the greatest problem among troops of the B.A.O.R. arose from the increasing number of very young, frequently immature and inexperienced, national servicemen who were posted for service in Germany:* one of the matters of concern to the military and civil authorities, in this connection, was the high incidence of V.D. amongst these soldiers, and Army psychiatrists once more stressed the important relationship which low morale and immaturity had been found to bear to the incidence of sexual promiscuity and V.D. When, however, there was subsequently a very great improvement in the provision of facilities for education, training, recreation and welfare, in the B.A.O.R., together with better selection and the exclusion of dullards, and the gradual amelioration and stabilization of the socio-economic condition of the German civilian population in the British Zone, this was very soon reflected in the general state of morale and, incidentally, in the decreasing incidence of V.D., delinquency and psychiatric breakdown among the occupation force.

It is also significant that, as a result of the general lowering of morale in S.E.A.C. among troops with long overseas service, the V.D. rate showed a marked increase in men who had been in India for some three years, as compared with those who had only been in that theatre for a relatively short period.[93]

Another problem of morale which was investigated by Army psychiatrists, was a rumour which arose and caused a minor panic amongst members of the A.T.S. at Training Schools, who feared that work in connection with radar would cause sterility. This incident recalls the widespread fear among British troops overseas, that the anti-malarial drug, mepacrine, would cause impotence and sterility. These are interesting instances of the unexpected repercussions which may occur, as a result of deep-seated psychosexual anxiety and conflict in individuals who suddenly, or for long periods, find themselves segregated in unisexual communities.[97]

---

* Indeed, the young serviceman, both during and after the war, was in many cases, at least emotionally, hardly more than a

". . . school-boy, with his satchel,
And shining morning face, creeping like snail
Unwillingly to school. . . .
Then a soldier,
Full of strange oaths, and bearded like the pard,
Jealous in honour, sudden and quick in quarrel. . . ."

SHAKESPEARE, *As You Like It*

PROBLEMS OF TRAINING AND MORALE

The causes of the low morale and poor mental health of men who accumulated at Depots and Transit Camps, were also investigated by Army psychiatrists. This type of unit, as an almost inevitable result of its function as a 'sorting stage' for many very different groups of men who were awaiting either postings or disposal, did not possess the permanence and stability necessary for the maintenance of good group morale. Men were nevertheless required at times to remain in such units for appreciable periods, even up to several months; and the high incidence of psychiatric disorders, and the 'depot deterioration', which occurred amongst them constituted a definite problem. Thus, during a four-week period in 1944, 28% of the total psychiatric out-patients in one district in the U.K. were referred from Depots. Suitable recommendations were made, with a view to improving, so far as possible, this state of affairs.

That this problem was of particular importance in the case of men serving in overseas theatres, or proceeding there as reinforcements, was confirmed by the observations of the Adviser in Psychiatry in the C.M.F., in 1944, which agreed substantially with the experience of Army psychiatrists in other theatres of operations. Col. MacKeith stated that, in general, the deterioration of the soldier's morale from any but the shortest of periods spent in a Transit Camp or Reinforcement Training Depot was considerable, or indeed disastrous. He recommended that a greater number, as well as a higher quality, of personnel be allotted to the permanent staff of such units. Corps Psychiatrists had repeatedly emphasized the deleterious effect of the mismanagement of reinforcements on individual and group morale, as shown by the incidence of psychiatric casualties and desertion in a given unit: a large number of psychiatric patients gave a history of a recent change of unit, either as a result of being sent on a draft from the U.K. or B.N.A.F. to C.M.F., or through having been ill or wounded.

It was noted that reinforcements of the 18–22 age-group who had not seen any action constituted a special problem. The officers and N.C.O.s of the unit receiving them needed to display considerable skill and care if these reinforcements were to be adequately assimilated by the unit; they also required time for the job. It was very wasteful to send 'green' reinforcements straight into the line in such a place as the Anzio Bridgehead, not knowing their fellow soldiers, their N.C.O.s or their officers, although in certain circumstances this might, of course, be quite unavoidable. Only when the reinforcement had become integrated in his new unit, had developed a natural loyalty to it, and had identified himself with it as a member and not an outsider, was he fully armoured against neurosis. The system of drafting reinforcements seemed to aggravate the difficulty: drafts often consisted of men drawn from many units—in one case, no less than sixteen; there appeared to be little attempt to make them into a coherent body, and there was at times no more than an N.C.O. in charge. Ideally, men should come out from the U.K. in compact groups with their own officers and N.C.O.s. This was probably impossible in practice, but at least the reinforcements should be moved up the line in accordance with a pre-arranged programme, and without unnecessary delays.

It is relevant here to refer briefly to two major 'lesions of group morale', the so-called 'Salerno mutiny' and 'Airborne mutiny', which occurred in the British Army, respectively during and following the recent war, in so far as they provide most significant evidence as to the aetiology of such potentially serious incidents.

The events which culminated in the 'Salerno mutiny' in September, 1943, and which were subsequently the subject of an important investigation by an Army psychiatrist (Lt.-Col. T. F. Main), were officially summarized as follows: "A party of reinforcements refused to join the units to which they had been ordered. It was impossible at the height of the battle, which was at a most critical stage, to send them to their own specific units or normal formations, and the men concerned refused to obey orders to join the other units where they were urgently needed." As a result of this incident, 192 British soldiers were tried by court-martial in October-November, 1943, and 191 were convicted and sentenced to from five to twelve years' penal servitude. "Except in two cases where the men were found to have had recent previous sentences of penal servitude, the sentences were suspended immediately or within a few weeks in all cases and the soldiers were despatched to 8th Army units as reinforcements."*

The significant data obtained by Col. Main as a result of his careful and detailed investigation were, as he emphasized in his report, built up and pieced together from information derived from individual interviews, which, however honestly given, was nevertheless subjective. The account so obtained was necessarily concerned, therefore, only with emotional events and points of view of the group involved, and did not argue the degree of rationality of attitudes nor

* *Parl. Deb.*, 5th ser., Commons, **410**: 61; 17 April, 1945.

attempt to pass judgement on them: it was merely a presentation of what was felt and thought by the men, and in this lies its full and considerable significance.*

The men comprising the draft which set out from Tripoli were from the start firmly convinced that it was formed to reinforce the divisions to which they had hitherto belonged: this view had been confirmed by the R.S.M. at the Transit Camp, and men eager to rejoin their divisions had seized this opportunity—including a few, not fit for full duty, who had found it easy in the general hurry to gain permission to join the draft. It may be said, therefore, that this draft consisted mainly of men willing and glad to face whatever the future might hold for them, in their own divisions—in the community to which they belonged, with their familiar officers and the comrades of their own unit. All were men who shared common experiences of past battles, similar immediate emotions, and a common prospect of rejoining in the field a division, brigade or battalion to which they felt bound by strong group loyalties.

However, through lack of precise information and for other reasons, by the time the men reached Salerno three features of importance had appeared: a growing doubt in extra-divisional authority, an anxious need for news and direction, and the discussion of illegal methods, should the need arise, of rejoining their own division. On arrival at Salerno, instructions were eventually given to the men, that the draft was to reinforce two other divisions. As recorded by Col. Main, the decision to refuse to join the drafts gained adherents among men of different calibre: the man of high divisional morale who hoped his action would be subsequently approved; the angry affronted patriot of high personal morale, who believed he was right whatever the consequences; the man whose sense of justice was outraged and who had been encouraged in this by the attitude and obvious sympathy of the draft officers and N.C.O.s, and by the number of his companions who were taking the same course; a few men whose anxiety about future battle in strange company led them to follow the firm lead given them; and a few useless men who preferred idleness to discipline and service in any formation. It should be noted that men in these latter two categories were few enough to have no directing influence on the others, and apparently, those of the highest divisional morale and a combative family spirit grouped

* The following summary is based on Col. Main's report on 'General Matters in the Salerno Mutiny' (1945).

themselves together in the decision to refuse all divisions but their own. They believed at that time that their actions were soldierly and they were content to wait, in the belief that a senior official would sooner or later support them.

The official mention of mutiny, at the formal parade which was held the same afternoon, at once alienated and alarmed the men. When the order was given, "Fall out on the road, pick up your kit and move to — divisional area", some men accepted the challenge angrily, and many, undecided and fearful, either obeyed or stood firm; when the order had been repeated attitudes hardened, and after the third order those men who remained were disarmed. There was still a belief that, now they had obtruded themselves forcibly on the notice of authority, the error of sending them 'on the wrong draft' would be fought and righted, but in general they were anxious or indignant that the charge, when it came, was so serious. As a result, the common defensive opinion arose that they had been tricked into a serious charge by a provocative and diffuse order. Many had hoped that they would get to their own divisions with a warning or a small award for disobedience. For a few, the formal parade had been the first opportunity they had had to make protest and they were astonished and frightened to find themselves suddenly under arrest as mutineers. Their disgrace was brought home to them when they were put in a P.O.W. 'cage' next to some Germans who jeered at them. The men were thus banded together in feeling, and behaved as well as possible in the hope of being vindicated at the court-martial. Men who missed the train at a station on the way from Bizerta to Constantine caught it up by lorry, determined to show they were not mutineers.

It is probable that the group morale of the men concerned was never higher than at the time of their trial at Constantine: they were now for the first time really united in a single group, by the same emotions and a common predicament. The trial seemed to them full and just, and they firmly believed that their actions at Salerno had been proper and in the tradition of their divisional teaching, and saw themselves—as they were rightly represented by the defence—as 'first-class fighting men' and old campaigners. The sentences were read out on a parade, and then immediately suspended, and it seemed to the men for a moment that the 'authorities' had, after all, supported them. These feelings, however, were short-lived, for the administrative officer who had announced the sentences, unwisely took the opportunity of delivering a speech on disgrace and cowardice, in which he emphasized that suspension did not mean full release but that the sentences could be reimposed for any minor act of indiscipline; the men were told that they would be sent to the 8th Army as a chance to retrieve their honour. This speech led to a widespread feeling of hopelessness and fear.

There can be little doubt that the subsequent desertions occurred very largely because of these reactions. The men were quickly marched to a ship at Philippeville and found that other soldiers on it would not speak to them: this badly damaged their self-esteem—authoritative disapproval was one thing, but contempt from the ordinary soldier was too much. They were shocked and dismayed, and began now to dislike the group in which they found themselves: its reputation was too unpleasant. Both personal and group morale were low, and in spite of mutual feelings of injustice and humiliation, the unity of the group had gone. In their gloom, some saw penal servitude as the only alternative to death in a strange and hostile unit, and few argued against such a deduction. These individual fears completed the disruption of the group spirit of the draft, and desertions began. Group disintegration and the destruction of personal dignity had thrown each man on his individual resources.

Reviewing this subjective evidence, Col. Main observed—it may be thought, with some degree of understatement—that one simple conclusion could be drawn: the plans for rehabilitation of the men after the first sentence had been suspended were not wholly successful; the opportunity to restore and stimulate morale was not taken, and this led to a rapid failure of discipline.

In fact, it may be said that the whole of this pitiful incident was a tragedy of errors. In the first place, the men were misled from the very beginning; secondly, there was a complete absence of clear direction, precise information, or firm leadership, throughout; thirdly, there was a total disregard (whether avoidable or not) of well-established group loyalties in experienced fighting men of previously high morale; and finally, when the trouble was well under way, the men were further demoralized—it would seem, almost beyond repair—by the humiliation and degradation which they suffered: it should not be forgotten that these experienced British soldiers, who together had been through previous battles and campaigns, were subjected to ridicule by German prisoners of war, and to the contempt of their comrades in arms. Incidentally, in this instance as on

PROBLEMS OF TRAINING AND MORALE

other occasions, the absence may be noted of any effective procedure to enable men to express collective grievances. The effect of these serious errors in man-management and leadership, was a gradual disintegration first of group morale, and then of individual morale. The consequences of ignoring certain basic principles essential to morale proved disastrous.

It remains only to add that the men who deserted had their sentences reimposed, and were for the most part brought to various civil prisons in the U.K. There was considerable uneasiness in these men's divisions as to their fate, and their officers held them to be good soldiers, and persisted in regarding their refusal to join other formations as evidence of good divisional spirit. The North-West European Campaign depleted these divisions of experienced soldiers, and requests were made by regimental officers that these men be released for fighting duties; and representations were made by the men's relatives, through the regimental officers, Members of Parliament and ministerial channels. In consequence, a few months after the commencement of the Campaign, the Adjutant-General was asked to investigate the matter, and decided that the men should be interviewed by a psychiatrist.

In April, 1944, General Montgomery—who was C.-in-C., 21 Army Group—informed the Adjutant-General of certain facts concerning the mutiny; and in particular, that reinforcements for British divisions on the Naples front had been urgently required by the 5th Army, who had therefore ordered up a number of men of the 8th Army from the Depots in Tripoli. Neither General Montgomery nor General Alexander had been consulted before this action was taken, and had they known what was intended they would both have refused. With the insight of the experienced commander, skilled in leadership, General Montgomery stated that the men's refusal to go into battle was of course quite inexcusable, and could not be condoned; but when soldiers got into trouble it was nearly always the fault of some officer who had failed in his duty.* The Adjutant-General similarly expressed the view that these men should never

---

* That the fault might lie with the officers and not with the men, in such failures of group morale, was already recognized in the seventeenth century: "A Regiment, or Company of Horse or Foot, that chargeth the Enemy, and retreats before they come to handy-strokes, shall answer it before a Councell of War; and if the fault be found in the Officers, they shall bee banished the Camp; if in the Souldiers, then everie tenth man shall bee punished at discretion, and the rest serve for Pioners and Scavengers, till a worthy exployt take off that Blot" (*Lawes and Ordinances of Warre, Established for the better Conduct of the Army by His Excellency the Earle of Essex*, London, 1642).

have been placed in the position which caused them to commit the offence. These authoritative opinions, and the B.L.A.'s urgent need for good reinforcements, led to the review of the men's sentences in September, 1944, and at long last, the majority were released to rejoin units of their original regiments; a few were discharged on medical grounds or transferred to the Pioneer Corps.

Although it was not the subject of a psychiatric investigation, the 'mutiny' of a Parachute battalion in Malaya, in May, 1946, may also be mentioned, as a further illustration of a serious and avoidable disturbance of group morale.

The battalion arrived at a tented camp in Malaya, from Java, some ten days before the incident occurred, and was shortly afterwards joined by a draft of 50 men straight from the U.K., and 70 men who had been away from the battalion for the previous six months due to illness. The bad conditions of the camp, together with such other factors destructive to morale as relative inactivity, lack of recreational and other facilities, and the petty enforcement of rigid discipline, rapidly caused widespread demoralization and discontent, and the men began to talk of the possibility of a 'strike'.*

On the day of the 'mutiny', 258 men congregated 'in a sullen mood'. The C.O. informed them that he could not entertain collective grievances, and that if they refused to return to duty they would be guilty of mutiny. The men twice refused to obey the C.O.'s orders to return to their companies, whereupon the divisional commander ordered another battalion to take them into custody. As a result of two courts of inquiry, the 258 men concerned were brought to trial, a process which lasted from mid-August to mid-September. Of the 258 men, only 3 were acquitted, and 12 more were subsequently released as their convictions were not confirmed. The remaining 243 men were sentenced to five or three years' penal servitude (later commuted to two years' imprisonment with hard labour), and to be discharged with ignominy.†

---

* The existence of these bad conditions was confirmed by the Secretary of State for War. On this occasion, one Member pointed out (correctly) that "conditions at the camp were so intolerable that the men, however much they might have wanted to conform to military discipline in regard to dress and bearing, found it impossible to do so" (*Parl. Deb.*, 5th ser., Commons, **427**: 34–42; 8 Oct., 1946). Cf. *ibid.*, 366–73; 10 Oct., 1946; and 780, 796–800; 15 Oct., 1946; **425**: 1058; 16 July, 1946; also, Lords, **143**: 967–72; 5 Nov., 1946.

† This news aroused considerable public protest, reflected in the press, and in Parliament where three public petitions were presented (signed by more than 45,000 people). All the convictions were subsequently quashed—because of 'irregularities'

PROBLEMS OF TRAINING AND MORALE

It is obvious that the low state of group morale which led to this unfortunate incident was a direct consequence of mismanagement, and of a failure on the part of the officers concerned to fulfil one of their most important and elementary duties—that of attending to the welfare of their men. Where the officers failed in this respect, the men were at a disadvantage, in that no satisfactory means were available whereby other ranks could put forward collective complaints, official provision having only been made for a complaint by an individual soldier.* Nevertheless, the position with regard to collective complaints, as opposed to actual 'mutiny', has been clearly stated as follows: "The combined complaint of several can never be permissible, but should not, if well founded, be treated as mutinous, where it is plain that the only object of those making the complaint is to procure redress of the matters by which they think themselves wronged." †

In March, 1947, it was officially stated that instructions had been issued, that 'welfare committees' should be set up in units: it was intended that such committees, on which other ranks would be fully represented, would provide the men with the necessary means of making 'collective complaints' or representations. ‡

It is not possible to mention here more than a few of the numerous other investigations and activities of military psychiatrists during the recent war, in connection with matters affecting the morale of the British Army.

At the request of the Director of Military Training, M.E.F., a psychiatrist (Lt.-Col. T. F. Main) was posted to the Middle East from October, 1942, to May, 1943, to advise on methods of improving morale in Base Depots and areas, and on related matters. In a report, in September, 1943, on the 'Psychological Problems of Troops Overseas', based on his investigations during this period, Col. Main discussed certain important factors destructive to the morale of men who had served overseas for a long time, and suggested possible ways of counteracting such adverse influences by the

---

in the trial, viz., "the evidence was neither elicited nor applied in such a way as to establish either the guilt of those who were really guilty or the innocence of all those who were really innocent" (*Parl. Deb.*, 5th ser., Commons, **427**: 797. Cf. *ibid.*, 366–7).

* Cf. *Army Act*, S. 43; *Army Act, 1955*, S. 181.

† *Manual of Military Law*, 7th ed., 1929, p. 462, n. 1. The Lewis Committee stated in their Report: "An attempt should be made to define the offence of mutiny. In the light of present-day conditions it is capable of too wide an interpretation." [104] Cf. also the views of the Select Committee on the Army Act.[105]

‡ Cf. *Parl. Deb.*, 5th ser., Commons, **435**: 1299–1324; 26 March, 1947.

PROBLEMS OF TRAINING AND MORALE

judicious use of films and radio. Many of his recommendations were subsequently implemented, and, on his return to the U.K., Col. Main was placed at the disposal of the B.B.C., to advise the Corporation on questions concerning broadcasts to troops overseas.

The Army Broadcasting Committee, of which the Director of Army Psychiatry was a member, worked in close liaison with the B.B.C., and dealt with the policy underlying broadcasts to the Army. As a result of experience and enquiries in the Middle East (including Col. Main's investigations), it was possible to devise specific programmes for broadcasting to troops overseas, intended to produce a 'corrective and tonic effect' on their morale, and mental attitudes and health.

Army psychiatrists soon became aware of the importance of films, both as a means of propaganda and of influencing morale, and, in certain circumstances, as a potential source of effects harmful to morale. Advice was, therefore, given by the Directorate of Army Psychiatry to the Directorate of Army Kinematography, on psychological aspects of film production. Thus, in July, 1942, it was pointed out that camera angles in military training films were of importance in their effect on the soldier's morale. "We, in some of our films, whether they were news reels or training films, were tending to show big guns pointing at the audience instead of encouraging the audience to visualize themselves behind the big guns; we showed tanks looming up like monsters in front of the camera, reminding one of the civilians and others who were crushed by tanks on the roads of France, tanks running over British soldiers instead of Germans." [97]

In September, 1942, it was pointed out that the emotional training of a recruit in military values might be helped by films. On advice given by psychiatrists to the Directors of Military Training and Army Kinematography, a film, *The New Lot*, was made. This film, intended for new recruits, "deliberately emphasized all their difficulties and grumbles, and gradually dissipated them. It showed the way in which the group spirit developed and the gradual mounting of morale amongst recruits, and managed to do this without any suspicion of propaganda".[97] It was suggested, at the same time, that a film intended for officer candidates would be useful, to illustrate the growth of an adequate officer-man relationship and the emotional rewards of the officer's duties. Such a film was eventually produced by a commercial firm, under the title, *The Way Ahead*: the broad themes had been outlined by a psychiatrist, and were faithfully followed by the scriptwriter, with a successful result.[97]

PROBLEMS OF TRAINING AND MORALE

The Director of Army Psychiatry also attended meetings of the Morale Committee which, under the Adjutant-General, considered matters connected with the morale of the Army. A few of the subjects which came under consideration by the Committee, and upon which psychiatric advice was sought, may be mentioned: the frequency and regularity of mails to soldiers serving overseas; the character of the news transmitted by press and radio to soldiers serving at home and overseas; the welfare problems affecting the relationship between the soldier and his family; and matters affecting morale, arising out of the relations between the British Army and the Allied and Dominion Armies.*

It became apparent, in the summer of 1942, that the morale of troops in A.A. formations was exceedingly low, and that this was responsible for a considerable wastage of personnel. This situation was largely due to the operational conditions at that time prevailing in most parts of the U.K. A further, contributory factor was the large number of troops in low medical categories present in A.A. groups. In addition, the environmental conditions and accommodation were probably less satisfactory in these formations than in other arms of the Service. The Command Psychiatrist, South-Eastern Command, discussed the entire problem with the Commander of No. 2 A.A. Group, and, as a result of his recommendations, 'No. 2 A.A. Group School' was opened at Storrington, Sussex, in July, 1942, for personnel of that formation whose contribution and effectiveness was felt to be inadequate because of poor morale. These troops were carefully sorted, from both the physical and the psychiatric point of view: appropriate recommendations were then made as to alternative employment, etc., and the men received a 'refresher course' in gunnery, after which they were returned to duty in accordance with the recommendations. This scheme provided a satisfactory solution to the problem, and the School, having fulfilled its function, closed in September, 1943.

In the course of a follow-up investigation of paratroop volunteers in various battalions, in 1944, with a view to improving methods of selection and thus reducing the wastage rate during training, Army psychiatrists were required to consider the problem of trained parachutists who refused to jump. The latter were, at that time, invariably

---

* Similarly, an Anglo-American Relations (Army) Committee was formed, to deal with some of the thorny problems, liable to influence morale, which from time to time arose in relations between British and American troops.

PROBLEMS OF TRAINING AND MORALE

court-martialled: these investigations, however, clearly indicated that such refusals were related to the low morale of the individual and the group concerned.

In their report, the psychiatrists stated that, in so far as all such cases had completed at least eight parachute descents, and few had been referred for psychiatric examination before court-martial, it was likely that the act of refusal was, in most instances, mainly a problem of morale. This was particularly evident from the considerable variation in the number of refusals occurring in the three battalions. The battalion with the lowest wastage rate also had the smallest number of refusals, and in general its morale seemed to be high: it was the policy of this battalion to sort out unsuitable personnel and get rid of them as quietly as possible, and thus the group was not disturbed. In another battalion, where it was believed that all men who refused to jump should be court-martialled and deprived of their 'wings', the refusal rate not only increased, but was accompanied by a good deal of disturbance in the battalion, and appreciable ill-feeling at the difference in treatment of members of the several units. While in one unit such a case might be discharged on medical grounds, in another he would be compelled either to jump, or to face a court-martial. It was found that refusals occurred mostly in those men who had been given the lower personality ratings in selection.

It was subsequently decided, at a time when an intensive training programme was being undertaken in view of important forthcoming airborne operations, that every parachutist who refused to jump should be interviewed by an Army psychiatrist who was himself a trained parachutist. The information derived from such examinations proved extremely valuable to those concerned with the maintenance of the military efficiency and morale of airborne units, and with the selection and training of parachutists.

In addition to their work on problems of morale in our own Forces, Army psychiatrists also investigated the psychological aspects of morale in enemy nations. In particular, Lt.-Col. H. V. Dicks carried out important research, based on extensive interviews of German prisoners captured at various stages of the war, on the psychological structure of the German Forces and of their morale. As a result of these and other investigations, Col. Dicks reached certain conclusions as to the social and psychological factors influencing the development of German, and Nazi, national characteristics, as well as individual personality traits.[41, 99] Consequently, he was able to give valuable advice on the question of psychological warfare, and to forecast some of the problems and reactions to be expected in various sections of the German population following defeat and during the period of occupation.* Lt.-Col. J. Kelnar similarly made a survey of the psychological and social effects of upbringing and education, in relation to Japanese morale.

* Col. Dicks became one of the Psychiatric Advisers to the Psychological Warfare Division, S.H.A.E.F.

IX

REHABILITATION AND CIVIL RESETTLEMENT OF REPATRIATED PRISONERS OF WAR

> ... 'Tis past, and all is victory.
> And, for our life in those long years, there were
> Doubtless some grievous days, and some were fair.
> Who but a god goes woundless all his way? ...
>   Oh, could I tell the sick toil of the day,
> The evil nights. . . .
> Our quarters close beneath the enemy's wall;
> And rain—and from the ground the river dew—
> Wet, always wet! Into our clothes it grew,
> Plague-like, and bred foul beasts in every hair.
>   AESCHYLUS, *Agamemnon*

FROM 1940 ONWARDS, those with specialized knowledge and personal experience (gained in the previous war) of the particular problems of repatriated prisoners of war, repeatedly drew attention to the situation which would arise with the return of over 100,000 such men from Germany at the end of hostilities, and urged that this question be given careful and sympathetic consideration by the appropriate authorities.

Experience in the First World War had already demonstrated that prisoners of war showed, after their release, evidence of psychological instability and maladjustment, and difficulties in resocialization and reintegration in the community.

On the other hand, in the early years of the Second World War, for emotional reasons related to the nature of the problems concerned, there were from all sides anxious denials of the need to offer help to the returned prisoner of war. As the war proceeded, however, the obvious difficulties of repatriated men and their families gradually led to a widespread realization of their need for assistance in resettlement. Within the Army itself, the attention of the authorities was drawn to the problem for entirely practical reasons. In 1942, a follow-up survey in the Army of a sample of repatriates confirmed the earlier impressions as to the reality and intensity of the difficulties experienced in rehabilitating and successfully employing these men, and it became evident that a comprehensive plan was necessary for dealing with all those prisoners of war who would eventually be released and return to this country.

As an increasingly large number of men returned to the United Kingdom, either after escaping, or as a result of repatriation on medical or other grounds, the high rate of sickness and of disciplinary offences among them began to cause considerable anxiety. In the course of 1943, the authorities became aware of the high invaliding rate among repatriated officers who had been back in the United Kingdom for some months, and the difficulties arising from the psychiatric breakdown of a number of these officers on return to duty. In the same year, various other problems, such as disciplinary incidents, arose in the course of retraining returned prisoners of war, including regular soldiers with previously excellent military records.[36, 133]

In an important article published in June, 1943, Captain G. F. Collie, who had been a prisoner of war from 1940 to 1942, described the special problems involved, and put forward suggestions for a scheme for the rehabilitation of the repatriate. He wrote: "It is to be hoped that it will be possible for the authorities to make their treatment of the returned prisoner of war a sympathetic one, and one which will show some understanding of the special requirements of those who have suffered long periods of enforced captivity. It is ... appreciated that the problem has difficulties and that the authorities have to consider many points of view. . . . Nevertheless, there is room for considerable improvement in the present attitude to the returned prisoner. It is essential that efficient arrangements are made for him on arrival in this country, and that he should be in a position to go to his home with the minimum of delay. . . . He should be free from financial worries. From the psychological aspect this is important.... Until quite recently the returned prisoner of war was sent to his home with an advance on his accumulated credits to the handsome sum of £2, and with no certainty as to when further finance would become available. The sympathetic treatment of prisoners on their return can, at best, only avoid any sense of bitterness: it cannot cure the prisoner of his malady as a result of his captivity.... It is suggested that there should be drawn up a comprehensive scheme for the psychological treatment of the prisoner." [31]

In particular, Captain Collie suggested that, after having been sent as soon as possible on three weeks' leave to his home, the returned prisoner should report to a special rest centre, where conditions were comfortable and congenial. On arrival at the centre, he would have a psychiatric examination: while in some cases it would be found that the man was completely fit, and could either be discharged or returned to duty, the majority would require treatment of some kind, which would be prescribed by a psychiatrist. "Most of the returned prisoners will be suffering from minor mental abnormality, and experience has shown that in dealing with such cases a psychiatrist can ... effect a complete and lasting cure.... It will be found that the time taken to effect a cure will vary greatly ..., and therefore no hard and fast rules should be laid down, but even in the most difficult cases, it is believed that three months will be found sufficient to complete the rehabilitation.... As an extension of the plan, it might be practicable in special cases to provide the necessary training for placement in industry. At the very least, it would be possible to provide authoritative and useful statements for the Ministry of Labour as to the condition of those about to be discharged, and as to types of work for which they would be suitable." While undergoing treatment at the rest centre, the men would be able to acquire knowledge of events which had happened during their captivity and of which they were ignorant—an important aspect of the problem.

In conclusion, Captain Collie stated: "The disabilities from which the returning prisoner of war suffers have been acquired in the service of his country, and it seems logical that the State should use its best endeavours to rehabilitate him for his successful return to civilian life, so that he may again become a useful member of the community. What has been suggested here is not intended to be anything but a tentative proposal. It is put forward in the hope that the necessity for having some such scheme may be appreciated in sufficient time to be put into practice on the return of the prisoners of war."[31]

REHABILITATION AND CIVIL RESETTLEMENT

In September, 1943, a meeting was held, under the chairmanship of the D.G.A.M.S. (Lt.-Gen. Sir Alexander Hood), to discuss the question of the rehabilitation of repatriated prisoners of war. Reference was made to an investigation which had been carried out on 90 British prisoners of war recently repatriated from Italy, from which it appeared that, three months after returning home, one-third of these men showed sufficient evidence of maladjustment and instability to warrant some action being taken. The Consulting Psychiatrist pointed out that there were no studies or statistical data on this problem, from the First World War, which were likely to provide guidance, and it was not possible to draw valid conclusions from this limited investigation which referred to R.A.M.C. personnel, the great majority of whom had been employed on their own job of nursing in their prison camps; it was possible that other soldiers who had not been employed on their own jobs might show even greater signs of abnormal reaction on returning home.

The Director-General stated that the question of the rehabilitation of repatriated prisoners of war had been brought to a head as a result of the recent publication of the article by Captain Collie, and that there was no doubt that the returned prisoner must be regarded as a 'Rip Van Winkle'. The Consulting Psychiatrist had proposed a scheme for rehabilitation which was similar to that put forward by Captain Collie, but differed in certain details. The preliminary investigation had shown that at first all symptoms of abnormality in these returned prisoners were masked by the initial elation consequent upon returning home, and that their real condition only became apparent when they were examined three months later. It had, therefore, been proposed, first, that the relatives of these men should have some instruction on the best way to look after and handle them on their immediate return; and, secondly, that when the initial period of four weeks' leave was over, these men be sent to special depots, for investigation and disposal. Their disposal would depend on whether they were repatriated during the war, in which case the majority would remain in the Service—(those who were medically unfit would be admitted to hospital or discharged to civil life)—or whether they were returned at the end of the war, when they would nearly all be demobilized and would require to be placed in civil employments.

The Director of Army Psychiatry stated that there was a considerable body of public opinion which considered that something along

REHABILITATION AND CIVIL RESETTLEMENT

these lines was required, and Major-General Sir Richard Howard-Vyse, representing the British Red Cross and Order of St. John, said that he was being very strongly pressed by the relatives of prisoners of war for the introduction of some scheme such as had been outlined. All those attending the meeting agreed that a scheme of rehabilitation was needed. There was some uncertainty as to which Government department should be responsible for the rehabilitation of prisoners returned at the end of the war, but, after discussion, it was generally agreed that the Army had a moral responsibility in this matter.

The Consulting Psychiatrist suggested that, after one month's leave, every prisoner repatriated at the end of the war could be asked to report to a centre near his home where his physical and mental condition would be investigated. Those who were fit, and had jobs to which they could go, would require no further assistance; in other cases, treatment would be provided if necessary, and those who were fit and had no jobs could go through a selection procedure, and then receive vocational training or be placed by the Ministry of Labour. The Consulting Psychiatrist pointed out that, in view of the temporary, initial masking of symptoms which had been observed it would only be possible to pick out what might be called the 'social problem' group, after a period of seven to ten days at a Selection Centre, one month after the man had first returned home. The Director-General said that the Army had a moral responsibility to see that these men were fit before they were returned to civil life, and that they should receive guidance in finding the most suitable employment.

As a result of this meeting, it was agreed that the Director of Army Psychiatry and Consulting Psychiatrist, together with the Director of Selection of Personnel, should draft a scheme for the rehabilitation of repatriated prisoners of war, for further consideration.

In October, 1943, the repatriation from Germany of some 1,200 protected personnel (principally of the R.A.M.C.) presented an opportunity for devising an experimental procedure for the rehabilitation and retraining of these men. It was hoped that this scheme of about four weeks' duration, which was carried out at No. 1 Depot, R.A.M.C., Crookham, Hants, would simultaneously provide information applicable to the larger problem which, it was anticipated, would arise from the return of the very considerable number of prisoners of war at the end of hostilities. A psychiatrist (Lt.-Col.

REHABILITATION AND CIVIL RESETTLEMENT

A. T. M. Wilson), who was attached to the Depot at this time and worked in conjunction with the medical officer, had the opportunity of studying some of the special problems which occurred.

It was found that, when the men returned from Christmas leave, sick parades became large, and while a small number required to be admitted to a psychiatric hospital because of severe neurosis, an appreciable proportion of the remainder complained of physical symptoms which were largely functional in origin. More important, however, was the evidence of difficulties in social readjustment. It was not easy to interpret the results of this investigation, because of the serious difficulties which arose in connection with such matters as pay, promotion, leave, and reallocation. Characteristically enough, these difficulties led to considerable tension between the repatriates and the authorities, and emphasized the necessity for those in the home community, whether military or civilian, to take into consideration the special problems of these men, and the fact that the emotional burden of readaptation fell, to a very great extent, on members of that community and not on the repatriates alone.[133]

In his report on the Crookham experimental rehabilitation scheme, in 1944, Col. Wilson noted in particular the following points of significance: a relatively large sick parade; minor psychological disturbances in at least 60% of the men; a poor prognosis of effective social readaptation in at least 20%; 'brittle' individual morale; widespread passive attitudes covering latent hostility; a widespread desire for discharge from the Service; uneasiness about possible future foreign service; and a relatively high absentee rate. From this experiment, he concluded that essential requirements of any rehabilitation scheme for repatriates would be a full medical examination, and special attention to welfare, questions of pay, re-education, future employment, reallocation in the Army, and a definite policy as to leave.

Col. Wilson commented that, in considering how much time and thought should be given to the problem of rehabilitating repatriated prisoners, weight should be given to the fact that public opinion was, for various reasons, peculiarly sensitive on this point and appeared to regard the handling of repatriates as a test case of the intentions and capacities of the authorities responsible for demobilization, and even reconstruction. For this reason, the post-war public attitude to the Army was directly involved, and it might be suggested that the problem concerning prisoners of war had an importance out of all

REHABILITATION AND CIVIL RESETTLEMENT

proportion to their actual numbers. In addition, there was reason to believe that the handling and fate of these repatriates was being anxiously watched by 180,000 men who still remained in Germany. Mishandling of this 'trial run' might, therefore, easily prejudice the solution of the larger problem by giving rise to reactions such as would eventually present almost insuperable difficulties.

Towards the end of 1943, the number of officer prisoners of war of all arms who returned to this country from Germany, on medical grounds or by escaping, began to rise very considerably, and a special Officer Reception Unit (at No. 21 W.O.S.B.) was set up to provide them with advice on military retraining and re-employment, and on other problems. An attempt was made by psychiatrists and psychologists to work out a practical technique for the rehabilitation of these officers for continued military service in a suitable form, to reach an opinion as to the proportion capable of such rehabilitation, and to follow up the results. From the results of this work, it was possible to formulate a number of principles which not only constituted a basis for the planning, by the Director of Selection of Personnel, of the military rehabilitation of officer prisoners of war in general, but also provided information of considerable importance concerning the readjustment of repatriates, whether officers or other ranks, in their relationship to the civil community.[133]

In November, 1943, the Director of Army Psychiatry suggested that repatriated prisoners of war who were retained in the Army should be subjected to personnel selection procedure at the earliest practicable opportunity after their return, and that this might conveniently be carried out at the Convalescent Depots, two or three of which could be set aside for the specific purpose of dealing with all repatriates. Area Psychiatrists would be available, to advise on the disposal of difficult cases. At a conference of C.O.s of Military Convalescent Depots, in the same month, the Director of Army Psychiatry outlined some of the particular problems presented by returning prisoners of war, and the psychological principles which should be observed in dealing with them. He pointed out that representations had been made by members of various organizations who were anxious to ensure that these men should receive proper attention, with a view to preventing the unfortunate results which followed the none too skilful handling of such cases in the First World War.

In January, 1944, an article by Major P. H. Newman, R.A.M.C., himself a repatriated prisoner of war, drew further attention to 'The

REHABILITATION AND CIVIL RESETTLEMENT

Prisoner-of-War Mentality', and the difficulties of readjustment after repatriation: "During this repatriation period, abnormal reactions are common; in fact, probably all prisoners of long standing will present symptoms to some degree. . . . Briefly, these symptoms are restlessness, irritability, disrespect for discipline and authority, irresponsibility, and even dishonesty. Other symptoms that occur are the fear of enclosed spaces, especially a fear of large crowds in confined spaces,* cynicism, embarrassment in society, rebellious views against any code which tends to restrict the repatriate's activities, and a tendency to quick and violent tempers. . . .

"This syndrome, when it exists, should pass off after six months to one year. . . . There are two types, however, which will give cause for anxiety: (i) the repatriate with exaggerated symptoms, (ii) the repatriate with persistence of symptoms. . . . The first type is associated with symptoms of severe restlessness, irritability, emotional outbursts, acute discontent, and possibly excessive alcoholism. The second type shows chronic apathy, loss of initiative, and loss of morale and of personal drive, resulting in the inevitable appearance of more serious neurotic symptoms. The returning prisoner of war is ill equipped for the difficult period of readjustment. He is temporarily without the sheet-anchor of his daily routine, he has laid aside his habits of recreational relaxation, and he has lost the art of working for his living. With these handicaps he must readjust himself to his return to normal life. Should domestic trouble and unemployment further burden him, he may succumb to his adversities and relinquish the struggle." Major Newman suggested that 'advice centres', and a rehabilitation centre with consultant psychologists and a trained staff, should be organized to assist repatriated prisoners of war.[85]

During the middle period of the war (1942–3) when prisoners who had escaped or been repatriated were returning in sufficient numbers to give rise to appreciable difficulties, Army psychiatrists, to whom the problem had been referred for general investigation by the military authorities concerned, conducted on a small scale several systematic follow-up enquiries which, in spite of their limitations, produced information of basic importance for all subsequent

---

* It is interesting to note that crowds, whether or not in confined spaces, may induce in the predisposed a reaction akin either to claustrophobia or to agoraphobia: one may be 'lost in a crowd' (through loss of individuality), or he may feel 'hemmed in' by a crowd that 'closes in on him'; the word 'swamped' is applicable to both cases—"The heterogeneous is swamped by the homogeneous" (G. Le Bon, *The Crowd*).

developments, both theoretical and practical, in connection with the rehabilitation of repatriates.

The conclusions reached by psychiatrists, at this early stage of their studies of the problem, have been summarized by Major A. Curle and Lt.-Col. E. L. Trist as follows: ". . . The standard psychiatric examination had, of course, established the fact that repatriated P.s O.W.—referred for examination in view of presenting symptoms of a psychological or psychosomatic kind, or in relation to disciplinary offences, or difficulties over retraining—were seldom to be regarded as suffering from neuroses in the accepted psychiatric sense; nor indeed were they individuals with personalities which specially predisposed them to neurotic or conduct disorders. Such a first result, however, was open to more than one interpretation. There was, for example, the possible inference that these post-repatriation states, however acute and difficult from the standpoint of morale and discipline, were nevertheless to be regarded from a psychiatric point of view as transitory and superficial disturbances. . . . This view was not uncommon among repatriates themselves; and their tendency to deny the seriousness of their difficulties was undoubtedly aggravated by the fear of being in any way regarded as psychiatric patients.

"The particular viewpoint which has been described, though superficially protecting men from the very real hostilities existing in their society towards those who suffered from psychological disabilities, did little either to relieve their suffering or to assist military authority in solving the awkward problems with which it was presented. Conclusive evidence against the accuracy of this viewpoint was yielded by the early follow-up studies. These showed that in a significantly high proportion of cases there were no signs of spontaneous and relatively rapid recovery with an automatic return of the personality to its previous level of adjustment and military effectiveness. Even when men had been back for 18 months or even longer, serious and persistent difficulties were reported in something like one-third of the men. Such findings pointed strongly to the need for special therapeutic measures. . . . This evidence . . . was strongly supported by the abundant testimony offered at this time by ex-P.s O.W. of World War I, many of whom gave accounts of distress and difficulties of an unusually pervasive kind which had over a period of many years influenced wide areas of their behaviour and disturbed personal relationships of the greatest importance to them. Wives and other members of the families of repatriated prisoners of World

REHABILITATION AND CIVIL RESETTLEMENT

War I also offered a wealth of material regarding the extent to which their husbands or brothers had often remained, for months or even years, apparently unaware either of their own unusual behaviour or of the distress they were causing to others." [37]

It may be mentioned that, of 90 repatriated men (protected personnel) examined initially at No. 1 Depot, R.A.M.C., at Crookham, in April, 1943, within four to five days of arrival in the U.K., not more than 12% showed evidence of psychological abnormality; it is, therefore, noteworthy that, on re-examination some three to four months later, more than 30% of this same group of men showed abnormal reactions. Analysis of the first 2,000 repatriates from Europe dealt with, from November, 1943, onwards, at Army Selection Centres showed that nearly 30% were referred to psychiatrists, and that some 8% were admitted to psychiatric hospitals. Of the total number of repatriates dealt with by 45 Division by the middle of 1945, some 20% were referred to psychiatrists either by the medical officer or by the Personnel Selection Officer.

It is of some interest that the prisoners of war in Japanese hands, subsequently released in the course of 1945, showed certain apparent differences in their psychological reactions, as compared with the repatriates from Europe. Some of the early reports on the mental state of prisoners of war released in S.E.A.C., commenting on this marked and unexpected contrast, were over-optimistic. It was reported, almost universally, that the mental health of these men was 'unbelievably good', that they were 'in excellent spirits' and had a very high group morale, and that they showed surprisingly little evidence of psychiatric instability. The principal reasons for this first impression were that the men were seen in the initial stage of excitement and euphoria, before the reaction set in, and that, in view of the tremendous contrast between the appalling conditions and suffering during their internment, and conditions on release, the reaction was much delayed as compared with repatriates from Europe. In fact, it has been recorded that the typical prisoner-of-war syndrome, in some of these men repatriated from S.E.A.C., did not manifest itself until some nine to twelve months after release from internment.

Nevertheless, the Army psychiatrists who examined the men released from Japanese camps and prisons gave a clear warning of probable psychological reactions and inevitable difficulties in the future, and drew attention to the presence of symptoms which gave definite support to this view. Thus, it was noted that the released

REHABILITATION AND CIVIL RESETTLEMENT

prisoners of war in S.E.A.C. showed such symptoms as 'elation, mild over-activity', 'overconfidence, and disregard for real danger', and much anxiety over their personal future, especially with regard to health and employment; significantly, "the thought of returning to the U.K. was not greeted with the enthusiasm one might expect".

Apart from the relatively low incidence of serious overt psychiatric illness (reported as varying from 0·5% to 2% in groups from different prisons constituting a total of some 7,000 men evacuated for medical reasons—including 36 psychotics), a number of cases showed 'psychological exaggeration' of their physical symptoms, and psychosomatic disorders would, in general, not have been separately diagnosed and recorded. Acute psychotic episodes were observed to occur when release was imminent, or after there had been a failure to effect anticipated evacuation. Among the first 1,000 repatriated prisoners of war and internees from Malaya and Singapore examined after release, some 60% 'showed some degree of anxiety' (marked in 5%), and there was evidence of 'underlying tension and anxiety'; about 50% showed minor degrees of apathy and depression (severe in 2%); and it was noted that there was considerable evidence of psychiatric difficulties in adjustment, in this group.*

As a result of experience gained from the Crookham experimental rehabilitation scheme, Col. Wilson forwarded to the War Office, in February, 1944, a general report on the 'Psychological Aspects of the Rehabilitation of Repatriated Prisoners of War', in which he made certain important recommendations. He pointed out that the successful rehabilitation of returned prisoners of war could only be achieved through an understanding of their special psychological problems, and required a unit with a certain kind of atmosphere and certain types of opportunity. A small experimental centre, with a specially selected staff, should be set up. Personnel to plan, organize and administer rehabilitation schemes should be selected by technical methods, and might with advantage include selected repatriates. It was important that careful consideration be given to the need for reassurance on questions of health, and for early assistance with personal, domestic and other problems. Immediate efforts, it was suggested, might be made through the Red Cross, to keep men who were still prisoners of war fully informed with regard to such matters as pay, welfare facilities, leave on repatriation, release and demobilization priorities, and the aims and methods of rehabilitation. Warning

* Cf. also the findings of D. A. Smith and M. F. A. Woodruff.[116]

REHABILITATION AND CIVIL RESETTLEMENT

of the high incidence of social problems in repatriates should be given to the social organizations concerned.

It was emphasized that the larger psychological and sociological aspects of resettlement should be more fully considered by the various Government departments concerned, and, before release or discharge, the soldier should be given more contact and, if possible, familiarity with the civil organizations which would take the place of the Army when he returned to civil life. Whatever the administrative position, military responsibility for such resettlement was held to be imperative on psychological grounds. It was suggested that the provision of military rehabilitation officers and of units with the function of preparing the repatriate for civil life and his resettlement there, not only might diminish that part of the embittered discontent of the demobilized soldier which arises from the loss of military group morale and leadership, but might, in addition, minimize the recurrence of an unfortunate public attitude towards the Army, which was not uncommon in time of peace.

In February, 1944, the War Office agreed to the introduction of a general scheme, similar to that outlined by Col. Wilson. The Ministries of Pensions and Labour also showed interest in the problem of returned prisoners of war, and, at an Inter-Departmental Meeting in the spring of 1944, the three Fighting Services accepted the responsibility for the rehabilitation and resettlement of their respective repatriates, whether the latter were returning to civil life or not.* At the same time, group discussions with repatriates proved of great value in planning, and later administering, a scheme for civil resettlement, as well as in relation to many other problems concerning prisoners of war; and an Advisory Panel on the Problems of the Repatriated was set up, in March, 1944, and held meetings in conjunction with representatives of the Directorate of Army Psychiatry.[36]

Rehabilitation and retraining of repatriated prisoners of war for further military service, as distinct from their civil resettlement, was undertaken by a large special organization: on being flown to England, the men passed through special reception camps administered by 45 Division, and then proceeded on leave. Men in Age-and-Service Groups not yet due for release, returned, after their repatriation leave, to 45 Division, where they were interviewed by selection teams.

* The continued concern and interest of the public, no less than the Government, in this respect, was shown by the questions and statements in Parliament from December, 1943, onwards. (Cf. *Parl. Deb.*, 5th ser., Commons, **395**: 1105; 9 Dec., 1943; **400**: 1484–5; 8 June, 1944; and *ibid.*, Lords, **132**: 1179; 26 July, 1944.)

REHABILITATION AND CIVIL RESETTLEMENT

For this work, 25 psychiatrists were attached to the Division, under the direction of Lt.-Col. R. F. Barbour, Adviser in Psychiatry to H.Q., 45 Division. Some 20% of prisoners of war repatriated from Germany were referred to Army psychiatrists working in the Division. All experience suggested that such military rehabilitation as was provided in 45 Division did little to remove the need of assistance in civil resettlement when the men subsequently left the Army.[37, 133]

The need for an experimental rehabilitation centre had been recognized as early as February, 1944, and the suggested functions of such a unit were the acquisition of experience, the planning of future developments, and the training of specialized staff for future work. For this purpose, therefore, a small 'pilot' Civil Resettlement Unit, known as No. 10 Special Reception and Training Unit, was set up in November, 1944, in a large hutted camp on the outskirts of Derby, and provided accommodation for 60 repatriates. These men were not volunteers, but they knew that at the end of the course they would be leaving the Army. Various handicaps to this experiment should be mentioned: it was not possible to submit the staff to selection procedure; the hutted camp bore a certain resemblance to a stalag, particularly in the wintry weather; there were no officer repatriates among the trainees; and the numbers of men on the two trial courses were only 24 and 30, respectively. The staff included a psychiatrist. There was a preliminary period of two months before the repatriates arrived at the unit. In this short period of time, the camp had to be equipped, the staff trained, and effective relationships established with the neighbouring civilian community and with the local military administration.

From this experiment it was possible to draw certain general conclusions, relevant to the planning of a policy in the immediate future, which were stated as follows: (*a*) All repatriates need assistance in reorientation for resettlement; but for psychological reasons any scheme for this purpose must be on a voluntary basis. (*b*) Civil liaison—the education and reorientation of families, next-of-kin, and employers—is an essential feature, as resettlement, both in families and communities, is a reciprocal process between two groups, military and civil. (*c*) In resettlement, diminution of the mistrust of authority, and restoration of a certain minimum of confidence in others and in oneself, are of fundamental importance. This can be achieved by the provision of a certain level of amenities, by manifest efforts to help, by tolerance and understanding; and by personal contact on matters of importance, between repatriates and members of the home community. (*d*) It appears probable that the length of such a resettlement course should, in most cases, preferably be between three and seven weeks—(on an average, five weeks). (*e*) The staff of resettlement units must be capable not only of understanding the problems of repatriates, but also of withstanding in themselves the emotional stresses arising in work where it is necessary to overcome suspicion or hostility. (*f*) The selection of staff, and the inclusion in the latter of a proportion of former repatriates, are of great importance. (*g*) Draft establishments, accommodation scales, and methods have been worked out for a standard unit with 250 trainees.* This is probably the maximum number for such units, having regard to the estimated 'saturation point' of essential local contacts, and other relevant factors. (*h*) Training of staff for units should be on the same scale as that of the experimental unit. It should include actual contact with civil bodies, with appropriate civilians, and with groups of repatriates leaving the Army, and should be under the guidance of officers with special experience of the psychological problems concerned. These needs could most easily be met through a period of 'apprenticeship' to a working unit. (*i*) In view of this last point, adequately trained new units can only be formed by a process of 'budding off', with a subsequent period of time allowed for the growth of civil contacts in a new locality.

The experimental pilot Civil Resettlement Unit proved sufficiently successful to justify the inauguration of a general civil resettlement scheme. The War Office decided, in March, 1945, to proceed, in planning the civil resettlement work, on the assumption that 20,000 eligible repatriates would volunteer under the scheme in the first six months after V.E.-Day, and that it might be necessary to provide a five weeks' course for as many as 5,000 men per month. For this purpose, twenty Civil Resettlement Units (C.R.U.s) would be required, which must, of necessity, be located within easy access of industrial areas, and be regionally planned in relation to the men's homes. The units would be controlled by the Director of Organization, advised by the Director of Army Psychiatry.

A Civil Resettlement Planning Headquarters was formed in April, 1945, and its staff included a psychiatrist (Lt.-Col. A. T. M. Wilson)

* In fact, it was proposed that a standard resettlement unit should take 16 officers and 240 other ranks.

REHABILITATION AND CIVIL RESETTLEMENT

and a psychologist (Lt.-Col. E. L. Trist). By the end of May, the first C.R.U. was functioning, and by October, the planning unit had become an executive headquarters. By January, 1946, twenty regional C.R.U.s had been established, each capable of taking some 250 repatriates for a period varying from a few days to three months, the average length of stay being about five weeks.*

The majority of repatriates from Europe had been dealt with by the time the ex-Japanese prisoners of war had reached this country, and thus there was a continuity in the activity of the C.R.U.s until this latter group had been successfully treated. The gradual closing down of C.R.U.s commenced in May, 1946, and the last Unit had closed by the end of June, 1947. It was, however, the expressed intention of the Army authorities to institute a permanent C.R.U. for the civil resettlement of regular soldiers leaving the Service. In all, a total of some 19,000 ex-European, and some 4,500 ex-Japanese, prisoners of war had attended C.R.U.s up to the end of March, 1947.

Attendance at C.R.U.s was entirely on a voluntary basis: men were free to enter them or not, and to leave at any time. All ex-prisoners of war were offered C.R.U. treatment. Among the repatriates from Europe, the initial volunteering rate was 83%, although subsequent cancellations averaged one-quarter of this number. That some 60% of ex-prisoners of war from Germany entered C.R.U.s was a sure index of the great popularity of the units with the soldiers, and of the need for them. Among repatriates from the Far East, the initial volunteering rate was 45%.

The purpose of the C.R.U. was to reintroduce the returned soldier to civil life, and consequently its atmosphere was largely civilian. Although the majority of men elected to wear their uniform, and although the majority of the officers on the staff were military, the usual discipline and routine of Army life were excluded from the units. Originally, repatriates invariably attended the C.R.U. while still in the Army (often, while on demobilization leave), but the scheme was subsequently extended to allow them to attend as civilians after the end of their terminal leave, and up to one year after repatriation.

The military officer staff of a C.R.U. consisted of a commanding officer, second-in-command, and adjutant, a medical officer (two in

* A pamphlet entitled 'Settling Down in Civvy Street', published in May, 1945, was distributed to all repatriated prisoners of war, and gave information on the nature and purpose of the C.R.U.s. A.C.I.s 1392/45 (December, 1945) and 396/46 (April, 1946) dealt with the subject of civil resettlement and C.R.U.s.

some cases), a vocational officer, a technical officer (R.E.M.E.) responsible for the workshops, and four 'syndicate officers' (comparable to company officers). Each syndicate comprised some 60 men, i.e. there were four sections of 15 from the successive weekly intakes of 60 to the whole C.R.U.; this 'staggered' intake ensured that each syndicate was evenly composed of repatriates at all stages of resettlement. It was not possible to provide a resident psychiatrist for more than a few C.R.U.s, so that in most units the psychiatrist was a part-time associate. The civil officer staff of the C.R.U. consisted of a Ministry of Labour Liaison Officer, and a 'Civil Liaison Officer' (a professional woman social worker).*

The aim of the C.R.U. was to enable men not only to learn about post-war civil life and receive the benefit of the specialist advice they required, but to live as members of a free society while they were in the unit, and to reintegrate themselves within the civilian community in general, and their home environment in particular. Opportunities were provided in the workshops for men to rediscover or practise skills which they might have feared they had lost, or to acquire and discover new skills. For those wishing to practise their former trade, but still lacking self-confidence, 'job rehearsals' were arranged at a local firm. Vocational guidance was given by the vocational officer and his selection team, with the aid of tests for aptitudes and abilities. The Ministry of Labour representative then gave assistance in placing the man in appropriate employment in a suitable locality.

In the not inconsiderable difficulties which were experienced by the men in domestic matters, assistance and advice were provided by the Civil Liaison Officer. Problems relating to pay and allowances, which were an important source of anxiety and worry to the men, were dealt with by R.A.P.C. staff.

The most important aspect of all, however, at the C.R.U., was the resocialization of the individual, pre-eminently by group discussions, aided where necessary by specialist psychotherapy. Careful examination by the medical officer was required, to exclude physical illness or treat such illness as might be present: the majority of complaints

* The civil resettlement scheme was the subject of a detailed and important study by A. Curle and E. L. Trist. Major Curle, an anthropologist, became Research Officer at the Civil Resettlement Headquarters; Col. Trist, who was Senior Psychologist at the Research and Training Centre, became Adviser in social psychology to the civil resettlement organization. Their paper on 'Transitional Communities and Social Reconnection' comprises two parts: a sociological survey of the problem of civil resettlement and how it was dealt with in C.R.U.s; and a follow-up investigation of the civil resettlement of returned prisoners of war.[36, 37]

were, however, those symptomatic of psychological maladjustment, and these were dealt with mainly by the medical officer, either in group discussions or by reassurance of the individual.

At one C.R.U. where there was a full-time psychiatrist, the proportion of men initially given psychiatric interviews was about 15% of other ranks, and about 25% of officers. Of the other ranks, two-thirds were referred through staff members (medical officer, vocational officer, social worker), and one-third came spontaneously. Officers came entirely on their own initiative. The proportion of other ranks attending spontaneously subsequently showed a gradual increase, and there were indications that a fair number of repatriates had insight into the psychological nature of their resettlement difficulties.[134]

In resettlement work it became obvious that, while there were many individual problems which could only be effectively dealt with in private interviews, there were others which, being common to a number of the repatriates, could with considerable advantage be discussed in small therapeutic groups of from six to ten men[133, 134]—a procedure which had already been found to be of value in the past, in the treatment and resocialization of psychiatric patients in civil and military hospitals.

"The pattern of the C.R.U. community proved an exceptionally rich field for the development of these discussion techniques. The many-sided activities of the programme and the frequent but yet discontinuous to and fro contact with civil life, whether through the weekends home, the factory visits, the entertainments, or the personal expeditions, stimulated the need to talk (since problems were continually being raised), while the syndicate and other groups, to which the repatriates belong, provided the occasion. In this way the 'activities' of individuals led spontaneously to a therapeutic discussion of their significance, and the process of 'acting out' or testing out of interests, plans and daydreams in relation to reality was linked to the process of evaluating and assimilating the significance of these activities—the process of 'working through', in the group discussions. Moreover, the raised insight and changed feeling resulting from this process of working through in the group led to further activity—but at a higher social level, e.g., group projects through which the repatriates attempted to express altruistic needs which were liberated in proportion as they minimized or resolved their own individual problems." [133]

REHABILITATION AND CIVIL RESETTLEMENT

An interesting illustration of the problem of internal and external discipline in a 'democratic' transitional community of this nature (as contrasted with the authoritarian military community), and its solution through such group discussions, has been given by Major M. Doyle:

"Some weeks after the first C.R.U. opened, a resident psychiatrist arrived to find an interesting problem. A group of about fifteen men had refused to co-operate in any communal activity and were using the C.R.U. as an easy-going hotel from which they could enjoy the neighbouring night-life. Two or three of this group were flagrantly antisocial and had already been in trouble with the civilian population and with the police. They all exhibited various psychosomatic disorders and reactive depressive features of moderate severity. The administrative staff had come to the end of their tether in their ability to deal with the situation, and expulsion from the unit was their only solution. It was obvious from the beginning that there was marked anxiety not only about this situation but also in relation to the psychiatrist. In consequence, the psychiatrist and his patients were first of all isolated in a consulting-room situated in a remote part of the building. And there was no doubt that by so doing the remainder of the community felt, firstly that they had rid themselves of a doubly dangerous group, and secondly that the delinquent group could thus be conveniently neutralized and later removed by the psychiatrist, via a hospital for psychoneurosis, or, if they were unwilling to accept treatment, by recommending termination of their stay in the C.R.U.

"For the C.R.U. to rid itself of its troubles in this way was most undesirable, for its essential function was to be tolerant of neurotic, antisocial, or destructive behaviour, and to provide a community setting in which the repatriate could act out his emotional difficulties. The first therapeutic duty of the psychiatrist was therefore towards the staff of the unit, and his first efforts had to be directed towards impressing the executive, both specialist and administrative, with the necessity to keep these disturbing elements within the C.R.U. and to tolerate their shortcomings. Previous efforts by the staff to deal with the situation had been unsuccessful, the manipulation of the neurotic 'attack' on the community being outside the scope of the ordinary individual, and needing the training and insight of a psychiatrist. This, therefore, pointed the way to the second main function of the psychiatrist, which was to tackle and, if possible, to canalize this neurotic force. This was undertaken both by individual interview and by group discussions. It can be well understood that these early group meetings, in which the psychiatrist had to face a tough body of repatriates thirsting to get even after five years of confinement in hostile hands, provided a considerable display of fireworks.

"The important topic thrown up in these discussions was the failure of the unit to provide discipline; without the discipline of authority there could be no punishment, and without punishment nobody knew where he was. Could they go on behaving in the way they were doing and, if they did, would not authority take action? Authority in the person of the psychiatrist assured them that, so far as the C.R.U. was concerned, no action would be taken; but the outside bodies, such as the War Office or the civil authorities, were less inclined to such tolerance, and their behaviour might so seriously reflect on the resettlement scheme as to bring it to a close. It was also brought to their notice that there were 385 other people in the C.R.U. who were affected by their behaviour and who would assert their authority in dealing with their antisocial acts, should these affect them adversely. They were made aware that they were up against not the authority of the executive but the wishes of the C.R.U. as a group. If necessary, a general meeting would be held and a vote taken on their conduct by all the members of the community. This approach proved immediately effective; after one memorable and stormy meeting in which this situation was made quite clear there was prolonged silence, and then, one by one, each member of the group gave an assurance that no further trouble would be experienced from his particular quarter.

"The effect was dramatic, and, needless to say, what was going on between the psychiatrist and the neurotic group was being closely watched by all the rest of the C.R.U. The outcome of this conflict was to decide the future pattern of 'government' within the C.R.U. Should the neurotic triumph, chaos would result with subsequent dissolution and destruction of the resettlement unit; if the neurotic was expelled, authoritarianism and intolerance would supplant the democratic atmosphere essential to the scheme. The recognition by the neurotic element of the effect they were producing on the rest of the community solved the immediate social problem. Their altered attitude and behaviour became reflected in the unit as a whole, which was now not only tolerant of the 'bad boys' but also took up a rather protective attitude, removing them from public places if drunk and likely to become a nuisance, and so shielding them and the unit as a whole from the outside world.

"Practically no further difficulty was experienced in disciplinary matters after this showdown; nor has one arisen later with similar intensity at any of the other C.R.U.s subsequently opened. The solution of this single 'psychiatric event' was important not only for the community but also for the growth of the whole scheme. So far as the psychiatrist was concerned, it brought him full community status, and his functional role became fully established; his services were sought as a valued aid to resettlement instead of being the last resort of a desperate authority. He emerged from his confinement into the general life of the community, taking a natural part in interviewing, discussion groups, or the highly important casual contacts that took place in the N.A.A.F.I., bar, grounds, or corridors, or at the dances. The staff conferences and informal discussions provided a rich channel of communication with the administration and other specialists.

"The increasing rate of the demand for psychiatric help is shown by the following figures: during the first month about 5% of the repatriates were seen, all referred through a medical or other officer; whereas in the third and fourth months some 60% were spontaneously seeking advice." [134]

From the very beginning of the civil resettlement scheme, the principle had necessarily been accepted by the authorities concerned, that the function of C.R.U.s was not to make or train soldiers but, on the contrary, to create good civilian citizens. It was, thus, almost inevitable that the decision of the Army to undertake responsibility for the rehabilitation of repatriates should lead to difficulties in fitting civil resettlement into a military framework.

In order to understand the serious difficulties which did, in fact, exist in the relations between the War Office and Civil Resettlement Headquarters, for some appreciable time after the formation of the latter in April, 1945, it is necessary to realize that by nature they were essentially sociological problems, derived from the organizational and administrative situation rather than from personalities.

The problem which had to be faced was that of the soldier's transition from the authoritarian military community, where his individual responsibility and initiative had been limited and he had necessarily become dependent (or, indeed, over-dependent) on authority for the

REHABILITATION AND CIVIL RESETTLEMENT

provision of his needs and the direction of his activities, to civil life in a democratic community, where he was expected suddenly to assume an appreciable degree of personal responsibility and initiative, and himself to become the figure of 'authority' who must direct and provide for himself and his family.

This situation was well described by Col. Wilson as follows: "The enthusiasm of the soldier for a return to the relative freedom of civil life carried with it, in a large proportion of men, an anxiety over the uncertainty and the suddenly increased responsibility of a strange new civilian world, and . . . some resistance to replacing the external authority of military life with the self-discipline necessary in the civilian. From the beginning it was, therefore, necessary to insist that Civil Resettlement Units would be transitional communities in which there was a gradual but maximum acceptance of responsibility and the maximum opportunity for the display of initiative, both by the permanent staff and by the men passing through to civil life. It will be appreciated that within a military framework there were inevitable difficulties in bringing about this changed emphasis in individual responsibility; and during its earlier life the Civil Resettlement organization found itself occasionally beset with what was commonly described as 'umpire trouble'. By this was meant that there was some difficulty in explaining to various parts of an organization as large as the Army that the purpose of Civil Resettlement Units was not to make soldiers but to make civilians, and that it was not possible to 'teach' anyone responsibility without 'giving' them real responsibility. The C.R.U.s were, so to speak, concerned in playing a curious game of civilian football on a military cricket pitch, and there were occasional misunderstandings as to the nature and rules of the game. The difficulties, however, diminished as soon as it became clear that the method of selecting and training staff and the programme laid down for repatriates did, in fact, adequately achieve its purpose of fostering a sense of responsibility." [133]

Some of the principal administrative difficulties which were encountered in relations with the War Office, in the course of 1945, may briefly be mentioned. The Civil Resettlement organization, although an essentially technical one (in much the same sense as the War Office Selection Boards were technical), was not primarily responsible to a technical directorate within the War Office. (In fact, a non-technical branch, under the Director of Organization, remained officially responsible for the C.R.U.s throughout their exist-

REHABILITATION AND CIVIL RESETTLEMENT

ence.) The right of Civil Resettlement Headquarters to be consulted with regard to changes of policy, and to administer instructions which had a bearing on policy, although it had been agreed to in principle at the outset, was not, in fact, conceded in practice. The fact that a voluntary attitude towards rehabilitation for civil life might be damaged by routine military administration, also did not receive recognition. Excellent liaison had been established by personal contact between civil resettlement staff and the civil ministries concerned, on the initiative of the latter; but, although it was an essential additional requirement, such liaison at departmental level did not exist in any effective form. The original agreement that all members of the staff should be carefully selected, and that the final decision as to their suitability for this special work should rest with the Commander, was not adhered to in practice, and thus it was necessary to retain on the staff certain unsuitable persons, who were not in sympathy with the basic principles of the scheme and impaired its efficiency.

By the beginning of 1946, the need had become apparent for more precise information as to the subsequent condition of ex-prisoners of war who had been released from the Service, in order to assess how far their condition had been modified by C.R.U. training. The Director of Selection of Personnel requested that a follow-up investigation be made, and accordingly a series of conferences, attended by many authorities, both military and civilian, in the fields of welfare, psychiatry and psychology, were held at the War Office to consider the general methods and lines of approach to be adopted. These and other discussions led, in March, 1946, to the initiation of various enquiries, including a 'pilot' survey, carried out by Major A. Curle, which comprised a fortnight of intensive field work and covered 37 cases—17 repatriated prisoners of war who had attended C.R.U.s, and 20 who had not. As a result of this preliminary survey, the specific methods for the subsequent investigation were worked out.

The field work for the main investigation was also undertaken, over a period of some six months, by Major Curle. In one particular area (Oxford), selected in accordance with carefully determined criteria, socially comparable samples of 50 repatriated prisoners of war who had attended C.R.U.s, and 100 others who had not done so, were intensively studied, both in relation to each other and in relation to a control group of 40 families in the same area, who represented the civilian norm at the socio-economic levels at which the repatriated groups were settling down some months after demobilization. Throughout this sociological survey the investigator remained in touch with the psychological staff at Civil Resettlement Headquarters, and frequent discussions of his material took place in the light of previous, more specifically psychiatric, studies of the same problem.[36, 37]

This investigation revealed that, of the men who had attended C.R.U.s, 26% showed evidence of 'unsettlement' (i.e. social maladjustment at home, at work, or in the community), whereas, of those who had not had C.R.U. training, 64% were unsettled. From data obtained through the application of criteria of social participation, it was possible to draw three conclusions: First, the level of adjustment of the C.R.U. sample was superior to that of the non-C.R.U. sample. Secondly, the level of adjustment of the C.R.U. sample was superior to that of the control group, in spite of the fact that persons reputed to be 'unsatisfactory' or 'difficult' had been excluded from the latter. Thirdly, the level of adjustment of the control group was between that of the C.R.U. and non-C.R.U. sample. This general superiority of the C.R.U. sample occurred in spite of the existence of individual cases in which treatment had been inefficacious, and in spite of the higher degree of current external stress to which the sample was found to be subjected.[37]

In their discussion of the significance of the findings of this investigation, Major Curle and Col. Trist stated: "The chief impression gained from this survey is this: unsettlement which is unspectacular —since it is far more widespread and much less easily identified— is in the long run a greater menace to the community than that which leads to broken marriages and crime. In the less obvious forms of unsettlement, not only is the man's own life, and particularly his family life, reduced to a far lower plane of efficiency and enjoyment, but the whole of the society to which he belongs will suffer by his withdrawal from active social participation. Such unsettled men are dead weights in society and, if their external situation deteriorates, through sickness, unemployment, or anti-social activity, they may become actual casualties to the community and liabilities to the state. This is all the more serious in view of the fact that unsettlement of this kind does not appear to be much reduced as time goes on, but rather to harden into a rigid and intractable mould. .... The man who had been to a C.R.U. had one advantage, which almost all freely admitted. He had learned, chiefly through group discussion, to understand the nature of the tensions which are almost bound to arise in resettlement and had some idea of how they might be dissipated. He appreciated the fact that unsettlement is not one-sided, and that even if he himself felt perfectly well integrated, the domestic balance achieved by his wife and children during his absence would inevitably be thrown out of gear by his return. . . .

"The significantly higher proportion of well-adjusted men in the sample who had attended a C.R.U. emphasizes the worth of the C.R.U. as a therapeutic community. The extent of social integration amongst those rated as 'settled' cannot be attributed entirely to C.R.U. experience of approximately one month's duration. It may be suggested that traumatic experience, where circumstances of personality and social setting are propitious, may lead to improved social participation. This suggestion is supported by the supra-norm social participation of 'settled' men in the non-C.R.U. group. The proportion of 'settled' men was, however, significantly higher in the C.R.U. group. The C.R.U. may, therefore, be regarded as an agency through which the potentially educative experiences of P.O.W. life may be released from tensions and anxieties which otherwise inhibit their assimilation and application in civil life." [37]

It should, perhaps, be mentioned in conclusion, that Army psychiatrists and others were well aware that similar psychological problems and difficulties in readjustment would occur, in some degree, in a large number of demobilized servicemen, and particularly in those who served for long periods overseas. Already in 1944, Major P. H. Newman, referring to the 'prisoner-of-war mentality', stated that "all men returning from overseas, and especially those who have been in isolated areas for long periods, will show these symptoms to a certain extent".[85] Some of the more common reactions were, on the part of such soldiers, restlessness and irritability, disillusionment, social anxiety and lack of self-confidence, and a mistrust of impersonal authority; and, on the part of the civilian population to which they returned, those arising from 'non-combatant guilt'. Thus, the psychiatrists were able to advise those who would have to deal with these problems in civil life, in social and welfare work, or in industry, and also in part to minimize the misunderstandings and difficulties which almost inevitably arose between civilians and ex-servicemen.[49, 75, 94, 133]

Lt.-Col. T. F. Main has well summarized the situation existing at the end of the war, as follows: "Prisoner repatriates have been studied intensively and there is agreement . . . that the basic problems they present are different *in no essential* from the problems presented by servicemen in general who have returned to home life after years in the Services. Civil Resettlement Units could not be created, however, for other than prisoners of war. Their numbers were too large, and in any case they do not arouse the same mixture of curiosity and compassion as was aroused by prisoner-repatriates. There is little public feeling now for the man leaving the Services. He may once have been treated by the public with propitiatory fêtes and rites, like a sacred sacrificial animal, but naturally, now the war is over, he is an anachronism, and any difficulties he may have in becoming a civilian he must handle as best he can, with few social agencies to help him. An estimate of the numbers who have not made a good adjustment must be a guess—a sample survey of non-prisoner repatriates suggests that a quarter are as unsettled as the most unsettled prisoners of war—certainly the majority will never come for medical diagnosis, and they must be regarded as a sociological as well as a medical problem, an incubus on the mental health of the nation. . . .

"Two warnings are relevant. Many of them have in the past come face to face with loneliness, death, destruction and horror. Their experiences will often have given them a conviction that they know more about life than civilians. The contrasting confidence of civilians often therefore irritates them, and leads them to feel that they can never be understood. The civilians are felt to be wrong and queer. On this account advice to a man to make an effort to pull himself together will meet with quiet hopeless contempt for his advisers. Secondly, sympathy shocks and hurts, for it sets them apart as 'different'. Almost universally they have compelling needs to feel integrated again with their own people, and in any case do not feel it is they who have changed. They need understanding and recognition of their distress on an adult basis, as a settlement problem. . . . We would be wise to recognize that our pre-war and wartime experiences do not wholly befit us to understand or treat them. Only a determination to grasp the emotional problems inherent in a change of community will enable us to bring therapeutic interest and understanding to this wide and important social problem." [75] *

* Cf. also the important American study by R. Hill, *Families under Stress*.[59]

X

CONCLUSION

UNWELCOMED AND REGARDED WITH SUSPICION, if not despised, psychiatrists—the Cinderellas of Medicine—entered the Army, where they had gradually to overcome prejudices, administrative resistance and executive inertia, while simultaneously caring for their patients and attempting to bring home the fundamental importance of preventive psychiatry in saving man-power and maintaining morale. Thus, they had to fight a battle on two fronts—against mental disease, and against opposition not only from certain military and civil authorities and a section of the public, but also from not a few members of the medical profession. Little by little, albeit reluctantly, the Army came to realize the importance of the preventive functions of military psychiatry, and that the treatment of actual mental illness was but one, somewhat negative, aspect of the whole field of modern psychological medicine and the allied disciplines.

The psychiatrist in the Army was at times not unlike a prophet or a missionary in a foreign, and perhaps rather hostile, country. Indeed, there come to mind in this connection some words attributed by Plato, in his *Apology*, to Socrates: "Someone will say: Yes, . . . but cannot you hold your tongue, and then you may go into a foreign city, and no one will interfere with you? Now I have great difficulty in making you understand my answer to this. . . . Yet I say what is true, although a thing of which it is hard for me to persuade you."

And if it be asked whether Army psychiatry, after the Second World War, has at least succeeded in maintaining the position which it reached, after great labours and after overcoming many obstacles,

CONCLUSION

some of which should never have been encountered, others inevitable, the answer is that the position has been safeguarded in part only. The urgency of the situation during the war compelled many, grudgingly or anxiously, to turn to Army psychiatry as a means of solving difficulties or obviating disasters. As it had been anticipated —and, through their psychological insight, no more clearly than by the psychiatrists themselves—when the urgency of the stress of active warfare, and of acute problems of morale and man-power, had subsided into the 'cold war' and the unsettled post-war period, the pendulum to some extent swung back, under the renewed momentum of an ambivalence which could once again receive more overt expression now the immediate danger had, it was felt, been overcome.

The lessons learnt in Army psychiatry during and following the First World War [124, 128] were largely ignored or forgotten, both in this country and in the United States.[78, 79, 121] It may be relevant, however, to summarize here very briefly the principal lessons learnt or rediscovered in the field of Army psychiatry during the Second World War.*

It is true of this country as of the United States, that "Many of the handicaps and obstacles which had to be overcome were the result of the lack of planning during peace-time and early in hostilities, along with the ignorance and prejudices of many people. Sometimes it seemed that we were trying to hew a foothold in solid granite and only by the dint of the tremendous effort of many people could we increase that hold by a fraction of an inch." [78]

It must, however, be fully admitted that psychiatrists themselves were not without some degree of responsibility for the unsatisfactory state of affairs which existed at the beginning of the recent war. In this connection, some general comments by two American psychiatrists appear to be largely applicable to both countries.

Brigadier General William C. Menninger has stated: "We, as psychiatrists, have talked about morale and prevention but . . . few had thought in concrete terms of which methods were applicable to the Army. We often failed in orienting our own medical officers, including psychiatrists, to the specific needs of the military, in which one must accept the group aim and needs as of paramount im-

---

* For an account of psychiatric experience in the U.S. Forces during the Second World War, some of the lessons learnt, and the post-war status and developments of military psychiatry, cf. F. J. Braceland,[22] J. M. Caldwell,[26, 27] A. Gregg,[53] W. C. Menninger,[78, 79] J. M. Murray,[83] A. A. Rosner and B. H. Balser,[111] H. M. Snyder,[118] and E. A. Strecker and K. E. Appel.[121]

CONCLUSION

portance instead of that of the individual. We felt acutely our lack of previous recruiting of capable men into the field of psychiatry. ... We were aware ... of the few undiplomatic or eccentric individual psychiatrists who unfortunately did much to slow the acceptance of our specialty. ... The most severe indictment that can be made must be laid at the feet of the psychiatric profession as a whole—we permitted the military to forget almost all the lessons that we learned in the last war." [78]

Captain F. J. Braceland, U.S.N.R., has also noted: "It is of course obvious that psychiatry in general was not prepared for the massive problem which the war was to present, but this indictment has to be qualified, for in the same fashion no one else was prepared, be they medical or non-medical. What is an indictment of psychiatry is, however, the fact that most psychiatrists entered the military services with insufficient knowledge of the normal reactions to the vicissitudes of everyday life and the slight deviations of young adults under stress, and thus they were unprepared for most of the situations which they were to encounter. The psychiatrists, as was expected, had no difficulty at all in diagnosing, understanding and treating the psychoses when they appeared, but the psychoses represented less than 10% of the hospital problem to say nothing of the overall psychiatric picture. ... The neuroses and psychopathies in general made up more than 90% of the problem which we encountered, yet the psychiatrists entering military service were in general poorly equipped to handle them. Allowing for the fact that there is a great difference in orientation between caring for the individual and looking out for the welfare of the group which is one of the corner-stones of military psychiatry, there were still additional deficiencies." [22]

It is not proposed here to refer to any possible lessons which might be drawn from experience in the Second World War for psychiatry in civil life in peace-time. Some of those which are of potential value to the community have been noted elsewhere.[79, 97] Other such lessons as might be salvaged from war-time experience could be applied only at the expense of individual liberty and initiative, in favour of expediency and of the increased efficiency and simplified sociological approach which are necessarily inherent in an authoritarian military community in time of grave national emergency. Nor does the author of this History possess the gift of prophecy—a deficiency for which he is truly grateful. All that can be said, then, is that certain lessons are apparent from our war-time psychiatric experience, which have

CONCLUSION

been proved beyond reasonable doubt to constitute a *sine qua non* for maximal military efficiency and utilization of man-power, the maintenance of morale—itself the only real basis of discipline, and the prophylaxis of psychiatric casualties, in the event of the general mobilization of the country's entire resources in total warfare.

1. *Personnel Selection.*—It is essential, and particularly so when it is necessary to mobilize the country's total resources of man-power, (*a*) that all men be subjected to a thorough medical (physical and psychological) examination before being accepted for military service, in order that the *degree* of their physical and mental fitness for such service may be determined (e.g. 'Pulheems assessment'); (*b*) that all those men who have been found fit for full or limited military duties should be subjected on enlistment to thorough scientific selection, on the basis of intellectual capacity, vocational aptitudes and experience, etc., in order that they may be allocated to duties in such a manner as to make the best possible use of the limited skilled man-power available, to ensure maximal efficiency and to avoid psychiatric breakdowns resulting from inappropriate allocation; (*c*) that facilities should exist at all times for the scientific reallocation of men who subsequently prove to have been wrongly allocated, of those who as a result of subsequent impairment of their physical or mental condition are rendered fit for limited military duties only, or in cases where the exigencies of the military situation require a widespread redistribution of man-power.

2. *Officer Selection.*—At a time when the number of officers required far exceeds the number who are normally available to the Army and the number of regular officers available on completion of their training, the introduction of scientific methods of selection of officer candidates renders possible the fullest and most economical utilization of the suitable officer material otherwise available. Experience has established beyond doubt that the scientific methods of selection, provided that they are efficiently organized and include a skilled psychiatric personality assessment as well as psychological and military tests, can at the least increase by one-third the number of suitable candidates discovered by the conventional, unscientific methods.

3. *Mental Dullness.*—Men of low mental capacity are of limited military value. Where, however, it is imperative to make the fullest possible use of available man-power, it is possible for the Army to employ *stable* dullards on simple labouring duties, provided that

CONCLUSION

they are organized into separate units (Pioneer Corps), according to their fitness to use arms in self-defence or, alternatively, for an unarmed unit only. Thus segregated, stable dullards maintain a high level of morale and do not constitute a disciplinary, medical and psychiatric problem as is in general the case when they are present as inadequate misfits in an ordinary military unit. Furthermore, their employment on simple labouring duties releases men of higher intelligence for more skilled duties. *Unstable* dullards, on the other hand, are not fit for any form of military service, and any attempt to employ them in the Army on the specious grounds that they should not be permitted to 'evade' military service inevitably results in the placing on the military medical and non-medical authorities of a burden out of all proportion to the numbers and practical value of these men.

4. *Treatment and Disposal of Psychiatric Cases.*—In general, experience tends to show that *military* psychiatric hospitals are best suited to deal with patients whom it is proposed to rehabilitate for further military service, at least in a limited capacity. The maintenance of a modified military organization and atmosphere not only is essential in order to bring about the greatest possible degree of military rehabilitation, but also greatly facilitates the continuity of treatment, rehabilitation, and the subsequent accurate assessment of the individual's capacity for military duties and his appropriate reallocation. Where it is apparent, on the other hand, that a patient is unfit for further military service, and requires either prolonged psychiatric treatment and hospitalization or rehabilitation for civil life, it would seem that these functions can be best fulfilled by *civil* psychiatric hospitals, which also have greater facilities with regard to staff, the more complex forms of therapy, and after-care. It appears that, in the Second World War, our efforts to rehabilitate for civil life psychoneurotics who were discharged from the Army, for some reason did not meet with that measure of success which might have been anticipated. The results of research and practical experience also emphasize the considerable importance of psychological factors in determining the course of the subsequent adjustment and vocational rehabilitation of the physically disabled: in many cases, a successful result can only be achieved by the fullest co-operation between surgeon, physician, and psychiatrist, in a combined psychosomatic approach.

5. *Forward Psychiatry.*—It has been established beyond doubt

CONCLUSION

that, however successful may be the prophylaxis of psychiatric breakdown, and however effective the promotion of positive mental health and morale, wherever fighting is in progress psychiatric casualties will occur, and that when the fighting is severe the number of these casualties becomes such as to constitute a military problem. (In the Second World War, psychiatric casualties constituted on an average some 10% of total battle casualties; depending on the type of battle, figures varied from 2% to 30%.) The military problem arising from this type of battle casualty resolves itself into: (*a*) Preventing psychiatric casualties from impeding (i) actual fighting operations, (ii) the evacuation and treatment of the wounded; (*b*) Selection and treatment of the proportion of men from the stream of psychiatric casualties who will be capable of early return to further effective fighting; (*c*) The prevention of deterioration in those unable to return early, or at all, to further fighting duty; (*d*) The factor of long-term conservation of man-power. With adequate triage at R.A.P. and M.D.S., and a properly constituted 'Exhaustion Centre' at C.C.S. level or its equivalent (e.g. one F.D.S. taken over for the purpose), it is possible to return the majority of cases to fighting within a week (in the recent war, figures varied from 70% to 56%, and only some 5% of these broke down again in the course of the same battle). The whole success of forward psychiatry depends on early treatment, the essentials of which are adequate sedation by the regimental medical officer immediately after the breakdown, and continuance of this sedation at the M.D.S. and Corps Exhaustion Centre. (The results were as good as those quoted only when treatment could be given first within a matter of hours.) Cases of poor prognosis alone should be evacuated to the base. It is essential that patients from psychiatric Rehabilitation Units should proceed direct to their future unit without an intermediate period of waiting in R.H.U.s, etc., if subsequent deterioration is to be avoided: it requires high morale to withstand boredom and inaction, and soldiers who have recently had a psychiatric breakdown are obviously not fit to withstand this kind of strain. It is essential that the whole progress from breakdown to final return to active, effective duty shall be continuous if the results of treatment are to be good. In the light of experience in the recent war, in appears certain that modern warfare imposes on the individual a strain so great that men involved in active fighting, however stable they may be, will break down in direct relation to the intensity and duration of their exposure. Thus, psychiatric casualties ('campaign

CONCLUSION

exhaustion') are as inevitable as gunshot and shrapnel wounds in modern warfare. American investigations in the recent war showed that, in the case of the infantryman who is exposed to the greatest danger and the greatest stress, the average point at which such breakdown occurred and the soldier became ineffective appears to have been in the region of 200 to 240 'aggregate combat days' (10 combat days being taken as equivalent to 17 calendar days). Experience shows that Corps and Divisional Psychiatrists are of proved value in the field, in an advisory and supervisory capacity, and the latter in particular serve an essential function in theatres of war where local conditions make it necessary for divisions to operate independently.

6. *Morale and Discipline.*—From the psychiatric point of view, essential factors in the maintenance of high individual and group morale are adequate selection and allocation (including the rejection or segregation of the immature, inadequate, unstable, and those of low mental capacity), thorough training, good leadership, and attention (particularly in overseas theatres) to such matters as good welfare facilities, regular mails, and the provision of frequent and adequate information. It has been clearly established that morale is the only real and permanent basis of discipline, and that there is a definite and direct relationship between low morale and a high incidence of military disciplinary and social problems such as absenteeism and desertion, sexual promiscuity and V.D. Experience suggests that the only satisfactory method of dealing with military delinquents, from the point of view of economy of man-power and money, is to subject them to a thorough scientific process of sorting principally based on a psychiatric personality assessment, in order that their further potential usefulness to the Army may be accurately determined. Men who, on the basis of personality and military record, are regarded as redeemable for further useful military service should be rehabilitated by the Army in suitable units or institutions, which must, however, be such as to foster in the men who are sent there high individual and group morale. Chronic offenders, men with long and serious criminal records in civil life, unstable and anti-social psychopathic types with severe personality disorders, are useless to the Army, exert an adverse effect on morale out of all proportion to their numbers, and involve the Service in a completely unjustifiable expenditure of money and man-power which it can ill afford. Such individuals, who are irredeemable for military service,

would better be dealt with, with respect to detention and rehabilitation for civil life, by the civil authorities (who, it is hoped, will gradually develop more progressive, constructive and scientific methods in their penal system). It is, in any case, essential that the Army should cease to be regarded by many as a suitable penal colony upon which may be unloaded such social misfits, on the specious grounds that the latter should not be permitted to 'evade' military service and that the Army can, or indeed has the time and resources to, 'make men of them'.

7. *Rehabilitation of Repatriated Prisoners of War.*—In view of the well-known psychological and social difficulties of repatriated prisoners of war, it is essential to provide special units with the specific function of aiding the psychological rehabilitation and civil resettlement of these men, if they are not subsequently to become a burden to the community. At the end of the recent war, such rehabilitation was successfully carried out by special 'transitional communities' (Civil Resettlement Units). Ex-servicemen who have been for prolonged periods in overseas theatres, frequently present similar problems in their readjustment to civil life and would benefit by similar provisions.

8. *Organization of Army Psychiatry at Home and Overseas.*—In order to co-ordinate the various important prophylactic and therapeutic activities of Army psychiatry in war-time, and to maintain necessary liaison with the several branches and departments of the War Office, it is essential that there be an independent central organization (Directorate of Army Psychiatry) as a part of the Army Medical Department. Equally important, from the psychiatric point of view, is the existence of a separate department in charge of personnel selection (Directorate of Selection of Personnel) as part of the Adjutant-General's branch of the War Office. In order to ensure effective measures of psychiatric prophylaxis and therapy in units and in the field, it is necessary to supply sufficient numbers of Command and Area Psychiatrists, Corps and Divisional Psychiatrists, and, in overseas theatres, Psychiatric Consultants and Advisers who must, however, in order that their work may be effective, be invested with sufficient rank and authority, and who must, together with the nucleus of a psychiatric organization, *accompany* any force which is being sent overseas.

In conclusion, it is well to bear in mind the words of the late Dr. Alan Gregg, who was Director, Division of Medical Services of

CONCLUSION

the Rockefeller Foundation: "... The lessons of the war are clear enough. They are so nearly trite that it will take special effort if they are not to be neglected, ignored, and forgotten. Many of the lessons are humiliating—a powerful reason for repressing them. Many call for unremitting work if the mistakes are not to be continued and repeated. Circumstances make a schizoid reaction all too easy for us—a flight from reality and the escape from responsibility. The greatest unpleasant surprise of the war for medical men was the importance of psychiatry and psychology. And yet so inconstant, evasive, or preoccupied are the majority of men that this greatest lesson can be disputed, evaded, and soon forgotten." [53]

APPENDIX A

PRACTICAL CONSIDERATIONS ON THE DISPOSAL OF DELINQUENTS IN THE ARMY

BY R. H. AHRENFELDT AND P. R. A. MAY*

DISCUSSION

1. *Selection and segregation of offenders*

ONE of the main defects of the present system is the inefficiency of the methods of selection and segregation of offenders, which, however well intentioned, can only be described as unscientific, antiquated and lamentably inadequate. This statement is in no way to be interpreted as a criticism of the individual commanding officer, who is faced with the impossible task of arriving at an accurate estimate of a man's potentiality for rehabilitation without any expert assistance, and who is liable to be unfairly criticized. The defect lies, not in the commanding officer, but in a system which normally leads him to make a decision without the benefit of advice by medical and non-medical experts who have made a special study of criminal behaviour, and who would enable him to arrive at a decision based on a scientific estimate of the man's personality and prognosis.

In practice, under the existing system, it is possible for a number of young psychopaths, and men of low intelligence or poor basic personality, who are irredeemable for military service, to be sent, even on two separate occasions, to a M.C.E., either because they have given a superficially favourable impression with regard to their military potentialities, or

* Excerpts from a Report submitted to the War Office in September, 1949. This material is published with the permission of the War Office. While indebted to several War Office Departments, viz., A.G.(P.M.)2, M.G.O.(F.), and F.1, for their friendly co-operation and invaluable assistance in providing the basic data for the financial and man-power study in this Report, the authors are to be held solely responsible for the presentation of the material, the accuracy of the statements, and the opinions and conclusions, contained therein. It should be stated that this Report refers, at least in matters of detail, to the situation at the above mentioned date, of which the authors had personal and first-hand knowledge both as military psychiatrists and as staff officers in the psychiatric section of the Army Medical Directorate.

APPENDIX A

because they have not yet committed a sufficient number of offences or incurred sufficiently long sentences of detention to ensure their segregation from essentially redeemable youths and their committal to a M.P. and D.B. with a view to their ultimate discharge from the Army. It is obvious that such men who are incapable of benefiting by methods designed to rehabilitate and train soldiers for further military service, can only exert a deleterious effect on the morale, and impair the chances of rehabilitation, of other soldiers at the M.C.E.

To attempt to redeem the irredeemable is a complete waste of the country's money and man-power, and to mix them with those who can be rehabilitated is, in addition, to jeopardize by their corrupting influence the latter's prospects of becoming useful soldiers. The essential practical point is that those who can be rehabilitated must be accurately picked out from those who cannot: this would be best done by a team that would consider fully all the aspects of the individual case. Of this team the psychiatrist must be an essential member because of his lengthy training in assessing and probing personality traits and potentialities, but the final decision would be the resultant of the contributions of all the members on the basis of their individual specialized knowledge.

Once the different types of offender had been segregated, they could be given the treatment appropriate to their potentialities. For those who were judged to be capable of becoming efficient soldiers, the emphasis would be on rehabilitation for military service in the true spirit implicit in the statement, "The proper amount of punishment to be inflicted is the least amount by which discipline can efficiently be maintained" (*Manual of Military Law*, 7th ed., 1929, Chap. V, § 78). In this connection, the Report of the Lewis Committee (§ 167) states:

"Ample powers exist under Section 57 of the Army and Air Force Acts to mitigate, remit or commute sentences which appear to higher Commanders to be unduly harsh, and under Section 57A of the same Acts to suspend sentences when it appears to the superior military authority that it is in the interests of the Service and of the person sentenced to do so.* ... Moreover, provision has now been made ... for Military Corrective Establishments, the purpose of which will be to make better soldiers and airmen, and better citizens, of those undergoing punishment. This development will, we think, meet the views of some of those who gave evidence before us to the effect that something in the nature of a probation system was required in the Services." [104]

However, it must be emphasized that obviously it will not be possible "to make better soldiers and airmen, and better citizens, of those undergoing punishment", without efficient selection and segregation.

2. *Consideration of previous record*

The paragraph in *King's Regulations, 1940* (§677) laying down the nature of the evidence as to character and former convictions by civil courts that may be given to Courts-Martial merits close study and attention.

---

* Cf. *Army Act, 1955*, SS. 110, 113, 114, and 120.

APPENDIX A

No one would question the underlying principle that no court should be prejudiced against a man because of his past record, and that, therefore, it is proper to place limitations upon what may and what may not be given in evidence; but once a verdict of guilty has been established and a decision has to be reached as to the appropriate disposal in a given case, evidence concerning the man's previous criminal behaviour becomes highly relevant and of extreme importance in determining the prognosis and, therefore, the proper treatment to be administered. No facts, favourable or unfavourable, should be withheld from those who have the serious responsibility of deciding on the correct sentence.

The present sophistical distinction between "offences of the same general nature committed in civil life" that may be disclosed to the Court-Martial, and "offences of a different nature" that may not (*King's Regulations, 1940*, § 677 (c) and (d)), can only be described as an unscientific anachronism that must necessarily result in the Court-Martial being seriously misled in its efforts to determine what sentence is appropriate. Clinical experience demonstrates that, in their careers, many chronic delinquents show a remarkable and characteristic variety of criminal offences and that any attempt to determine prognosis on the basis of one particular class of offence would, therefore, be quite invalid.

Pedantic verbal distinctions cannot alter the fact that a man who, for example, has been convicted of homosexuality, burglary, larceny, petty theft, robbery with violence and absence without leave—to refer to an actual case—is quite obviously in a different psychiatric and prognostic class, from a man whose only offence has been absence without leave.

It may be noted, in this connection, that the Report of the Lewis Committee (§ 133 (iii)) states: "A Court-Martial should be given, wherever possible, after finding but before sentence, the same kind of record of the accused's career as is now given at that point in a civil criminal trial." [104]

Thus there is at present adequate precedent for providing the Court with full information as to the accused's past record, military and civil, after finding but before sentence. This information might also properly be provided to any of the authorities concerned with review or confirmation of sentence.

3. *The consequences of retaining chronic military offenders in the Army*

There is no doubt that many chronic delinquents are retained in the Army long after their uselessness has become obvious to the psychiatrist, and that the country's money and man-power are wasted in vain and futile attempts to return to duty men who are manifestly incapable of giving useful military service under normal conditions.

In the light of the facts described above, it is relevant here to consider the expenditure of man-power and money consequent upon the retention of delinquents in the Army.

From the point of view of man-power, a comparison between the establishments of military disciplinary institutions on the one hand, and an infantry battalion on the other, demonstrates clearly that segregation of delinquents involves a relatively heavy drain on man-power, not only

APPENDIX A

with respect to staff as a whole, but particularly in the senior Non-Commissioned Officer and Warrant Officer class.

Thus, from a comparison between the size of the staff required, and the number of soldiers under sentence, in military disciplinary institutions, it would appear that it is necessary to employ, on an average, one member of the staff for every two soldiers under sentence. Similarly, from a comparison between the number of officers and N.C.O.s required in military disciplinary institutions on one hand, and in an infantry battalion on the other, proportionately to the number of soldiers under sentence, and to the number of privates in the battalion, respectively, it was found that to maintain soldiers in a M.C.E. or M.P. and D.B.—during which time they are not giving any effective reckonable service—it is necessary to provide, on an average, as many officers and N.C.O.s, and from three to five and a half times as many senior N.C.O.s and Warrant Officers, as are required in an infantry battalion.

From the financial point of view, a careful evaluation of relevant data shows that it costs the country approximately half as much again to keep a soldier under sentence in a M.P. and D.B., and one-third as much again in the case of a soldier under sentence in a M.C.E., as it costs to keep a private in an ordinary unit. Moreover, the prisoner is performing no useful reckonable service, whilst the private in an ordinary unit is undergoing full military training.

The following examples relating to sentences commonly imposed will perhaps serve to emphasize the importance of these figures concerning the expenditure of money and man-power:—(i) The admission of a soldier to a M.C.E. to serve a sentence of 56 days' detention is the equivalent of sanctioning an expenditure of £43 and 478 Staff-Man-Hours. (ii) The admission of a soldier to a M.P. and D.B. to serve a sentence of six months' detention is the equivalent of sanctioning an expenditure of £160 and 2,440 Staff-Man-Hours.

Even the striking data summarized above do not convey an adequate impression of the cost to the Army of retaining a chronic delinquent: it would, indeed, be impossible in a short paper such as this to detail every source of wastage of money and man-power. The figures do not take into account the corrupting influence of these men on their comrades. In the M.C.E. and after their return to a normal unit, their irresponsibility and negativistic, anti-social behaviour are detrimental to morale and good discipline; their bad example undoubtedly leads others astray and by so doing seriously interferes with the efficiency of the unit as a whole. Nor do the figures give any indication of the expenditure involved either before ever the man is brought to trial (e.g. keeping him under guard, taking a Summary of Evidence, holding a Court of Inquiry, etc.), or subsequently in holding a Court-Martial (e.g. as a result of attendance of the members of the Court, witnesses, escort, etc.).

No one, medical or non-medical, psychiatrist or non-psychiatrist, would deny that the urgent practical necessity is to decide quickly and accurately whether or not a man is of any use to the Army, i.e. whether he is capable of giving useful military service without involving the country in unnecessary

APPENDIX A

expenditure.* Yet, in spite of the fact that there is well-nigh universal agreement on this point, there is still a certain amount of irresponsible criticism of the psychiatrist by non-medical personnel, and of non-medical personnel by psychiatrists who are not familiar with the administrative and non-medical aspects of disposal of delinquents.

It seems clear that in order to arrive at a proper decision as to the disposal of a delinquent, it is necessary to assess his military usefulness on a scientific basis. The fact cannot be over-emphasized that such selection should be the work of a team, of which it is essential, however, that the psychiatrist should be a member (as has been stated above).

4. *Difficulties arising out of present methods of disposal of delinquents unsuitable for retention in the Army*

In December, 1945, all existing regulations concerning the discharge of 'habitual bad characters' and 'psychopathic delinquents' were consolidated and amended, and incorporated in an Army Council Instruction. In particular, this A.C.I. provided that all applications to the War Office for discharge of such men, whether for misconduct or as psychopathic delinquents, would be accompanied by a recent report by an Army psychiatrist. It was stated: "The psychiatrist's report is necessary in order to ensure that soldiers suffering from psychiatric disabilities are not wrongly disposed of and that the fullest information will be available to the authorities on whom the final decision will rest", the object being that a man whose chronic anti-social behaviour was primarily due to definite psychiatric disability would be discharged from the Army on medical grounds, whilst if his delinquency was primarily due to a psychopathic personality defect but disposal on purely medical grounds was not considered justifiable he would be discharged as a 'psychopathic delinquent'. In cases where it was considered that there was no psychiatric disability, discharge would be carried out on administrative, disciplinary grounds. This A.C.I. was replaced, in June, 1946, by a revised and amended version.

The psychiatrist's function at present is only to report on the medical aspects of these cases, i.e. to state whether or not a man is a psychopathic personality or suffering from some other psychiatric disability. If a psychiatric diagnosis is made, the psychiatrist can recommend disposal, either as a purely medical case (under an A.C.I. of January, 1949), or as a psychopathic delinquent (under the A.C.I. of 1946). Recommendations as to discharge on purely disciplinary grounds are not considered to be within the province or competence of the psychiatrist. Thus, in practice, psychiatrists have two alternative methods of disposal of psychopathic personalities with anti-social trends.

While there can be little doubt that the A.C.I. of 1946 provides an expedient method of dealing with psychopathic delinquents, it nevertheless represents a compromise. From the purely medical, psychiatric point of view, an individual who is diagnosed as a psychopathic personality is

* It is not proposed here to discuss the advisability or otherwise of retaining delinquents in the Army for labour under supervision in times of grave National Emergency.

APPENDIX A

ipso facto deemed to be suffering from a psychiatric disorder and, in many cases, it would be hard to justify scientifically the differentiation of delinquents who, being also psychopaths, should be disposed of under the A.C.I. of 1946, from psychopaths who, showing chronic anti-social behaviour as one of the symptoms of their condition, should be discharged as medically unfit for military service under the A.C.I. of 1949. It is, indeed, often a somewhat arbitrary decision as to whether a man should be placed in the 'purely medical', or in the 'half medical, half disciplinary' category. At the other end of the scale, the decision as to whether a man is a 'psychopathic personality with anti-social trends' or whether there is 'No psychiatric disability' often depends only on the particular viewpoint of the examining psychiatrist Thus the latter often finds himself in a somewhat invidious position, in which the onus is placed upon him of drawing an arbitrary line between 'habitual criminals and bad characters' (an administrative and social diagnosis), psychopathic or other unstable personalities (a medical diagnosis), and 'psychopathic delinquents' (a hybrid and equivocal diagnosis).

Clinical experience shows that every chronic delinquent has certain peculiarities of temperament that underlie his adoption of a career of delinquency: these temperamental peculiarities vary from case to case but tend to fall into two classes:

(1) Those tending to result in an inability to settle down to a steady occupation, e.g. restlessness, impulsiveness, inability to concentrate, wanderlust, overactivity, irritability, shiftlessness, passivity, insecurity.
(2) Those tending to result in rebellion against authority, e.g. feelings of revenge and persecution, resentment, frustration, aggression, hostility, cruelty, destructiveness, self-assertion, and attention-seeking.

The critical question is whether a delinquent with these behaviour characteristics but with no gross neurotic or psychotic symptoms should be called 'normal' or a 'psychopath', and the dilemma is reinforced by the lack of any consistent and satisfactory definition of these two terms.

A survey of the medical literature on 'psychopathic personality' reduces the reader to a state of cynical despair: to one author any delinquent is *ipso facto* a psychopath; to another any person suffering from any form of mental disorder or, indeed, it would seem any person at all except the author concerned, is a psychopath. Definitions are innumerable and contradictory and there is clearly little hope of agreement on this matter in the near future.

One is forced to the conclusion that in the present circumstances, even although all were agreed that a man was quite unsuitable for further military service, there would almost inevitably be as many different diagnoses as there were individual psychiatrists examining the case. The function of the psychiatrist might, therefore, properly be confined to the essentially practical issue of determining whether, in the absence of a psychotic or gross neurotic disorder such as would justify the man's admission to hospital or medical discharge from the Service, the chronic offender is, in his opinion, 'irredeemable' for military service or not. This opinion

APPENDIX A

would be formed by the psychiatrist, on the basis of an assessment of the man's personality, mental capacity and emotional stability, and he would, as a result of his examination, make a recommendation to the disciplinary authorities. A convenient practice might be for all such cases to be considered by a special board, of which the psychiatrist would be one member, adopting a procedure similar to that of the original Review of Sentences Boards of B.A.O.R., which were composed of two non-medical members (a president and vice-president) and a psychiatrist.

At these Review Boards all relevant documents were studied, and then the man under consideration was brought in and questioned by each member. The president dealt with military matters, the vice-president with domestic affairs and questions of upbringing, and the psychiatrist with the medical side. The great importance of this interview, which was made as informal as an interview between a bench of officers and a private can be, was that the Board got a personal contact with the man, and its members were able to study all the evidence, and so come to a reasoned conclusion as to the correct disposal of his case.

Should the special Board which has been proposed above decide that the soldier is irredeemable from a military point of view, the latter could be discharged on administrative, non-medical grounds, e.g. under *King's Regulations, 1940,* § 390, (xviii)(*a*).

From the psychiatric standpoint, all men of the so-called chronic or psychopathic delinquent types may be regarded as belonging to one diagnostic group—anti-social or 'psychopathic' personalities, disorders of character and conduct, call them what we may. It would seem that neither from the point of view of military psychiatry, nor from that of the Army in general, and the administrative and disciplinary authorities in particular, is there very much to be gained by perpetuating the present system of somewhat arbitrary differentiation between individual types; provided of course, that the psychiatric examination and personality assessment of all such cases is ensured and is taken into consideration in deciding upon the man's disposal.

If the men who could be rehabilitated for further useful military service under ordinary conditions could be adequately selected as described above, there would be no cause for anxiety about their treatment after sentence has been passed, for there already exists adequate provision for the mitigation and suspension of sentences by the Confirming and Reviewing Authorities: if these authorities could call upon the advice of a Board of Experts as to the precise action indicated in each particular case there can be no doubt that more men would be restored to full military efficiency with the expenditure of less time and money.

However, if a man is recommended for discharge as useless to the Army, the question will arise as to what sentence he should serve prior to his discharge. From a financial point of view, retention in the Army of a man adjudged useless is quite unjustifiable, unless the country gets value for the money and man-power expended. It should be noted in this respect that current psychiatric opinion is in favour of keeping a chronic delinquent who is liable to commit further anti-social offences, in preven-

APPENDIX A

tive detention under medical observation, and with medical advice available, for an indeterminate period until he has been rehabilitated so that he is no longer a potential menace to the community—in much the same way as socially irresponsible and harmful insane and mentally defective persons are committed to an institution under certificate. Unfortunately there is at present no legal authority for such treatment, and until it exists psychiatrists can only observe with regret the inadequate and pathetically short sentences that are commonly awarded to chronic, often dangerous, delinquents from whose depredations the community should be protected.

In this respect two quotations from recent reports are apt:

(1) The Report by the Scottish Advisory Council on the Treatment and Rehabilitation of Offenders (§ 31, (v)–(ix)) contains the following recommendations:

- "(v) Cases which might respond to treatment, but which also require restraint, should be committed to prison for a length of time sufficient to ensure that the course of treatment is completed before the offender is released.
- (vi) Offenders committed to prison for treatment should be sent to a special psycho-therapeutic treatment centre, to be set up within the prison system, and ought not to live under the usual prison conditions.
- (vii) Where treatment would have no reasonable chance of success, the offender should either (*a*) be sentenced to a period of preventive detention not exceeding fourteen years; or (*b*) be detained in a State Mental Hospital, administered by the General Board of Control, on the certificate of two qualified medical psychiatrists.
- (viii) Conditions of preventive detention under (vii) (*a*) above should include frequent contacts with the outside world, varied and creative work, the minimum amount of solitary confinement, skilled observation and psycho-therapeutic treatment, and a measure of unsupervised liberty.
- (ix) Detention under (vii) (*b*) above should provide for re-examination of the detainee at stated intervals, resulting either in recommittal or in conditional or unconditional liberation." [114]

(2) The Report of the Joint Committee on Psychiatry and the Law, appointed by the British Medical Association and the Magistrates' Association, states:

"The East-Hubert report suggested . . . a 'special institution' within the Prison Service where some of those needing residential psychiatric treatment would be obliged to stay for a period. Provided that there is power in the Home Secretary to discharge offenders regardless of the length of their sentences, when safe for life at liberty, this proposal is strongly supported. . . . Such special facilities need not be restricted to sex offenders and could provide simultaneously for many other types of delinquent and non-delinquent psychopaths" (§ 60).

"Courts sending cases to such an institution should be empowered to impose, within limits, longer sentences than those hitherto provided by law. Until such institutions are established the Committee would not

APPENDIX A

oppose longer sentences in prison provided that psychiatric treatment is being given. Otherwise the Committee is strongly opposed to any lengthening of sentences to places of custody" (§ 62).

"The Committee is strongly opposed to the use of short sentences of imprisonment. They are too short to permit of any curative treatment and are inadequate as a deterrent" (§ 64).*

Until the advent of the millennium, psychiatrists can only recommend again and again that these principles should be followed, and that if it is considered necessary to retain in custody a soldier who is useless to the Army and who is liable to commit further anti-social offences, he should receive the maximum sentence permissible by the law.

Indeed, when making a decision as to the 'necessity' for retaining a soldier in military custody, it would seem advisable to consider, in each individual case, whether there is sufficient justification for the heavy financial burden and expenditure of man-power that would be involved; it might also be a matter for further consideration, whether long-term detention and rehabilitation for civil life is not properly a civil rather than a military responsibility. In this connection it may be pointed out that it is accepted policy that men who are of no further use to the Army for medical reasons (whether physical or mental) may only be retained in the Service for treatment for a limited period; and that medical treatment upon a long-term basis is rightly regarded as a civil responsibility.

PROPOSALS

In an effort to make our criticisms constructive, we put forward the following tentative proposals:

1. A man sentenced by a Court-Martial to a period of detention, corrective training or imprisonment, for a military offence should be subjected to a medical, physical and psychiatric, examination, and his correct 'Pulheems assessment' † determined. If he is unfit for further service on medical grounds, for reasons other than delinquent or anti-social behaviour, whether 'psychopathic' or otherwise, he should be brought before a Medical Board with a view to his discharge on medical grounds (under *King's Regulations, 1940*, § 390, (xvi)(*b*)).

2. If, however, he is not medically unfit, so as to justify discharge on medical grounds as in paragraph 1 above, he should be brought before a special Board consisting of at least two non-medical members and a psychiatrist (comparable to the original Review of Sentences Boards of B.A.O.R., which consisted of a president, a vice-president and a psychiatrist).

The following types of case should also be examined by the special Board as described above:

(*a*) Men considered by their commanding officer or by a military psy-

---

* 'The Criminal Law and Sexual Offenders', *Brit. med. J., Supplement*, 1949, 1: 139.
† Cf. R. T. Fletcher, 'Pulheems: A New System of Medical Classification', *Brit. med. J.*, 1949, 1: 83–8.

APPENDIX A

chiatrist to be chronic delinquents, unlikely to give further useful military service.
  (b) Men sentenced by a commanding officer to undergo a period of detention or corrective training in a M.P. and D.B. or a M.C.E.
  (c) Men sentenced by the Civil Power to a period of Borstal training, or imprisonment.

3. This special Board should interview the man and consider the following evidence:
  (a) The man's previous military record.
  (b) His previous record of civil offences *of all types*.
  (c) The nature and quality of his present offence.
  (d) Medical and psychiatric reports.
  (e) A Social Welfare Worker's report on his family background and home circumstances (if deemed relevant and necessary).
  (f) Reports from his unit as to his efficiency, influence and behaviour in the unit. Obviously, the most desirable procedure would be for this evidence to be given direct to the Board, where practicable, rather than as a written statement.

4. The Board should have the power to advise the Confirming Authority (or the Personnel Branch concerned, in the case of men sentenced by the Civil Power) as to:
  (a) Whether the man is of any further use to the Army.
  (b) Except in cases sentenced by the Civil Power, the type of sentence appropriate (including suitability for suspension of sentence, corrective training and rehabilitation).
  (c) Whether the man should be discharged from the Army after completion of his sentence.

5. If discharge is recommended by the Board, it should be carried out administratively, e.g. under *King's Regulations, 1940*, § 390, (x), (xi), (xii), (xiii), or (xviii)(a). In practice, this would mean that normally no chronic delinquent would be discharged through medical channels unless he were suffering from a physical defect or mental disorder necessitating invaliding for reasons other than delinquent behaviour, and that the procedure laid down in the A.C.I. of 1946 could be dispensed with (provided, of course, that it were replaced by a procedure such as that outlined in this paper).

6. During sentence the case should be reviewed by the same Board (if possible) every 3 months; at the Review Board a report on the man's progress by the Commandant of the M.C.E. or M.P. and D.B. and further medical (including psychiatric) reports should be available.

7. If the man is returned to a unit for further service, either after completion of sentence or under suspended sentence, his military record should be submitted for review by a Board after successive periods of 1 year, 3 years, 5 years, and thereafter if indicated. If at the review there is any reason to doubt his military efficiency, he should be brought before a special Board again for review of his case.

8. It is considered highly desirable that if the members of a Board disagree as to whether a man is fit for further service, either the case should be referred to a higher board (analagous to the War Office Medical

APPENDIX A

Board) or the man should be returned to his unit, even despite a majority of opinion. Such cases should always be followed up by the same Board; this would have the salutary effect of demonstrating mistakes in prognosis to those who have made them.

9. The relevant A.C.I.s* should be amended to ensure that all delinquents recommended for discharge from the Army, who are both mentally backward and considered liable to commit further anti-social offences in *civil life*, should be effectively notified to the Ministry of Health.

In this way, all those who should be certified as mentally deficient would be so dealt with; and aftercare and other supervision could be provided where necessary, either under Section 30 of the Mental Deficiency Act, 1913, or under the provisions of the National Health Service Act, 1946.†

It is suggested that a practical definition of 'Mentally Backward' should be adopted, such as the following:

(a) All men who are rated S.G. 5 on the Dominoes or Matrix test, and who are also rated Summed S.G. 5, i.e. those who, in intelligence, are in the lower 4% (approximately) of the Army population.

(b) Men who have been dealt with previously under the Mental Deficiency Act, 1913.

(c) Any others who are considered by the psychiatrist to be suitable for disposal under Section 30 of the Mental Deficiency Act, 1913.

In practice, acceptance of this definition would result in the notification of those delinquents who, in intelligence, are in the lower 10% (approximately) of the population as a whole, which includes those Mental Defectives who are segregated in Institutions or under statutory supervision or guardianship, and those who have been rejected for military service because of mental backwardness. This lower 10% of the population corresponds with the group generally regarded as Mentally Deficient or Borderline Mentally Deficient.‡

* Viz., an A.C.I. published in November, 1944 (as amended by an A.C.I. of 1949), which provided for the notification to the Ministry of Health of certain delinquents discharged from the Army on grounds of mental backwardness.

† In particular, *National Health Service Act, 1946*, S. 28. Cf. also *Provisions Relating to the Mental Health Services*, London (H.M.S.O.), 1948, § 66, pp. 22–3.

‡ Cf. D. Wechsler, *The Measurement of Adult Intelligence*, 3rd ed., Baltimore, 1944, p. 190.

APPENDIX B

THE INCIDENCE OF DESERTION IN THE BRITISH ARMY IN THE FIRST AND SECOND WORLD WARS, IN RELATION TO THE DEATH PENALTY AND ITS ABOLITION

DURING the First World War, the death penalty could be awarded by courts-martial for the offences of desertion and 'cowardice', and for certain other offences. According to the official statistics, from 4 August, 1914, to 31 March, 1920, the total number of death sentences passed by courts-martial on officers and men, in all theatres of war, was 3,080. The total number of men actually executed was 346 (i.e. 11%), of whom 322 were executed in France and Belgium, and the remainder in other theatres overseas. Of these 346 men, 18 were executed for 'cowardice' and 266 for desertion.

Among those executed, 91 men were under suspended sentences (including 9 under two suspended sentences). Of these 91 men, 40 had been previously sentenced to death (in 38 cases for desertion). One soldier had been sentenced to death for desertion on two previous occasions.[129] Yet these men had deserted again, in spite of the 'deterrent' effect of the death penalty.

The death penalty for 'cowardice' and desertion was abolished in April, 1930.*

In 1942, the relatively high incidence of desertion in the Middle East seriously affected the man-power situation in that theatre. This state of affairs prompted the Commander-in-Chief, Middle East (General Sir Claude Auchinleck), with the unanimous agreement of his Army Commanders, not to order an extensive investigation into the state of morale in the M.E.F., but to forward to the War Office, in May, 1942, a strong recommendation for the reintroduction of the death penalty for desertion in the field. In making his recommendation, he expressed the opinion that no less a deterrent was proved to be required from time to time, not merely in the interests of discipline but for the conduct of operations in conditions

---

* By amendments to SS. 4, 6, and 12 of the *Army Act*, introduced by the *Army and Air Force (Annual) Act, 1930*. The death penalty for military offences was, and still is, retained as a maximum penalty for aiding the enemy, and mutiny (*Army Act*, SS. 4, 6, and 7; *Army Act, 1955*, SS. 24, 25, 31 and 32).

APPENDIX B

of strain and stress, and that the knowledge that the death sentence was within his powers would have proved a salutary deterrent to those men to whom the alternative of prison to the hardships of battle conveyed neither fear nor stigma.*

The Executive Committee of the Army Council, while agreeing unanimously that, in the interests of discipline, there could be no question as to the military desirability of the death sentence for desertion in the field and 'cowardice in the face of the enemy', did not think that it would be possible to reintroduce the death sentence during the war, for political reasons as well as for considerations affecting security.

In November, 1942, in reply to an enquiry by the Secretary of State for War, General Alexander, who had taken over command in the Middle East, stated that, although in his opinion the morale of the Army was, at that time, high and was improving, and cases of desertion and 'cowardice' were comparatively few in number, and therefore there was no immediate need for reintroducing the death penalty for desertion, he was, in fact, in favour of its reintroduction; he felt, however, that the time was then inopportune.†

The official figures representing the average strength of the British Army, and the total number of deserters, per year during the First and Second World Wars are given in the accompanying table, and the incidence of desertion per year, per 1,000 strength, is shown in the table (p. 273) and the graph (p. 274). It should thus be evident that the average incidence of deserters per year, per 1,000 strength, for the period 1914–19, was 10·26—(the yearly incidence varying from 6·03 to 20·70); and the

---

* There is ample evidence, not only that an increase in the incidence of desertion and absenteeism, as well as of sick parade attendance and psychiatric casualties, was already apparent in the M.E.F. by the middle of 1941, but that it occurred concurrently with a general lowering of morale. In this connection, the importance and significance of the poor selection and inadequate training of recruits arriving in the Middle East in 1941, and in 1942 (when this state of affairs was at its worst), cannot be overemphasized. In addition, the year 1941 was a very arduous one for the M.E.F.: the men were exhausted by the fighting and worried about conditions in the U.K.; welfare problems increased, and news from home and mail were totally inadequate. By the summer of 1942, the men were utterly weary and dispirited, demoralized by our reverses and the chronic shortage of effective arms and equipment. In the light of these facts, it may be permitted to question the opinion that the general morale and discipline of the M.E.F., in 1941–2, would have been notably increased by adding to the very great stresses to which this much-tried Force was subjected, the further burden of the threat of the death penalty for desertion.

† The conviction that the death penalty was a highly effective, if not indeed the only, deterrent to desertion in war, has been strongly held and expressed by many persons in influential or prominent positions, particularly in the Army. Cf. the opinion of Gen. G. S. Patton;[89] and a statement by Lord Blackford, which may serve as a 'type specimen': "In the First World War desertion was punishable by death. There were very few desertions. In the Second World War capital punishment for this offence was abolished. There were scores of thousands of deserters" (*The Times*, 5 Dec., 1947). Brigadier Rees has observed that, in the few cases where there have been desertions by a number of men at one time, the explanation was to be found "usually in faulty handling by N.C.O.s or officers. . . . The fire-eater who regards all nerves as 'fiddlesticks' and anxiety as malingering . . . in practically every case that I have met is recognizable without much difficulty as a man carrying a considerable load of personal anxiety, and shame about it."[97]

APPENDIX B

average incidence, for the period 1939–45, was 6·89 (the yearly incidence varying from 4·48 to 10·05). It would, therefore, seem that the 'deterrent' value of the death penalty for desertion in the First World War was, at the least, somewhat dubious.*

Incidence of Desertion in the British Army in the First and Second World Wars

Period	Average Strength $(Army)^a$	Total No. Deserters	Incidence (p. yr. 0/00)
World War I:			
1/10/14–30/9/15	1,949,871	40,375	20·70
1/10/15–30/9/16	2,886,978	26,520	9·19
1/10/16–30/9/17	3,621,378	21,838	6·03
1/10/17–30/9/18	3,829,834	28,372	7·41
1/10/18–30/9/19	2,586,085	20,668	7·99
World War II:			
1/10/39–30/9/40	1,538,675	6,889	4·48
1/10/40–30/9/41	2,211,547	22,248	10·05
1/10/41–30/9/42	2,455,720	20,834	8·49
1/10/42–30/9/43	2,681,697	15,824	5·90
1/10/43–30/9/44	2,729,480	16,892	6·19
1/10/44–30/9/45	2,830,831	17,663	6·24

^{a} Calculated as the mean of the monthly or quarterly figures for each period of 12 months (1st October–30th September).

In more than one respect, these figures tend to corroborate military psychiatric experience that the problem of desertion is primarily a problem of selection and morale. By thorough medical examination and scientific selection, it is possible to exclude from the Army those who, through mental instability or dullness, are particularly liable to break down or desert under stress, and incidentally prove, in any event, harmful to unit morale.† By attention to morale, i.e. by careful training, suitable employment, good leadership, adequate welfare, etc., it is also possible to avoid

---

* It should also be borne in mind that the stress to which men were subjected in the Second World War—with its high degree of speed and mechanization, dive-bombing and armoured warfare, simultaneous bombing of the civilian population at home, and many other similar features—was incomparably greater, in the long run, than that experienced during the First World War. To acknowledge this fact is in no sense to minimize the appalling conditions under which soldiers were obliged to fight and exist in the First War, nor to underestimate the impact on these men of the first widespread application of modern warfare, but merely to recognize that at the outset of the recent war—in the striking words of Sir Winston Churchill—"Four or five millions of men met each other in the first shock of the most merciless of all the wars of which record has been kept." It is unnecessary to insist further on this point, which has frequently been stressed. Cf., for example, J. W. Appel, G. W. Beebe and D. W. Hilger;[14] and E. A. Strecker and K. E. Appel.[121]

† It is evident from the figures provided, that the extremely high incidence of desertion during the first year of the 1914–18 War has never been approached at any subsequent period, whether in the First or in the Second World War. If any further evidence be required, that this was no mere coincidence but bore a direct relationship to the

APPENDIX B

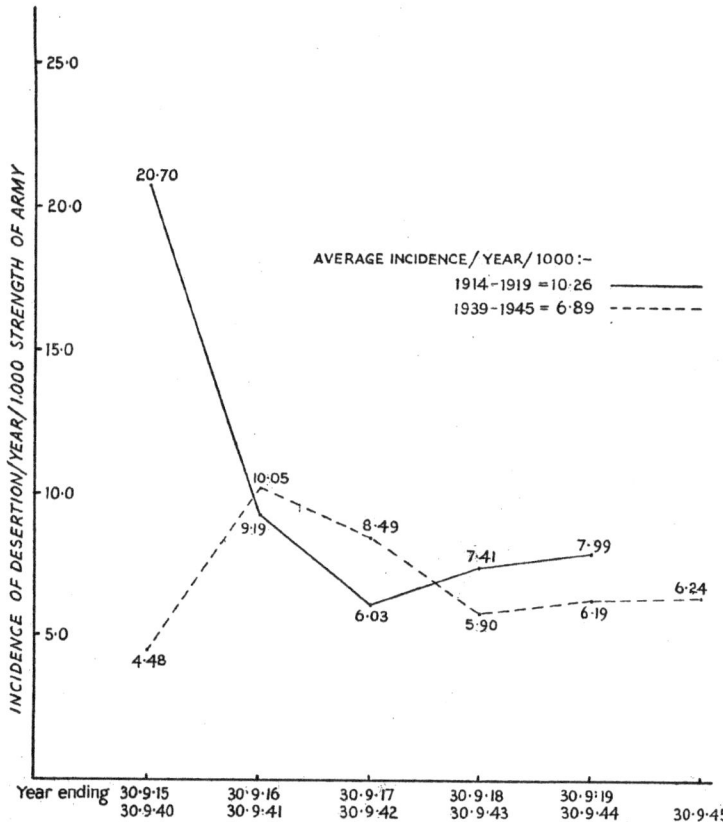

many of the precipitating factors which contribute to mental breakdown or desertion.

question of selection, it is surely to be found in the following description by the Southborough Committee of the situation immediately following the outbreak of war in August, 1914; "Immediately there was a tremendous rush of recruits to the Colours, and it was inevitable that they should be dealt with on the existing, almost ingenuously simple, system. . . . The result was chaos. . . . Tens of thousands of recruits were besieging the recruiting offices to get into the Army; the Army was in urgent need of men. . . . In these circumstances, thousands of men were passed 'fit' into the Army every week without any medical examination worth the name. . . . As the weeks went on, the Army itself began, as was inevitable, to realize that they were confronted with a new problem. . . . They were being flooded with men who, after a few weeks or months of military service, broke down and contributed an ever-growing quota to the sick returns and casualty lists. . . . During the period (18 months) in which enlistment was voluntary it is clear that there was no real check upon the enlistment of men who were unsuitable for military service owing to mental or nervous instability." [128] The high rate of desertion amongst young volunteers in B.L.A. has been discussed elsewhere in the present work.

APPENDIX B

Without attention to these fundamental prophylactic measures, in vain may the Army hold this sword of Damocles—as it were, a suspended death sentence—over the heads of fighting men already labouring under the intense stresses of modern warfare: they will prevent neither psychiatric breakdown nor desertion and other lesions of morale. Indeed, the figures indicate with great clarity the fact that the alleged 'deterrent' effect of the death penalty for desertion is no more than a delusion.

APPENDIX C
STATISTICS RELATING TO BRITISH ARMY PSYCHIATRY IN THE SECOND WORLD WAR

SUCH detailed statistical information as is available, concerning the incidence and disposal of psychiatric cases in the British Army during the Second Word War, is collected in the *Statistical Report on the Health of the Army, 1943-1945*, together with excellent illustrative charts.*[130]

A few of the broad general conclusions set forth, on the basis of the data presented, in this Report may briefly be mentioned here.

Psychiatric disorders are by far the largest cause of medical discharge among military personnel (O.R.s): they constituted, in 1943, over one-third of all discharges with respect to disease; and in 1944, their contribution rose to two-fifths. About one-half of all psychiatric disorders comprised *anxiety neuroses*, the incidence of which rose steadily throughout the three years, 1943-5. The second largest medical cause of discharge is *peptic ulcer*, which accounted for 13% of all such discharges in 1943, although its contribution fell substantially in subsequent years.†

Referring to the relation of age to medical discharge, it has been recorded that, "Broadly speaking we may thus summarize the experience of the war years: (i) if the youngest age groups of an Army population predominate, the two chief sources of wastage are psychiatric disorders and tuberculosis; (ii) if the middle age groups predominate, the two chief sources of wastage are psychiatric disorders and peptic ulcers; (iii) if the oldest age group were to predominate, the two chief sources of wastage would be bronchitis and psychiatric disorders." [62; cf. 130]

With respect to morbidity and man-day wastage, the statistics show that psychiatric disorders constitute the largest single cause of wastage resulting from disease, in both sexes: they comprise one-seventh of the total among males (O.R.s), and more than one-ninth among females (A.T.S.).[130]

---

* Cf. in particular Part IX of this Report, which, as stated in a foreword by the (former) D.G.A.M.S., Lt.-Gen. N. Cantlie, "draws attention to the magnitude of the psychiatric problems of modern Army medicine and presents a much needed record of the contribution made by Army psychiatry".

† It is hardly necessary to point out the psychiatric significance of peptic ulcer. E. Weiss and O. S. English have stated: "The term psychosomatic can be used without hesitation in connection with peptic ulcer because today even the most organically minded physician recognizes the importance of 'emotional factors' in ulcer cases." [131] Cf. also F. Dunbar.[43]

APPENDIX C

The accompanying tables and diagrams summarize in convenient form available data as to the relative importance of psychiatric disabilities in relation to the Medical Services of the British Army as a whole, during the Second World War. For purposes of rough comparison, some general statistics of a similar nature, relating to the United States Army during the Second World War, are also included.

It should be noted, however, that the statistical data available with respect to the British and U.S. Armies are, unfortunately, not strictly comparable, partly because of the different manner in which they have been collected and analysed, and partly because of the different periods to which they relate. In so far as possible, these data have been adapted to permit some degree of useful comparison, and the U.S. statistics concerning neuropsychiatric cases have been adjusted, by excluding neurological cases, in order to obtain comparable figures referring to psychiatric disorders only. The statistics here summarized may be taken, in general, as referring to white male subjects.*

The nature of the material summarized in the accompanying tables, and the periods to which the respective data refer, are as follows:

Table I: Rejections at intake (induction), (p. 278).

(a) U.K.—Examinations by Ministry of Labour and National Service Medical Boards (under the National Service Acts), June, 1939–March, 1947. The relative percentages of cases rejected for physical defects and psychiatric disorders were calculated from data obtained from a sample of 60,000 men, between 1939 and 1942.

(b) U.S.—Preinduction examinations (white recruits), October, 1945–April, 1946.

Table II: Rejections at intake (induction), and discharges from the Army on medical grounds—Distribution by diagnostic groups (p. 279).

(a) U.K.—Average figures (R.O.D.R.s)† for discharges on medical grounds, 1943–5. Figures for rejection at intake are derived from a sample of 60,000 men examined and rejected between 1939 and 1942.—It should be noted that available statistics for the British Army are, for the most part, not classified in the broad diagnostic groups indicated in the table, but by individual diagnoses. The figures here given are, therefore, in many cases approximations, obtained from the figures available with respect to the principal *individual* conditions which fall into, and constitute the main part of, the several broad diagnostic groups.

(b) U.S.—Disability discharges, 1941–5. Rejections at induction, November, 1940–August, 1945.

---

* The statistical material here given is adapted from data obtained from the following sources: *U.K.*—Official statistics,[130] and Brigadier A. E. Richmond;[107] additional data for Table II were kindly supplied by Major R. B. Stalbow, A.M.D.5 (Stats.), War Office. *U.S.*—Maj.-Gen. R. W. Bliss,[21] and Brig.-Gen. W. C. Menninger.[79] The author wishes, in particular, to acknowledge the fact that the accompanying tables are very largely based on those reproduced in Dr. Menninger's book.[79]

† R.O.D.R. = Relative Overall Discharge Rate—i.e. percentage of discharges of the type specified among *total* (medical) discharges.

APPENDIX C

TABLE I

Rejections at Intake (Induction)

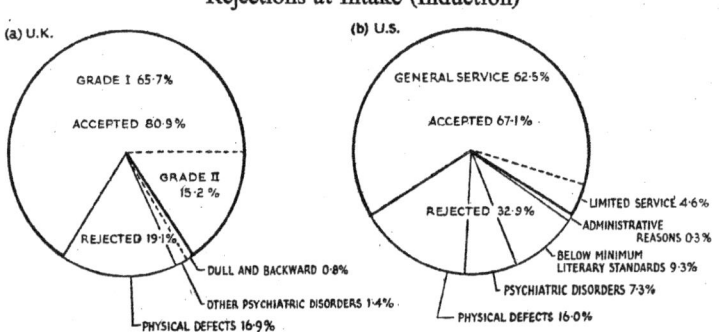

REJECTIONS AT INTAKE (INDUCTION)

	(a) U.K.		(b) U.S.	
ACCEPTED:	GRADE I	65·7%	GENERAL SERVICE	62·5%
	GRADE II (a)* 6·2% GRADE II 9·0%	15·2%	LIMITED SERVICE	4·6%
	TOTAL, GRADES I & II	80·9%	TOTAL	67·1%
REJECTED:	PHYSICAL DEFECTS	16·9%	PHYSICAL DEFECTS	16·0%
	PSYCHIATRIC DISORDERS { Nervous instability and Mental Disease 1·4% Dull and backward 0·8% }	2·2%	PSYCHIATRIC DISORDERS FAILURE TO MEET MINIMUM LITERARY STANDARDS ADMINISTRATIVE REASONS	7·3% 9·3% 0·3%
	TOTAL, GRADES III & IV	19·1%	TOTAL	32·9%

* Grade II (*a*) relates to persons in Grade II who could not be placed in Grade I solely on account of defects of visual acuity or on account of deformities of the lower extremities.

TABLE II

Rejections at Intake (Induction), and Discharges from the Army on Medical Grounds. Distribution by Diagnostic Groups

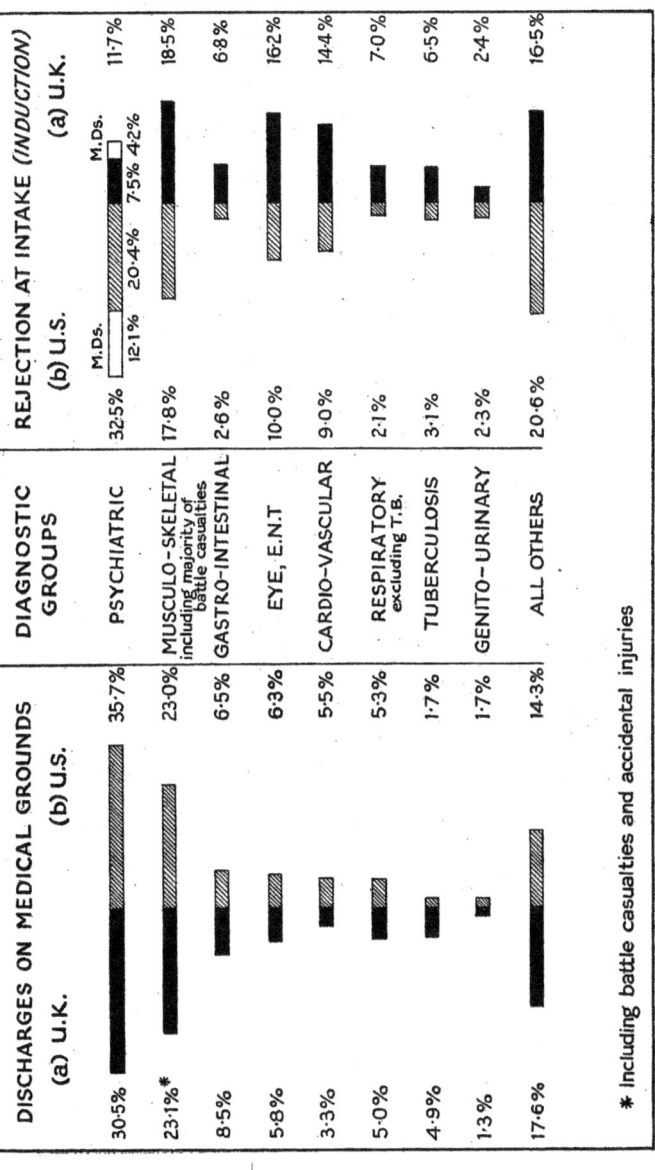

* Including battle casualties and accidental injuries

APPENDIX C

Table III: The magnitude of the psychiatric problem—British and U.S. Armies (p. 281).

(*a*) U.K.—All figures given in this table are approximations, adapted for comparison with U.S. data available only as integral numbers.— Figures relating to rejections at intake are derived from general statistics for Ministry of Labour and National Service Medical Boards, June, 1939– March, 1947, and from a sample of 60,000 men examined and rejected between 1939 and 1942. Figures relating to admission to hospital are based on the average R.C.R.* for hospitalized cases in the U.K., January, 1943– June, 1944 (and, with respect to R.C.R.s according to the *type* of hospital, the figures are for the year 1943). Figures relating to discharge from the Army on medical grounds (R.O.D.R.s) are average figures for 1943–5. Figures with respect to the number of other ranks and officers discharged from military psychiatric hospitals to civil employment are average figures for the period, April, 1942–December, 1944.

(*b*) U.S.—The figures available are approximations, in that they are integral numbers, and relate to the period, 1942–5.

* R.C.R. = Relative Casualty Rate—i.e. percentage of casualties of a given specification among *all* cases in a given period, including injuries (in addition to sick, in the more restricted sense).

Footnotes to Table III (opposite).

* These figures refer to cases treated *exclusively* in military hospitals. For *all* cases treated in hospitals (military, E.M.S., etc.), the corresponding average figures are: Psychiatric cases = 5% of total admissions. Of these, psychoneurosis = 71%; psychosis = 15%; other psychiatric disorders = 14%.

** Psychopathic personality = 9%; mental deficiency = 4%; other psychiatric disorders = 10%.

† These figures do *not* include *administrative* discharges of dullards, nor of 'psychopathic delinquents'.—The 21% comprise: psychopathic personality = 15%; mental deficiency = 6%.

‡ These figures *include administrative* discharges of dullards and psychopaths (for 'inaptness, lack of adaptability', etc.).—The 33% consist almost entirely of such administrative discharges.

§ Psychoneurosis = 29%; psychosis = 1%; psychopathic personality = 20%; other psychiatric disorders = 6%.

APPENDIX C

TABLE III
The Magnitude of the Psychiatric Problem—British and U.S. Armies

REJECTIONS

PSYCHIATRIC REJECTIONS FOR MILITARY SERVICE AT INTAKE (INDUCTION).
U.K. 2%
U.S. 10% } of all examined
U.K. 12%
U.S. 32% } of all rejections for all causes

	U.K.	U.S.
MENTAL DEFICIENCY	36%	44%
OTHER PSYCHIATRIC DISORDERS	64%	56%§

"Screening" excludes those unsuited for military service: many are not handicapped for civilian life

ADMISSIONS

PSYCHIATRIC ADMISSIONS TO MILITARY HOSPITALS DURING THE WAR
U.K. 6%*
U.S. 5-6% } of total admissions

	U.K.	U.S.
PSYCHONEUROSIS	65%*	70%
PSYCHOSIS	18%*	7%
OTHER PSYCHIATRIC DISORDERS	7%**	23%**

Stress of active military service is often so severe that psychiatric reactions develop in men of "NORMAL" stability

DISCHARGES

DISCHARGES FROM SERVICE FOR PSYCHIATRIC DISORDERS
U.K. 31%†
U.S. 45%‡ } of all discharges for mental and physical defects

	U.K.	U.S.
PSYCHONEUROSIS	67%	52%
PSYCHOSIS	10%	11%
PSYCHOPATHIC PERSONALITY MENTAL DEFICIENCY	21%‡	33%‡
OTHER PSYCHIATRIC DISORDERS	2%	4%

Soldiers obtain maximal benefit from Army hospitalization before discharge
U.K. { 75% other ranks
88% officers } discharged to civil employment
U.S. 80% gainfully employed after discharge

281

LIST OF ABBREVIATIONS

N.B.—In abbreviations in the text, plurals are indicated by the addition of *s* to the appropriate initial (e.g. C.O.s, O.sC., D.D.sM.S., P.sO.W., etc.).

'A' STAFF   Adjutant-General's Branch (War Office).
A.A.   Anti-Aircraft.
A.A.G.   Assistant Adjutant-General.
A.C.I.   Army Council Instruction.
A.D.M.S.   Assistant Director of Medical Services.
A.D.S.   Advanced Dressing Station.
A.G.   Adjutant-General's Branch (Departments of War Office).
A.L.F.S.E.A.   Allied Land Forces, South-East Asia.
A.M.D.   Army Medical Directorate (Departments of War Office).
A.M.P.C.   Auxiliary Military Pioneer Corps.
A.T.S.   Auxiliary Territorial Service (Women).
A.W.O.L.   Absent Without Leave.

B.A.O.R.   British Army of the Rhine.
B.B.C.   British Broadcasting Corporation.
B.E.F.   British Expeditionary Force.
B.L.A.   British Liberation Army.
B.N.A.F.   British North Africa Force.
B.T.N.I.   British Troops Northern Ireland.

CAMERONS   Queen's Own Cameron Highlanders.
C.B.   Confined to Barracks.
C.C.S.   Casualty Clearing Station.
C.-IN-C.   Commander-in-Chief.
C.M.F.   Central Mediterranean Force.
C.O.   Commanding Officer.
C.R.A.   Commander Royal Artillery.
C.R.U.   Civil Resettlement Unit.
C.S.S.B.   Civil Service Selection Board.

D.A. AND Q.M.G.   Deputy Adjutant and Quarter-Master General.
D.A.G.   Deputy Adjutant-General.
D-DAY   Date of Allied landing in Normandy (6 June, 1944).
D.D.M.S.   Deputy Director of Medical Services.
D.D.S.T.   Deputy Director of Supplies and Transport.

ABBREVIATIONS

D.G.A.M.S. Director-General, Army Medical Services.
D.G.I.M.S. Director-General, Indian Medical Service.
D.M.S. Director of Medical Services.

E.M.S. Emergency Medical Service.
E.N.T. Ear, Nose and Throat.

F.D.S. Field Dressing Station.
F.R.S. Fellow of the Royal Society.

'G' STAFF General Staff Branch (War Office).
G.H.Q. General Headquarters.
G.O.C.-IN-C. General Officer Commanding-in-Chief.
GORDONS Gordon Highlanders.

H.M.S.O. H.M. Stationery Office.
H.Q. Headquarters.

I.A.M.C. Indian Army Medical Corps.
i/c In charge.
I.T.C. Infantry Training Centre.

L.C.C. London County Council.
L. OF C. Lines of Communication (Area).

M.C.E. Military Corrective Establishment.
M.D. Mental Defective.
M.D.S. Main Dressing Station.
M.E.F. Middle East Force.
M.E.L.F. Middle East Land Force.
M.O. Medical Officer.
M.P. AND D.B. Military Prison and Detention Barracks.
M.P.S.C. Military Provost Staff Corps.

N.A.A.F.I. Navy, Army and Air Force Institutes.
N.C.O. Non-Commissioned Officer.
'N.Y.D.N.' 'Not Yet Diagnosed—Nervous'.

O.C. Officer Commanding.
O.C.T.U. Officer Cadet Training Unit.
O.R. Other Rank (as opposed to Officers).
O.T.S. Officer Training School (India).

Parl. Deb. Hansard's *Parliamentary Debates* (H.M.S.O., London).
'P.B.I.' 'Poor Bloody Infantry'.
P.O.W. Prisoner of War.
'PULHEEMS' System of medical classification: i.e. P = Physical capacity (physique); U = Upper limbs (functional efficiency); L = Locomo-

ABBREVIATIONS

tion (locomotor efficiency of lower limbs); H = Hearing (acuity); EE = Eyesight (visual acuity, right and left eye); M = Mental capacity; S = Stability (emotional).

Q.A.I.M.N.S.   Queen Alexandra's Imperial Military Nursing Service.

R.A.   Royal Artillery.
R.A.C.   Royal Armoured Corps.
R.A.F.   Royal Air Force.
R.A.M.C.   Royal Army Medical Corps.
R.A.O.C.   Royal Army Ordnance Corps.
R.A.P.   Regimental Aid Post.
R.A.P.C.   Royal Army Pay Corps.
R.A.S.C.   Royal Army Service Corps.
R.C.A.M.C. Royal Canadian Army Medical Corps.
R.C.R.   Relative Casualty Rate.
RECCE   Reconnaissance Corps.
R.E.M.E.   Royal Electrical and Mechanical Engineers.
R.H.U.   Reinforcement Holding Unit.
R.M.O.   Regimental Medical Officer.
R.O.D.R.   Relative Overall Discharge Rate.
R.S.M.   Regimental Sergeant-Major.

S.   Section (of Act, etc.).—(SS. = Sections).
S.E.A.C.   South-East Asia Command.
SEAFORTHS Seaforth Highlanders.
S.G.   Selection Group.
S.H.A.E.F. Supreme Headquarters, Allied Expeditionary Forces.
S.S.G.   Summed Selection Group.
S.T.U.   Special (Young Soldiers') Training Unit.

T.B.   Tuberculosis.

U.K.   United Kingdom (of Great Britain and Northern Ireland).
U.S.   United States.
U.S.N.R.   United States Naval Reserve.

V.D.   Venereal Disease.
V.E.-DAY   ('Victory in Europe')—Official end of war in Europe (9 May, 1945).

W.A.C.   Women's Army Corps (India).
W.O.S.B.   War Office Selection Board.
W. YORKS. West Yorkshire Regiment.

Y.S.T.U.   Young Soldiers' Training Unit.

GENERAL BIBLIOGRAPHY

N.B.—Only *published* works, referred to in the present History, are listed below. In addition to these and other material, the author consulted over 300 unpublished reports covering the years 1939–49, which had been submitted to the Directorate of Army Psychiatry or other War Office departments: as these unpublished documents are not, however, generally available, and indeed, many of them have since been destroyed or mislaid, no useful purpose would appear to be served by their inclusion in the present bibliography.

For convenience, the usual British convention has been adopted, of quoting volume numbers of *The Lancet* and the *British Medical Journal* as *half-yearly* volumes—(1 and 2, respectively)—for any given year.
H.M.S.O. = H.M. Stationery Office (British Government publishers).

Numbers in italics in parentheses refer to the pages in the text on which the following works are respectively mentioned or quoted.

1 ABRAHAMS, J., & MCCORKLE, L. W. 1946. Group psychotherapy of military offenders. *Amer. J. Sociol.*, **51**: 455-64. (*140*)
2 ABRAHAMS, J., & MCCORKLE, L. W. 1947. Group psychotherapy at an Army Rehabilitation Centre. *Dis. nerv. Syst.*, **8**: 50–62. (*140*)
3 ADAM, R. F. 1948. Lessons from the Army's experience in selection. *Psychol. at Work*, **1**, No. 2 (May): 2–5. (*66*)
4 AICHHORN, A. 1936. *Wayward Youth*; London (Putnam); p. 149. (*116 n.*)
5 ALLEN, E. P., & SMITH, P. 1931. *Selection of Skilled Apprentices for the Engineering Trades: Report of Research*; Birmingham (Education Ctee.). (*31 n.*)
6 ALLEN, E. P., & SMITH, P. 1932. *The Value of Vocational Tests as Aids to Choice of Employment: Report of Research*; Birmingham (Education Ctee.). (*31 n.*)
7 ANON. 1941. Mental fitness of U.S. recruits. *Lancet*. **2**: 103-4. (*95*)
8 ANON. 1942. Murder no killing—(from our Military Correspondent). *Time and Tide*, **23**, (9 May): 383 ff. (*200 n.*)
9 ANON. 1942. The military implications of psychiatry. *J.R. Army med. Cps.*, **78**: 138–40. (*6, 23, 24*)
10 ANON. 1948. [Editorial]. *Lancet*, **1**: 524–5. (*25*)
11 ANSBACHER, H. L. 1941. German military psychology. *Psychol. Bull.*, **38**: 370–92. (*38 n.*)
12 APPEL, J. W. 1950. *In:* Discussion; *Epidemiology of Mental Disorder*; New York (Milbank Memorial Fund); pp. 52–5. (*3*)
13 APPEL, J. W., & BEEBE, G. W. 1946. Preventive psychiatry: an epidemiologic approach. *J. Amer. med. Ass.*, **131**: 1469–75. (*3, 171, 173*)

GENERAL BIBLIOGRAPHY

14 APPEL, J. W., BEEBE, G. W., & HILGER, D. W. 1946. Comparative incidence of neuropsychiatric casualties in World War I and World War II. *Amer. J. Psychiat.*, **103**: 196–9. (*273 n.*)

15 *Australia in the War of 1939–1945*: Ser. 5 (Medical), I—*Clinical Problems of War*, by A. S. Walker; Canberra (Australian War Memorial), 1952; Psychiatry, pp. 674–707. (*15 n.*)

16 BARTEMEIER, L. H., KUBIE, L. S., *et al.* 1946. Combat exhaustion. *J. nerv. ment. Dis.*, **104**: 358–89, 489–525. (*171 n.*)

17 BENNET, E. A. 1945. Army psychiatry in India. *J. Indian Army med. Cps.*, **1**, No. 1: 21–25. (*191 n., 192, 193, 194*)

18 BENNET, E. A. 1948. Psychiatry in India and Pakistan. *Ment. Health, London*, **8**: 2–5. (*191, 191 n.*)

19 BION, W. R. 1946. The Leaderless Group Project. *Bull. Menninger Clin.*, **10**: 77–81. (*60, 61*)

20 BION, W. R., & RICKMAN, J. 1943. Intra-group tensions in therapy: their study as the task of the group. *Lancet*, **2**: 678–81. (*151*)

21 BLISS, R. W. 1948. The Army's part in the health program of the nation. *Bull. U.S. Army med. Dep.*, **8**: 341–9. (*277 n.*)

22 BRACELAND, F. J., 1947. Psychiatric lessons from World War II. *Amer. J. Psychiat.*, **103**: 587–93. (*252 n., 253*)

23 BRIDGER, H. 1946. The Northfield Experiment. *Bull. Menninger Clin.*, **10**: 71–6. (*152*)

24 BRODY, M. W. 1954. Venereal disease. *In: Recent Developments in Psychosomatic Medicine*, ed. E. D. Wittkower & R. A. Cleghorn; London (Isaac Pitman); pp. 364–80. (*213*)

25 BURT, C. 1942. Psychology in war: the military work of American and German psychologists. *Occup. Psychol.*, **16**: 95–110. (*38 n.*)

26 CALDWELL, J. M. 1948. The present status of neuropsychiatry in the Army. *Milit. Surg.*, **102**: 479–82. (*252 n.*)

27 CALDWELL, J. M. 1949. Current developments and problems in military neuropsychiatry. *Amer. J. Psychiat.*, **105**: 561–6. (*252 n.*)

28 CANTLIE, N. 1948. Forward psychiatry: address delivered . . . to a Conference on Psychiatry, August 8, 1944. *J.R. Army med. Cps.*, **91**: 93–5. (*183 n.*)

29 CHAPMAN, F. S. 1949. *The Jungle is Neutral*; London (Chatto & Windus); pp. 125–6. (*209*)

30 CHAPPELL, E. S. 1947. The role of the psychiatrist in the United States Disciplinary Barracks. *In: Handbook of Correctional Psychology*, ed. R. M. Lindner & R. V. Seliger; New York (Philosophical Library); pp. 333–48. (*140*)

31 COLLIE, G. F. 1943. Returned prisoners of war: a suggested scheme for rehabilitation. *The Fortnightly*, new ser., **153** (June): 407–11. (*228*)

32 *Courts-Martial Procedure and Administration of Justice in the Armed Forces* (Cmd. 8141); London (H.M.S.O.), 1951. (*139 n.*)

33 CRAIGIE, H. B. 1942. Physical treatment of acute war neurosis. *Brit. med. J.*, **2**: 675. (*179*)

34 CRAIGIE, H. B. 1943. Early recognition and treatment of psychiatric battle casualties. *Army med. Dep. Bull.*, Supplement No. 5 (June). (*179*)

35 CRAIGIE, H. B. 1944. Two years of military psychiatry in the Middle East. *Brit. med. J.*, **2**: 105–9. (*177, 178*)

36 CURLE, A. 1947. Transitional communities and social reconnection: a follow-up study of the civil resettlement of British prisoners of war; Part I. *Human Relations*, **1**: 42–68. (*227, 237, 241 n., 248*)

GENERAL BIBLIOGRAPHY

37 CURLE, A., & TRIST, E. 1947. Transitional communities and social reconnection; Part II. *Human Relations*, **1**: 240–88. (*235, 238, 241 n., 248, 249*)
38 CUTLER, E. C. 1944. A surgeon looks at two wars. *Lancet*, **2**: 429 (*188 n.*)
39 DAVIS, P. J. R. 1946. Divisional Psychiatry: report to the War Office. *J.R. Army med. Cps.*, **86**: 254–74. (*192*)
40 DAVIS, P. J. R., MILLER, J. W., & WILLIAMS, A. H. 1945. [Divisional] Psychiatry in Burma. *J.R. Army med. Cps.*, **84**: 66–9. (*192, 195*)
41 DICKS, H. V. 1950. Personality traits and National Socialist ideology. *Human Relations*, **3**: 111–54. (*224*)
42 DUKE-ELDER, P. M., & WITTKOWER, E. D. 1946. Psychological reactions in soldiers to loss of vision of one eye, and their treatment. *Brit. med. J.*, **1**: 155–8. (*161*)
43 DUNBAR, F. 1946. *Emotions and Bodily Changes*; New York (Columbia Univ. Press); 3rd ed., pp. 294–7. (*276 n.*)
44 *Expert Committee on Mental Health: Report on the First Session; World Health Org. techn. Rep. Ser.*, No. 9; Geneva, 1950; pp. 6–9, 32. (*3 n., 25 n.*)
45 FITTS, P. M. 1946. German applied psychology during World War II. *Amer. Psychologist*, **1**: 151–61. (*38 n.*)
46 FITZPATRICK, G. 1945. War Office Selection Boards and the role of the psychiatrist in them. *J.R. Army med. Cps.*, **84**: 75–8. (*63*)
47 FOULKES, S. H. 1948. *Introduction to Group-Analytic Psychotherapy*; London (Heinemann). (*151, 152, 153*)
48 FRASER, R. 1947. *The Incidence of Neurosis among Factory Workers; Med. Res. Council: Industr. Health Res. Board Rep.*, No. 90; London (H.M.S.O.). (*31 n.*)
49 FROST, F. [*pseud.* 'F. Beaumont']. 1946. 'Rip Van Winkle—1946.' *Transatlantic*, No. 30 (Feb.): 41–6. (*249*)
50 GALVIN, J. 1950. German psychiatry during the war. *Amer. J. Psychiat.*, **106**: 703–7. (*38 n.*)
51 GINZBERG, E. 1951. *Conservation of Human Resources: Progress Report, June, 1951*; New York (Graduate School of Business, Columbia University). (*4 n.*)
52 GLOVER, E. 1948. Freud or Jung. *Horizon*, **18** (Oct.): 242. (*6 n.*)
53 GREGG, A. 1947. Lessons to learn: psychiatry in World War II. *Amer. J. Psychiat.*, **104**: 217–20. (*252 n., 259*)
54 GRINKER, R. R., & SPIEGEL, J. P. 1943. *War Neuroses in North Africa: the Tunisian Campaign* (*January–May, 1943*); New York (Josiah Macy, Jr. Foundation); pp. 7, 95–6. (*5 n., 183 n., 184*)
55 GUTTMAN, E., & THOMAS, E. L. 1946. *A Report on the Re-Adjustment in Civil Life of Soldiers discharged from the Army on account of Neurosis; Ministry of Health Rep. Public Health med. Subjects*, No. 93; London (H.M.S.O.). (*161*)
56 HARRELL, T. W., & CHURCHILL, R. D. 1941. The classification of military personnel. *Psychol. Bull.*, **38**: 331–53. (*54 n.*)
57 HARRIS, H. 1949. *The Group Approach to Leadership-Testing*; London (Routledge & Kegan Paul). (*76 n.*)
58 HEWITT, M. 1949. The unemployed disabled man. *Lancet*, **2**: 523–6. (*162 n.*)
59 HILL, R. 1949. *Families under Stress: Adjustment to the Crisis of War Separation and Reunion*; New York (Harper & Bros.). (*250 n.*)
60 *History of the Great War: Medical Services—Diseases of the War*, Vol. 2; London (H.M.S.O.), 1923; Neurasthenia and War Neuroses, pp. 1–67. (*6, 7, 117*)

GENERAL BIBLIOGRAPHY

61 *History of the Second World War: United Kingdom Medical Series—Medicine and Pathology*, ed. V. Z. Cope; London (H.M.S.O.), 1952; R. J. Rosie, Psychiatry in the Army, pp. 357–71; and G. W. B. James, Psychiatry in the Middle East Force 1940–1943, pp. 371–81. *(15 n., 178 n.)*
62 HOGBEN, L., & JOHNSTONE, M. M. 1947. Relation of morbidity to age in the Army population. *Brit. J. soc. Med.*, 1: 149–81. *(276)*
63 HOME OFFICE. 1946. *Report of the Commissioners of Prisons, 1939–1941* (Cmd. 6820); London (H.M.S.O.); pp. 46–7. *(117 n.)*
64 HUNTER, H. D. 1946. The work of a Corps Psychiatrist in the Italian Campaign. *J.R. Army med. Cps.*, **86**: 127–30. *(185, 186)*
65 JAMES, G. W. B. 1945. Psychiatric lessons from active service. *Lancet*, 2: 801–5. *(180)*
66 JONES, E. 1945. Psychology and war conditions. *Psychoanal. Quart.*, **14**: 1–27. [Reprinted in: *The Yearbook of Psychoanalysis*, London (Imago Publishing Co.), 1946, **2**: 169–94.] *(27)*
67 KENTON, C. 1946. *In*: Discussion: forward psychiatry in the Army. *Proc. R. Soc. Med.*, 39: 137–40. *(169, 170)*
68 KNAPP, J. L., & WEITZEN, F. 1945. A total psychotherapeutic push method as practised in the Fifth Service Command Rehabilitation Centre. *Amer. J. Psychiat.*, **102**: 362–6. *(140)*
69 L'ETANG, H. J. C. J. 1951. A criticism of military psychiatry in the Second World War. *J.R. Army med. Cps.*, 97: 192–7, 236–44, 316–27. *(26 n.)*
70 LEWIS, A. 1943. Social effects of neurosis. *Lancet*, 1: 167–70. *(160)*
71 MACKEITH, S. A. 1946. Lasting lessons of overseas military psychiatry. *J. ment. Sci.*, **92**: 542–50. *(183, 184, 185, 186, 187, 207)*
72 MCLAUGHLIN, F. L., & MILLAR, W. M. 1941. Employment of air-raid noises in psychotherapy. *Brit. med. J.*, 2: 158–9. *(202)*
73 MAIN, T. F. 1946. *In*: Discussion: forward psychiatry in the Army. *Proc. R. Soc. Med.*, 39: 140–2. *(167)*
74 MAIN, T. F. 1946. The hospital as a therapeutic institution. *Bull. Menninger Clin.*, **10**: 66–70. *(152)*
75 MAIN, T. F. 1947. Clinical problems of repatriates. *J. ment. Sci.*, **93**: 354–63. *(249, 250)*
76 MARTEL, G. 1949. *An Outspoken Soldier*; London (Sifton Praed); pp. 324–6. *(65 n.)*
77 MEERLOO, J. A. M. 1952. Contribution of the psychiatrist to the management of crisis situations. *Amer. J. Psychiat.*, **109**: 352–5. *(28 n.)*
78 MENNINGER, W. C. 1947. Psychiatric experience in the War, 1941–1946. *Amer. J. Psychiat.*, **103**: 577–86. *(9 n., 252, 252 n., 253)*
79 MENNINGER, W. C. 1948. *Psychiatry in a Troubled World*; New York (Macmillan). *(252, 252 n., 253, 277 n.)*
80 MILLER, E. (ed.). 1940. *The Neuroses in War*; London (Macmillan). *(13, 14, 15)*
81 MIRA, E. 1944. *Psychiatry in War*; London (Chapman & Hall); Psychiatry in the Nazi Army, pp. 51–62. *(38 n.)*
82 MOLL, A. E. 1954. Psychosomatic disease due to battle stress. *In: Recent Developments in Psychosomatic Medicine*, ed. E. D. Wittkower & R. A. Cleghorn; London (Isaac Pitman); pp. 436–54. *(164 n.)*
83 MURRAY, J. M. 1947. Accomplishments of psychiatry in the Army Air Forces. *Amer. J. Psychiat.*, **103**: 594–9. *(252 n.)*
84 MYERS, C. S. 1940. *Shell Shock in France, 1914–18*; Cambridge (University Press). *(4, 5, 6, 8, 13, 14)*
85 NEWMAN, P. H. 1944. The prisoner-of-war mentality: its effect after repatriation. *Brit. med. J.*, 1: 8–10. *(233, 249)*

GENERAL BIBLIOGRAPHY

86 *Official History of the Canadian Medical Services 1939–1945*, ed. W. R. Feasby: Vol. 2, *Clinical Subjects*; Ottawa (Edmond Cloutier, Queen's Printer), 1953; Psychiatry in the Army, pp. 56–94. *(15 n.)*

87 *Official History of New Zealand in the Second World War 1939–45 — War Surgery and Medicine*, by T. D. M. Stout; Wellington (War History Branch, Dept. of Internal Affairs), 1954; Neurosis, pp. 630–57. *(15 n.)*

88 PALMER, H. A. 1945. Military psychiatric casualties: experience with 12,000 cases. *Lancet*, **2**: 454–7, 492–4. *(168, 169, 187)*

89 PATTON, G. S. 1947. *War as I Knew It*; Boston (Houghton Mifflin); pp. 340, 362, 381–2. *(5 n., 164 n., 272 n.)*

90 PENTON, J. C. 1946. Lessons from the Army for penal reformers. *Howard J.*, (1946–7), **7**: 81. *(140 n.)*

91 PRIVY COUNCIL OFFICE. 1947. *Report of an Expert Committee on the Work of Psychologists and Psychiatrists in the Services*; London (H.M.S.O.). *(10, 25, 26, 32)*

92 *Psychological Examining in the United States Army*, Washington, D.C. (U.S. Govt. Printing Office), 1921: *Mem. nat. Acad. Sci.*, **15**. *(38 n.)*

93 RATCLIFFE, T. A. 1947. Psychiatric and allied aspects of the problem of venereal disease in the Army: with particular reference to S.E.A.C. *J.R. Army med. Cps.*, **89**: 122–31. *(213)*

94 RATCLIFFE, T. A. 1947. The psychological problems of the returned ex-serviceman. *Ment. Health, London*, **7**: 2–5. *(249)*

95 READ, C. S. 1920. *Military Psychiatry in Peace and War*; London (H. K. Lewis). *(12, 99)*

96 REES, J. R. 1943. Three years of military psychiatry in the United Kingdom. *Brit. med. J.*, **1**: 1–6. *(9 n., 15, 32, 50, 98, 147)*

97 REES, J. R. 1945. *The Shaping of Psychiatry by War*; London (Chapman & Hall). *(6, 7, 10, 24, 28, 29, 29 n., 31, 32, 51, 52, 63, 64, 76, 82, 117, 144, 154, 156, 159, 164, 200, 213, 222, 253, 272 n.)*

98 REES, J. R. 1946. The development of psychiatry in the British Army. *In: Military Neuropsychiatry*, Baltimore (Williams & Wilkins): *Res. Publ. Ass. nerv. ment. Dis.*, **25**: 48–53. *(16)*

99 REES, J. R. (ed.) 1947. *The Case of Rudolf Hess*; London (Heinemann); pp. 195–202. *(224)*

100 REES, J. R. 1950. *In*: Discussion; *Epidemiology of Mental Disorder*; New York (Milbank Memorial Fund); pp. 51–2, 127. *(3)*

101 REES, J. R. 1957. The thirty-first Maudsley Lecture: psychiatry and public health. *J. ment. Sci.*, **103**: 314–25. *(3)*

102 *Report of the Prime Minister's Committee of Enquiry into Detention Barracks, 1943* (Cmd. 6484); London (H.M.S.O.), 1943. *(129, 131, 131 n., 135 n.)*

103 *Report of the Health Survey and Development Committee*; Calcutta (Govt. of India Press), 1946; Vol. **1**, pp. 130–2; Vol. **2**, pp. 206–17; Vol. **3**, Appendix 21, pp. 44–74 (Report by Col. M. Taylor, I.M.S., on his tour of mental hospitals), and Appendices 22–23, pp. 75–8; Vol. **4**, pp. 48–50. *(191 n.)*

104 *Report of the Army and Air Force Courts-Martial Committee, 1946* (Cmd. 7608); London (H.M.S.O.), 1949. *(139 n., 221 n., 261, 262)*

105 *Report from the Select Committee on the Army Act and Air Force Act*; London (H.M.S.O.), 1953. *(139 n., 221 n.)*

106 *Report from the Select Committee on the Army Act and Air Force Act, Session 1953–54*; London (H.M.S.O.), 1954. *(139 n.)*

107 RICHMOND, A. E. 1947. Positive health: its attainment in the soldier and the Army's contribution to it in the civilian. *J.R. Army med. Cps.*, **89**: 274–89. *(277 n.)*

GENERAL BIBLIOGRAPHY

108 RODGER, A. 1937. *A Borstal Experiment in Vocational Guidance; Med. Res. Council: Industr. Health Res. Board Rep.*, No. 78; London (H.M.S.O.) (*31 n.*)
109 RODGER, T. F. 1948. Personnel selection. In: *Modern Trends in Psychological Medicine*, ed. N. G. Harris; London (Butterworth); pp. 347–62. (*50 n., 76 n.*)
110 ROSIE, R. J. 1948. The early days of Army psychiatry. *J.R. Army med. Cps.*, **90**: 93–100. (*143 n.*)
111 ROSNER, A. A., & BALSER, B. H. 1950. Research in military neuropsychiatry, September 1945 to September 1947. *Amer. J. Psychiat.*, **106**: 808–11. (*252 n.*)
112 SARGANT, W. 1957. *Battle for the Mind: A Physiology of Conversion and Brain-Washing*; London (Heinemann); pp. 21–41 (and *passim*). (*164 n.*)
113 SARGANT, W., & SLATER, E. 1940. Acute war neuroses. *Lancet*, **2**: 1–2. (*164 n., 175*)
114 SCOTTISH HOME DEPARTMENT. 1948. *Psycho-Therapeutic Treatment of Certain Offenders, with special reference to the case of persons convicted of Sexual and Unnatural Offences*; Edinburgh (H.M.S.O.). (*139 n., 267*)
115 SEMRAD, E. V. 1944. Rehabilitation of military offenders. In: *Manual of Military Neuropsychiatry*, ed. H. C. Solomon & P. I. Yakovlev; Philadelphia (W. B. Saunders); pp. 570–5. (*140*)
116 SMITH, D. A., & WOODRUFF, M. F. A. 1951. *Deficiency Diseases in Japanese Prison Camps; Spec. Rep. Ser. med. Res. Council*, No. 274; London (H.M.S.O.); pp. 48–9. (*236 n.*)
117 SMITH, M., & LEIPER, M. A. 1936. *Sickness Absence and Labour Wastage*; Part I: Sickness absence: its measurement and incidence in clerical work and light occupations; *Med. Res. Council: Industr. Health Res. Board Rep.*, No. 75; London (H.M.S.O.). (*31 n.*)
118 SNYDER, H. M. 1947. Observations of psychiatry in World War II. *Amer. J. Psychiat.*, **104**: 221–5. (*252 n.*)
119 SPENCER, J. C. 1954. *Crime and the Services*; London (Routledge & Kegan Paul). (*136 n., 140 n.*)
120 STANBRIDGE, R. H. 1936. The occupational selection of aircraft apprentices of the Royal Air Force. *Lancet*, **1**: 1426–30. (*31 n.*)
121 STRECKER, E. A., & APPEL, K. E. 1946. Psychiatric contrasts in the two World Wars. In: *Military Neuropsychiatry*, Baltimore (Williams & Wilkins); *Res. Publ. Ass. nerv. ment. Dis.*, **24**: 38–44. (*252, 252 n., 273 n.*)
122 TRENAMAN, J. 1952. *Out of Step*; London (Methuen). (*112 n.*)
123 TUNBRIDGE, R. E. 1945. Psychiatric experiences of a general physician in Malta, 1941–3. *Lancet*, **2**: 587–90. (*189, 190*)
124 U.S. SURGEON GENERAL'S OFFICE. 1929. *The Medical Department of the United States Army in the World War*: Vol. **10**, *Neuropsychiatry*; Washington, D.C. (U.S. Govt. Printing Office); pp. 7–8, 26–7, 72–4; and T. W. Salmon, The Care and Treatment of Mental Diseases and War Neurosis ('Shell Shock') in the British Army, pp. 497–523. (*7, 9, 10, 11, 117, 170 n., 252*)
125 VERNON, P. E., & PARRY, J. B. 1949. *Personnel Selection in the British Forces*; London (Univ. of London Press). (*38 n., 50 n., 74, 76 n.*)
126 VON STORCH, T. J. C., PRATT, G. O., et al. 1941. Observations and suggestions concerning neuropsychiatric examinations for the Army of the United States. *New Engl. J. Med.*, **224**: 890–7. (*94 n.*)
127 WAR DEPARTMENT (INDIA). 1945. *Finding Officers for the Services*; Calcutta (War Dept., Govt. of India). (*69 n.*)

GENERAL BIBLIOGRAPHY

128 WAR OFFICE. 1922. *Report of the War Office Committee of Enquiry into 'Shell-Shock'* (Cmd. 1734); London (H.M.S.O.). (*13, 13 n., 22, 30, 40 n., 198 n., 252, 274 n.*)

129 WAR OFFICE. 1922. *Statistics of the Military Effort of the British Empire during the Great War: 1914–1920*; London (H.M.S.O.). (*271*)

130 WAR OFFICE. 1948. *Statistical Report on the Health of the Army, 1943–1945*; London (H.M.S.O.). (*183 n., 210 n., 276, 277 n.*)

131 WEISS, E., & ENGLISH, O. S. 1943. *Psychosomatic Medicine*; Philadelphia (W. B. Saunders); pp. 238–51. (*276 n.*)

132 WEISS, I. I. 1946. Rehabilitation of military offenders at the Ninth Service Command Rehabilitation Centre. *Amer. J. Psychiat.*, **103**: 172–8. (*140*)

133 WILSON, A. T. M. 1946. The serviceman comes home. *Pilot Papers*, **1**, No. 2 (April): 9–28. (*227, 231, 232, 238, 242, 246, 249*)

134 WILSON, A. T. M., DOYLE, M., & KELNAR, J. 1947. Group techniques in a transitional community. *Lancet*, **1**: 735–8. (*242, 245*)

135 WITTKOWER, E. D. 1945. The war-disabled: their emotional, social and occupational situation. *Brit. med. J.*, **1**: 587–90. (*161*)

136 WITTKOWER, E. D. 1947. Rehabilitation of the limbless: a joint surgical and psychologic study. *Occup. Med.*, **3**: 20–44. (*161, 162*)

137 WITTKOWER, E. D. 1949. Psychosomatic medicine. In: *Modern Practice in Psychological Medicine*, ed. J. R. Rees; London (Butterworth); pp. 103–34. (*161, 213*)

138 WITTKOWER, E. D., & COWAN, J. 1944. Some psychological aspects of sexual promiscuity. *Psychosom. Med.*, **6**: 287–94. (*213*)

139 WITTKOWER, E. D., & DAVENPORT, R. C. 1946. The war-blinded: their emotional, social, and occupational situation. *Psychosom. Med.*, **8**: 121–37. (*161*)

140 WITTKOWER, E. D., & LEBEAUX, L. 1943. The Special Transfer Scheme: an experiment in military psychiatric vocational re-employment. *Med. Press*, **209**: 366–8. (*155*)

141 YOAKUM, C. S., & YERKES, R. M. 1920. *Mental Tests in the American Army*; London (Sidgwick & Jackson). (*38 n., 78 n.*)

SUPPLEMENTARY BIBLIOGRAPHY

SUPPLEMENTARY (TECHNICAL) BIBLIOGRAPHY OF PUBLISHED WORKS ON BRITISH ARMY PSYCHIATRY AND RELATED SUBJECTS

N.B.—Works referred to in the text and listed in the General Bibliography are *not* here included.

For the purpose of providing a convenient source of reference, every attempt has been made to render this supplementary bibliography as comprehensive as possible, with respect to the subject matter under consideration: it is, therefore, in no way critically selective. Although it covers the period 1939–June 1957, it is not primarily concerned with material relating to post-war problems and developments, and such references are included only in so far as they appear to be more immediately relevant to the present work.

A. ARMY PSYCHIATRY—GENERAL WORKS

GILLESPIE, R. D. 1942. *Psychological Effects of War on Citizen and Soldier*; London (Chapman & Hall).
JAMES, G. W. B. 1945. The future of psychiatry in the Army Medical Service. *J.R. Army med. Cps.*, **84**: 51–3.
KRAPF, E. E. 1944. Wartime psychiatry in Britain. *Britannica*, **31**, No. 4: 11; No. 5: 15. [Abstracted in: *Psychoanal. Quart.*, 1946, **15**: 410–11.]
LEWIS, M. M. 1951. The promotion and maintenance of mental health in the military community. *J.R. Army med. Cps.*, **96**: 17–40, 102–14.
PENFIELD, W. 1942. Clinical notes from a trip to Great Britain. *Arch. Neurol. Psychiat., Chicago*, **47**: 1030–6.
POZNER, H. 1950. Some aspects of post-war Army psychiatry. *J.R. Army med. Cps.*, **94**: 38–47.
REES, J. R. 1944. Brief impression of British military psychiatry. *Bull. Menninger Clin.*, **8**: 29–35.
REES, J. R. 1944. Psychiatry in the British Army. *Amer. J. Psychiat.*, **101**: 20–2.
REES, J. R. 1945. Development of psychiatry in the British Army. *Dig. Neurol. Psychiat.*, **13**: 27–30.
SARGANT, W., & SLATER, E. 1952. The influence of the 1939–45 War on British psychiatry. *C.R. Ier Congrès mondial Psychiatrie, 1950*, Paris (Hermann); **6** (Psychiatrie Sociale): 180–96.

B. NEUROSES AND PSYCHOSES; CLINICAL PSYCHIATRY
(see also: C, D, E)

ANDERSON, C. 1942. Chronic head cases. *Lancet*, **2**: 1–4.

SUPPLEMENTARY BIBLIOGRAPHY

ANDERSON, C., JEFFREY, M., & PAI, M. N. 1944. Psychiatric casualties from the Normandy beach-head: first thoughts on 100 cases. *Lancet*, 2: 218–21.
ANON. 1939. Neuroses in war-time: memorandum for the medical profession. *Brit. med. J.*, 2: 1199–1201.
BECCLE, H. C. 1942. War psychoses: their nature and treatment. *Med. Press*, 208: 136–9.
BELLAMY, W. A. 1945. Battle exhaustion. *Med. Press*, 214: 155–6.
BENNET, E. A. 1941. Anxiety states in war. *Med. Press*, 205: 128–30.
BERG, C. 1940. Emergence of unsuspected war neurosis. *Practitioner*, 145: 345–8.
BERG, C. 1942. Clinical notes on the analysis of a war neurosis. *Brit. J. med. Psychol.*, 19: 155–85.
BROOKE, E. M. 1946. Battle exhaustion: review of 500 cases from Western Europe. *Brit. med. J.*, 2: 491–3.
CAROTHERS, J. C. 1953. *The African Mind in Health and Disease; World Health Org. Monogr. Ser.*, No. 17; Geneva; pp. 145–6, 150–1, 153–5, 159. [African troops.]
CULPIN, M. 1940. A week-end with the war neuroses. *Lancet*, 2: 257–9.
DEMBOVITZ, N. 1945. Psychiatry amongst West African troops. *J.R. Army med. Cps.*, 84: 70–4.
DIXON, H. B. F., & HARGREAVES, W. H. 1944. Cysticercosis (*Taenia solium*): a further ten years' clinical study, covering 284 cases. [Servicemen in India.] *Quart. J. Med.*, new ser., 13: 107–21.
DOUGLAS-WILSON, I. 1943. Minor psychological disturbances in the Services. *J.R. Army med. Cps.*, 81: 283–8.
EMANUEL, E. 1947. Transient abnormal behaviour in Indian troops. *J. Indian Army med. Cps.*, 3: 76–9.
EYSENCK, H. J. 1944. Types of personality: factorial study of 700 neurotics. *J. ment. Sci.*, 90: 851–61.
FAIRBAIRN, W. R. D. 1943. Repression and return of bad objects [in war neuroses]. *Brit J. med Psychol.*, 19: 327–41.
FAIRBAIRN, W. R. D. 1943. The war neuroses: their nature and significance. *Brit. med. J.*, 1: 183–6.
FRASER, R., LESLIE, I. M., & PHELPS, D. 1943. Psychiatric effects of severe personal experiences during bombing. *Proc. R. Soc. Med.*, 36: 119–23.
FREEMAN, A. G. 1946. Effect on troops of the 'V' weapon bombardment of Antwerp. *Brit. med. J.*, 1: 58–9.
GARMANY, G. 1946. Schizophrenia in the Forces. *J. ment. Sci.*, 92: 802–7.
GILLESPIE, W. H. 1944. The psychoneuroses. *In: Recent Progress in Psychiatry*, London (J. &. A. Churchill); *J. ment. Sci.*, 90: 287–306.
GOOD, R. 1942. Malingering. *Brit. med. J.*, 2: 359–62.
GUTTMAN, E. 1946. Late effects of closed head injuries: psychiatric observations. *J. ment. Sci.*, 92: 1–18.
HADFIELD, J. A. 1942. War neurosis: a year in a neuropathic hospital. *Brit. med. J.*, 1: 281–5, 320–3.
HALL, S. B., & HALL, M. B. 1942. Prognosis in mental instability: adolescent and service cases. *Lancet*, 1: 376–8.
HEMPHILL, R. E. 1941. Importance of the first year of war in mental disease. *Bristol med.-chir. J.*, 85: 11–18.
HEPPENSTALL, M. E., HILL, D., & SLATER, E. 1945. The E.E.G. in the prognosis of war neurosis. *Brain*, 68: 17–22.
HILL, D. 1941. Head injury and war neurosis. *Med. Press*, 205: 140–3.
HUBERT, W. H. de B. 1941. Acute nervous illness in active warfare. *Lancet*, 1: 306–8.

SUPPLEMENTARY BIBLIOGRAPHY

IRONSIDE, R. 1940. Feigned epilepsy in wartime. *Brit. med. J.*, **1**: 703–5.
JAMES, G. W. B. 1940. Anxiety neurosis. *Lancet*, **2**: 561–4.
JOHNSON, A. S. 1946. Some observations on the psychiatric casualties amongst I.O.Rs. [Indian other ranks]. *J. Indian Army med. Cps.*, **2**: 24–6.
KENNEDY, A. 1941. Hysteria in war conditions. *Med. Press*, **205**: 135–40.
LAUDENHEIMER, R. 1940. Predisposition in neuroses of war. *Med. Press*, **204**: 43–5.
LEIGH, A. D. 1941. Neurosis as viewed by a regimental medical officer. *Lancet*, **1**: 394–6.
LEWIS, A. 1942. Incidence of neurosis in England under war conditions. *Lancet*, **2**: 175–83.
LEWIS, A. 1943. Mental health in war-time. *Publ. Health, London*, **57**: 27–30.
LOGAN, W. R. 1941. Mental disease among the Services in Singapore. *J. ment. Sci.*, **87**: 241–55.
MACLAY, W. S., & GUTTMAN, E. 1940. The War as an aetiological factor in psychiatric conditions. *Brit. med. J.*, **2**: 381–3.
MATAS, J. 1945. A note on psychiatry in Indian troops—(Psychiatry in Burma). *J.R. Army med. Cps.*, **84**: 69.
MAYER-GROSS, W. 1939. Practical psychiatry in war-time. *Lancet*, **2**: 1327–30.
MILLER, E. 1945. Psychiatric casualties among officers and men from Normandy: distribution of aetiological factors. *Lancet*, **1**: 364–6.
MINISTRY OF PENSIONS. 1940. *Neuroses in War-Time: Memorandum for the Information of the Medical Profession*; London (H.M.S.O.).
MINSKI, L. 1944. War neurosis. *Med. Press*, **212**: 100–3.
MULLINDER, E. K. 1945. Psychotic battle casualties. *Brit. med. J.*, **1**: 733.
NEUSTATTER, W. L. 1942. The role of mild cerebral commotion in war neurosis. *Proc. R. Soc. Med.*, **35**: 549–52.
NEUSTATTER, W. L. 1943. Hysterical amnesia in soldiers, and some medico-legal implications. *Practitioner*, **150**: 35–9.
NEUSTATTER, W. L. 1945. What is a 'black-out'?—study of 50 cases. *J.R. Army med. Cps.*, **85**: 139–42.
NEUSTATTER, W. L. 1946. 750 psychoneurotics and ten weeks' fly-bombing. *J. ment. Sci.*, **92**: 110–17.
NICHOLS, L. A. 1944. Neuroses in native African troops. *J. ment. Sci.*, **90**: 862–8.
O'MEARA, F. J. 1951. B.A.O.R. medicine 1946–1949. *J.R. Army med. Cps.*, **97**: 38–40 (Psychiatry).
PAI, M. N. 1946. Sleep-walking and sleep activities. *J. ment. Sci.*, **92**: 756–65.
PALMER, H. A. 1944. Case report of psychosis following heat stroke. *J.R. Army med. Cps.*, **82**: 186–9.
PATERSON, A., REYNELL, W. R., & KREMER, M. 1944. Discussion on disorders of personality after head injury. *Proc. R. Soc. Med.*, **37**: 556–66.
PEARCE, J. D. W. 1945. Clinical aspects of psychiatric problems in the Army. *Practitioner*, **154**: 33–8.
PERK, D. 1947. Mepacrine psychosis. *J. ment. Sci.*, **93**: 756–71.
PETRIE, A. A. W. 1942. Types of psychopathic personality. *J. ment. Sci.*, **88**: 491–3.
RICKMAN, J. 1941. A case of hysteria: theory and practice in two wars. *Lancet*, **1**: 785–6.
ROBERTS, W. W. 1943. The death-instinct in morbid anxiety. *J.R. Army med. Cps.*, **81**: 61–73.
ROBERTS, W. W., &. MOORE, J. N. P. 1947. Mental illness among Army officers: a survey of admissions to a military psychiatric hospital. *Brit. J. soc. Med.*, **1**: 135–47.

SUPPLEMENTARY BIBLIOGRAPHY

ROSENBERG, E. 1943. A clinical contribution to the psychopathology of the war neuroses. *Int. J. Psychoanal.*, **24**: 32–41. [Reprinted in: *The Yearbook of Psychoanalysis*, London (Imago Publishing Co.), 1945, **1**: 237–55.]

RUDOLF, G. de M. 1946. 'Night nurse's paralysis': a temporary tonic motor paralysis. *Bristol med.-chir. J.*, **63**: 132–5.

RUDOLF, G. de M. 1946. Psychological aspects of a conscious temporary generalized paralysis. *J. ment. Sci.*, **92**: 814–16.

RUDOLF, G. de M. 1947. Brief retrograde amnesia. *J. ment. Sci.*, **93**: 342–53.

SARGANT, W., & SHORVON, H. J. 1945. Acute war neurosis: special reference to Pavlov's experimental observations and the mechanism of abreaction. *Arch. Neurol. Psychiat., Chicago*, **54**: 231–40.

SARGANT, W., & SLATER, E. 1941. Amnesic syndromes in war. *Proc. R. Soc. Med.*, **34**: 757–64.

SILVERMAN, M. 1950. Causes of neurotic breakdown in British service personnel stationed in the Far East in peacetime. *J. ment. Sci.*, **96**: 494–501.

SIM, M. 1945. The N.C.O. as a psychiatric casualty: study of 627 cases admitted to a psychiatric hospital. *J.R. Army med. Cps.*, **85**: 184–6.

SIM, M. 1946. A comparative study of disease incidence in admissions to a Base Psychiatric Hospital in the Middle East. *J. ment. Sci.*, **92**: 118–27.

SIM, M. 1946. Quantitative estimation in psychiatric diagnosis. *J.R. Army med. Cps.*, **87**: 281–5.

SLATER, E. 1941. War neuroses: general symptomatology and constitutional factors. *Med. Press*, **205**: 133–5.

SLATER, E. 1943. The neurotic constitution: a statistical study of 2,000 neurotic soldiers. *J. Neurol. Psychiat.*, new ser., **6**: 1–16.

SLATER, E. 1947. Neurosis and religious affiliation. *J. ment. Sci.*, **93**: 392–6.

SNOWDEN, E. N. 1939. Prevention of war psychoneurosis in soldiers. *Lancet*, **2**: 1130–2.

SODDY, K. 1946. Some lessons of wartime psychiatry. *Ment. Health, London*, **6**: 30–5, 66–70.

STOCKINGS, G. T. 1944. Acute neurotic depression as seen in military psychiatry and its differential diagnosis from depressive psychosis. *J. ment. Sci.*, **90**: 772–6.

STOCKINGS, G. T. 1945. Schizophrenia in military psychiatric practice. *J. ment. Sci.*, **91**: 110–12.

STOCKINGS, G. T. 1945. The syndrome of hystero-encephalopathy in military psychiatric casualties. *J. ment. Sci.*, **91**: 104–9.

STUNGO, E. 1946. Psychiatric casualties in Burma, 1945. *J. ment. Sci.*, **92**: 585–94.

SUTHERLAND, J. D. 1941. A survey of 100 cases of war neuroses. *Brit. med. J.*, **2**: 365–70.

SUTHERLAND, J. M., & ROSIE, J. M. 1955. Cerebral cysticercosis with mental symptoms. [Servicemen in India.] *J. ment. Sci.*, **102**: 343–4.

SYMONDS, C. P. 1943. Anxiety neurosis in combatants. *Lancet*, **2**: 785–9.

SYMONDS, C. P., & LEWIS, A. 1942. Discussion on the differential diagnosis and treatment of post-contusional states. *Proc. R. Soc. Med.*, **35**: 601–14.

SYMONDS, C. P., & RUSSELL, W. R. 1943. Accidental head injuries: prognosis in service patients. *Lancet*, **1**: 7–10.

TORRIE, A. 1944. Psychosomatic casualties in the Middle East. *Lancet*, **1**: 139–43.

TREDGOLD, R. F. 1941. Depressive states in the soldier: their symptoms, causation, and prognosis. *Brit. med. J.*, **2**: 109–12.

TREDGOLD, R. F. 1942. Invalidism from the Army due to mental disabilities: aetiological significance of military conditions. *J. ment. Sci.*, **88**: 444–8.

SUPPLEMENTARY BIBLIOGRAPHY

TREDGOLD, R. F. 1944. The importance of failure of concentration in the acute war neurosis syndrome. *J.R. Army med. Cps.*, **82**: 177–82.
TREDGOLD, R. F. 1947. Manic states in the Far East. *Brit. med. J.*, **2**: 522–5.
TREDGOLD, R. F., KELLY, G., et al. 1946. Serious psychiatric disability among British officers in India. *Lancet*, **2**: 257–61.
TRONCHIN-JAMES, R. N. 1945. Sociological aspects of psychoneurosis. *Practitioner*, **154**: 307–11.
WAR OFFICE. 1943. Confusional mental states. *Army med. Dep. Bull.*, No. 24: 1–3.
WITTKOWER, E. D., & SPILLANE, J. P. 1940. Neuroses in war. *Brit. med. J.*, **1**: 223–5, 265–8, 308–10.
WRIGHT, M. B. 1939. Psychological emergencies in war-time. *Brit. med. J.*, **2**: 576–8.
YELLOWLEES, H. 1940. Anxiety states. *J.R. Army med. Cps.*, **74**: 327–34.
ZANGWILL, O. L. 1945. A review of psychological work at the Brain Injuries Unit, Edinburgh, 1941–5. *Brit. med. J.*, **2**: 248–51.

C. TREATMENT OF PSYCHIATRIC DISORDERS (see also: B, E)

BLAIR, D. 1943. Group psychotherapy for war neuroses. *Lancet*, **1**: 204–5.
BRAMWELL, E. 1940. Treatment of wartime neuroses in combatants. *Practitioner*, **145**: 124–31.
CAMERON, K. 1940. Occupation therapy for war neuroses. *Lancet*, **2**: 659–60.
COSSA, P., AUGUIN, P., & CHIPPONI, P. 1946. Traitements anglo-saxons des névroses de guerre. *Presse méd.*, **54**: 394–5.
DEBENHAM, G. R. 1941. Psychotherapy and occupation therapy in war neuroses. *Med. Press*, **205**: 143–5.
DEBENHAM, G. R., SARGANT, W., et al. 1941. Treatment of war neurosis. *Lancet*, **1**: 107–9.
DEWAR, M. C. 1946. The technique of group therapy. *Bull. Menninger Clin.*, **10**: 82–4.
DICKS, H. V. 1940. Hypnotics in psychotherapy [Report of paper]. *Brit. med. J.*, **1**: 865.
EDKINS, J. R. P. 1948. Further developments in abreaction. *In: Modern Trends in Psychological Medicine*, ed. N. G. Harris; London (Butterworth); pp. 265–86.
FOULKES, S. H. 1946. Group analysis in a Military Neurosis Centre. *Lancet*, **1**: 303–6.
FOULKES, S. H. 1946. On group analysis. *Int. J. Psychoanal.*, **27**: 46–51.
FOULKES, S. H. 1946. Principles and practice of group therapy. *Bull. Menninger Clin.*, **10**: 85–9.
FOULKES, S. H., & LEWIS, E. 1944. Group analysis: a study in the treatment of groups on psycho-analytic lines. *Brit. J. med. Psychol.*, **20**: 175–84.
GOOD, R. 1941. Convulsion therapy in war psychoneurotics. *J. ment. Sci.*, **87**: 409–18.
HALDANE, F. P., & ROWLEY, J. L. 1946. Psychiatry at the Corps Exhaustion Centre. *Lancet*, **2**: 599–601.
JONES, M. 1942. Group psychotherapy. *Brit. med. J.*, **2**: 276–8.
JONES, M. 1944. Group treatment, with particular reference to group projection methods. *Amer. J. Psychiat.*, **101**: 292–9.
MINSKI, L. 1941. Emergency Medical Service: the organization of a neurological clinic. *Med. Press*, **205**: 131–3.
MURRAY, H. S. E., & HALSTEAD, H. 1947. Head injuries: a new treatment for the post-concussive syndrome. *J. ment. Sci.*, **93**: 303–17.

SUPPLEMENTARY BIBLIOGRAPHY

NEUSTATTER, W. L. 1942. Hysterical stupor recovering after cardiazol treatment. *J. ment. Sci.*, **88**: 440–3.
PALMER, H. A. 1945. Abreactive techniques—ether. *J.R. Army med. Cps.*, **84**: 86–7.
PALMER, H. A., KENTON, C., et al. 1946. Discussion: forward psychiatry in the Army. *Proc. R. Soc. Med.*, **39**: 137–42.
RICKMAN, J. 1957. The factor of number in individual and group dynamics. *Selected Contributions to Psycho-Analysis*; London (Hogarth Press); pp. 165–9. [Reprinted, with additions, from *J. ment. Sci.*, 1950, **96**: 770–3.]
ROBINSON, J. T. 1948. Group therapy and its application in the British Army to-day. *J.R. Army med. Cps.*, **91**: 66–79.
SARGANT, W. 1941. Some physical treatments of war neuroses. *Med. Press*, **205**: 145–8.
SARGANT, W. 1942. Physical treatment of acute war neuroses: some clinical observations. *Brit. med. J.*, **2**: 574–6.
SARGANT, W. 1943. Physical treatments of acute psychiatric states in war. *War Med., Chicago*, **4**: 557–81.
SARGANT, W., & CRASKE, N. 1941. Modified insulin therapy in war neuroses. *Lancet*, **2**: 212–14.
SARGANT, W., & STEWART, C. M. 1947. Chronic battle neurosis treated with leucotomy. *Brit. med. J.*, **2**: 866–9.
SHORVON, H. J., & SARGANT, W. 1947. Excitatory abreaction: with special reference to its mechanism and the use of ether. *J. ment. Sci.*, **93**: 709–32.
STOCKINGS, G. T. 1944. Shock-therapy in psychoses: a possible rational basis and its clinical applications, based on 3 years' experience of its use in military psychiatry. *J. ment. Sci.*, **90**: 550–3.
THORNER, H. A. 1946. The treatment of psychoneurosis in the British Army. *Int. J. Psychoanal.*, **27**: 52–9.
WEBER, H. 1943. The treatment of fear in recruits. *Med. Press*, **210**: 157–9.
WILDE, J. F. 1942. Narcoanalysis in the treatment of war neuroses. *Brit. med. J.*, **2**: 4–7.
WILDE, J. F., & MORGAN, C. J. 1943. Occupational therapy for psychoneurotics in hospital. *J.R. Army med. Cps.*, **81**: 24–31.

D. PSYCHOSOMATIC RELATIONSHIPS (see also: B)

BACKUS, P. L., & MANSELL, G. S. 1944. Investigation and treatment of enuresis in the Army: preliminary report on 277 cases. *Brit. med. J.*, **2**: 462–5.
BAKER, D., & TEGNER, W. S. 1945. Effort syndrome at an Army Physical Development Centre. *J.R. Army med. Cps.*, **84**: 232–4.
COOK, G. T., & SARGANT, W. 1942. Neurosis simulating organic disorder. *Lancet*, **1**: 31–2.
DANSON, J. G. 1942. The effort syndrome. *Med. Press*, **208**: 185–8.
DOUGLAS-WILSON, I. 1944. Somatic manifestations of psychoneurosis. *Brit. med. J.*, **1**: 413–15.
FRASER, F. R. 1940. Effort syndrome in the present war. *Edinb. med. J.*, new ser., **47**: 451–65.
GILSENAN, B. M. C. 1946. Dyspepsia of peptic ulcer type and its relationship to personality type and anxiety. *Practitioner*, **156**: 456–8.
GODDARD, D. L. H. 1945. Effort syndrome in the West African soldier. *Brit. med. J.*, **1**: 908–10.
GRAHAM, J. G., & KERR, J. D. O. 1941. The effort syndrome. *Glasg. med. J.*, new ser., **18**: 55–71.

SUPPLEMENTARY BIBLIOGRAPHY

GRANGER, G. W. 1954. The night visual ability of psychiatric patients. *Dioptric Rev. & Brit. J. physiol. Optics*, **11**: 226–32.

GRANGER, G. W. 1957. Night vision and psychiatric disorders: a review of experimental studies. *J. ment. Sci.*, **103**: 48–79.

GUTTMAN, E., & MAYER-GROSS, W. 1940. Psychology of mutilation and disablement. *Lancet*, **2**: 185–6.

HARROWES, W. M. 1946. Psychological reactions in war-blinded. *Brit. med. J.*, **2**: 129–30.

HILL, I. G. W., & DEWAR, H. A. 1945. 'Effort syndrome.' *Lancet*, **2**: 161–4.

HIMMELWEIT, H. T., DESAI, M., & PETRIE, A. 1946. An experimental investigation of neuroticism. *J. Personality*, **15**: 173–96.

HURST, A. 1941. Hysterical contractures following injuries in war. *Clinical J.*, **70**: 29–40.

JONES, M., & LEWIS, A. 1941. Effort syndrome. *Lancet*, **1**: 813–18.

JONES, W. L. 1942. Psychogenic illness in regimental practice. *Brit. med. J.*, **2**: 338–40.

LEWIS, A. 1941. Psychiatric aspects of effort syndrome. *Proc. R. Soc. Med.*, **34**: 758–60.

LINDSAY, S. F. 1946. Fatigue syndromes in West Africa. *Brit. med. J.*, **1**: 758–60.

LIVINGSTON, P. C., & BOLTON, B. 1943. Night visual capacity of psychological cases. *Lancet*, **1**: 263–4.

MCGREGOR, H. G. 1944. Physical examination of 2,000 cases of neurosis. *J. Neurol. Psychiat.*, new ser., **7**: 21–6.

MACKENNA, R. M. B. 1944. Psychosomatic factors in cutaneous disease. *Lancet*, **2**: 679–81.

MICHAELSON, I. C. 1943. Ocular manifestations of neuroses commonly found among soldiers. *Brit. med. J.*, **2**: 538–41.

MINSKI, L. 1942. Psychological reactions to injury. *Proc. R. Soc. Med.*, **35**: 195–9.

MINSKI, L. 1945. Psychological reactions in the wounded. *Brit. med. J.*, **1**: 444–5.

MITCHELL, S. D., & MULLIN, C. S. 1944. The neurotic dyspeptic soldier. *J. ment. Sci.*, **90**: 869–74.

OSBORNE, J. W., & COWEN, J. 1945. Psychiatric factors in peripheral vasoneuropathy after chilling. *Lancet*, **2**: 204–6.

REES, W. L. L. 1944. Physical constitution, neurosis and psychosis. *Proc. R. Soc. Med.*, **37**: 635–8.

REES, W. L. L. 1945. Night visual capacity of neurotic soldiers. *J. Neurol. Psychiat.*, **8**: 34–9.

REES, W. L. L. 1945. Physique and effort syndrome. *J. ment. Sci.*, **91**: 89–92.

REES, W. L. L., & EYSENCK, H. J. 1945. A factorial study of some morphological and psychological aspects of human constitution. *J. ment. Sci.*, **91**: 8–21.

RODGER, D. E. 1943. Effort syndrome in Iceland. *Brit. med. J.*, **1**: 351–2.

SPILLANE, J. D. 1940. Observations on effort syndrome. *Brit. med. J.*, **2**: 739–41.

STEADMAN, B. St. J. 1942. An investigation of night vision among personnel in an A.A. unit. *J.R. Army med. Cps.*, **78**: 14–24.

WITTKOWER, E. D. 1946. Psychological aspects of psoriasis. *Lancet*, **1**: 566–9.

WITTKOWER, E. D. 1947. Psychological aspects of seborrhoeic dermatitis. *Brit. J. Derm.*, **59**: 281–93.

WITTKOWER, E. D., RODGER, T. F., & WILSON, A. T. M. 1941. Effort syndrome. *Lancet*, **1**: 531–5.

WITTKOWER, E. D., RODGER, T. F., et al. 1941. 'Night blindness': a psychophysiological study. *Brit. med. J.*, **2**: 571–5, 607–11.

WOOD, P. 1941. Da Costa's syndrome. *Brit. med. J.*, **1**: 767–72, 805–11, 845–51.

SUPPLEMENTARY BIBLIOGRAPHY

E. RESETTLEMENT AND REHABILITATION; PSYCHIATRIC AFTER-CARE; PSYCHOLOGY OF PRISONERS OF WAR (see also: D)

BAVIN, M. G. 1947. A contribution towards the understanding of the repatriated prisoner of war. *Brit. J. psychiatr. soc. Work*, Sept., 1947: pp. 29–35.

BODMAN, F. 1946. Psychiatric cases referred by After-Care Officers in Region 7. *Brit. med. J.*, **2**: 59–60.

BOOTLE-WILBRAHAM, L. 1946. Civil resettlement of ex-prisoners of war. *Ment. Health, London*, **6**: 39–42.

COCHRANE, A. L. 1946. Notes on the psychology of prisoners of war. *Brit. med. J.*, **1**: 282–4.

DAVIDSON, S. 1946. Notes on a group of ex-prisoners of war. [Group therapy.] *Bull. Menninger Clin.*, **10**: 90–100.

DEARLOVE, A. R. 1945. Enforced leisure: a study of the activities of officer prisoners of war. *Brit. med. J.*, **1**: 406–9.

GAUTREY, B. 1946. Social work in a [Psychoneurotic] Military Hospital. *Ment. Health, London*, **6**: 62–5.

JEFFREY, M., & BRADFORD, E. J. G. 1946. Neurosis in escaped prisoners of war. *Brit. J. med. Psychol.*, **20**: 422–35.

JONES, M. 1946. Rehabilitation of Forces neurosis patients to civilian life. *Brit. med. J.*, **1**: 533–5.

KIRMAN, B. H. 1946. Mental disorder in released prisoners of war. *J. ment. Sci.*, **92**: 808–13.

LACK, C. 1946. The management of convalescent neurotics at the Neurosis Wing, 101 Military Convalescent Depot. *J.R. Army med. Cps.*, **86**: 32–4.

LEWIS, A., & GOODYEAR, K. 1944. Vocational aspects of neurosis in soldiers. *Lancet*, **2**: 105–9.

LEWIS, A., & SLATER, E. 1942. Neurosis in soldiers: a follow-up study. *Lancet*, **1**: 496–8.

MILLER, E. 1945. Psychiatric aspects of rehabilitation. *J.R. Army med. Cps.*, **84**: 54–65.

MINSKI, L. 1943. Rehabilitation of the neurotic. *J. ment. Sci.*, **89**: 390–4.

PETHER, G. C. 1945. The returned prisoner of war. *Lancet*, **1**: 571–2.

RADCLIFFE, R. A. C. 1943. The ex-serviceman in industry. *Industr. Welfare*, **25**: 99–101.

RATCLIFFE, T. A., & JONES, E. V. 1949. Regional community care. *Ment. Health, London*, **8**: 67–70, 92–4.

RICKMAN, J. 1945. [Anon.] First fruits of peace. *Lancet*, **1**: 565–6.

RODGER, A. 1943. The man and his job from war to peace. *Lancet*, **2**: 298–9. [Reprinted in: *Occup. Psychol.*, 1944, **18**: 63–8.]

STALKER, H. 1944. Psychiatric states in 130 ex-service patients. *J. ment. Sci.*, **90**: 727–38.

TORRIE, A. 1945. The return of Odysseus: the problem of marital infidelity for the repatriate. *Brit. med J.*, **2**: 192–3.

WALKER, E. R. C. 1944. Impressions of a repatriated medical officer. *Lancet*, **1**: 514–15.

WHILES, W. H. 1945. A study of neurosis among repatriated prisoners of war. *Brit. med. J.*, **2**: 697–8.

WITTKOWER, E. D., & MAYO, P. E. 1945. The employment of the blind in industry. *Industr. Welfare*, **27**: 10–13.

SUPPLEMENTARY BIBLIOGRAPHY

F. PERSONNEL SELECTION (INCLUDING OFFICERS); MENTAL TESTING; MENTAL DULLNESS (see also: B)

BENNETT, E., & SLATER, P. 1945. Some tests for the discrimination of neurotic from normal subjects. *Brit. J. med. Psychol.*, **20**: 271–82.

COSTEDOAT, A. L. D. 1947. La sélection psychologique dans l'Armée [britannique]. *Rev. Cps. Santé milit.*, **3**: 565–72.

ESHER, F. J. S. 1941. The mental defective in the Army. *Brit. med. J.*, **2**: 187–90.

ESHER, F. J. S. 1942. Military service for mental defectives. *Ment. Health, London*, **3**: 14–18.

ESHER, F. J. S., RAVEN, J. C., & EARL, C. J. C. 1942. Discussion on testing intellectual capacity in adults. *Proc. R. Soc. Med.*, **35**: 779–85.

EYSENCK, H. J. 1947. Screening-out the neurotic, *Lancet*, **1**: 530–1.

GARFORTH, F. I. de la P. 1945. War Office Selection Boards. *Occup. Psychol.*, **19**: 97–108.

GILLMAN, S. W. 1947. Methods of officer selection in the Army. *J. ment. Sci.*, **93**: 101–11.

GROVES, H. J. 1951. Medical aspects of selection procedure. *J.R. Army med. Cps.*, **96**: 115–25.

HALSTEAD, H. 1943. Analysis of Matrix test results on 700 neurotic subjects: comparison with the Shipley vocabulary test. *J. ment. Sci.*, **89**: 202–15.

HALSTEAD, H., & CHASE, V. E. 1944. Review of a verbal intelligence scale on military neurotic patients. *Brit. J. med. Psychol.*, **20**: 195–201.

HORDER, CURRAN, D., REES, J. R., et al. 1943. Discussion on functional nervous states in relation to service in the Armed Forces. *Proc. R. Soc. Med.*, **36**: 253–60.

KELLEY, D. M. 1943. Classification of personnel in the British Army: preliminary survey of methods. *War. Med., Chicago*, **3**: 386–92.

MAYER-GROSS, W., MOORE, J. N. P., & SLATER, P. 1949. Forecasting the incidence of neurosis in officers of the Army and the Navy. *J. ment. Sci.*, **95**: 80–100.

MILNE, J. 1946. Some medico-social problems of mental dullness in the Army. *J.R. Army med. Cps.*, **86**: 26–7.

RAVEN, J. C. 1942. Testing adults. *Lancet*, **1**: 115–17.

REES, J. R. 1946. 'Unfit on psychiatric grounds.' *Occup. Psychol.*, **20**: 125–31.

REYNELL, W. R. 1944. A psychometric method of determining intellectual loss following head injury. *J. ment. Sci.*, **90**: 710–19.

STALKER, H. 1941. Rejection of psychiatrically unfit recruits. *Lancet*, **1**: 535–6.

STALKER, H. 1943. Conscientious Objectors with psychiatric states. *J. ment. Sci.*, **89**: 52–8.

STRAKER, D. 1944. Difficulties of psychological field research in a fighting service. *Occup. Psychol.*, **18**: 133–41.

SUTHERLAND, J. D., & FITZPATRICK, G. 1945. Some approaches to group problems in the British Army. *In: Group Psychotherapy*, New York (Amer. Sociometric Ass.); *Sociometry*, **8**: 443–55. [Also, separate page numbers for this issue: pp. 205–17.]

TUCK, G. N. 1946. The Army's use of psychology during the war. *Occup. Psychol.*, **20**: 113–18.

VERNON, P. E. 1946. Statistical methods in the selection of Navy and Army personnel. *J.R. statist. Soc.*, **8**: 139–53.

VERNON, P. E. 1947. Psychological tests in the Royal Navy, Army and A.T.S. *Occup. Psychol.*, **21**: 53–74.

VERNON, P. E. 1947. Research on personnel selection in the Royal Navy and the British Army. *Amer. Psychologist*, **2**: 35–51.

SUPPLEMENTARY BIBLIOGRAPHY

WAR OFFICE: DIRECTORATE FOR SELECTION OF PERSONNEL. 1947. Personnel selection in the British Army. *8th int. Management Congress: Papers*, Stockholm (Esselte); **1**: 450–66.
WILSON, N. A. B. 1953. Applications of psychology in the Defence Departments. *In: Current Trends in British Psychology*, ed. C. A. Mace & P. E. Vernon; London (Methuen); pp. 22–33.

G. SOCIOLOGICAL PROBLEMS (INCLUDING ADJUSTMENT TO SERVICE LIFE; DISCIPLINARY PROBLEMS; ETC.) (see also: B, E)

ANDERSON, C. 1944. On certain conscious and unconscious homosexual responses to warfare. *Brit. J. med. Psychol.*, **20**: 161–74. [Reprinted in: *The Yearbook of Psychoanalysis*, London (Imago Publishing Co.), 1945, **1**: 215–36.]
BACKHOUSE, T. M., ANDERSON, E. W., *et al.* 1942. Discussion on the assessment of criminal responsibility in the Armed Forces. *Proc. R. Soc. Med.*, **35**: 723–32.
BROWN, J. A. C. 1945. Frustration and aggression. *J.R. Army med. Cps.*, **85**: 101–4.
HARRISSON, T. 1945. The British soldier: changing attitudes and ideas. *Brit. J. Psychol.*, **35**: 34–9.
MACKEITH, S. A. 1945. Psychological aspects of the problem of anti-malarial precautions. *J.R. Army med. Cps.*, **84**: 79–80.
RICKMAN, J. 1939. [Anon.] On conscription. *Lancet*, **1**: 830–1.
RUDOLF, G. de M. 1944. Reaction to military life and criminal behaviour. *In: Mental Abnormality and Crime (English Studies in Criminal Science*, ed. L. Radzinowicz & J. W. C. Turner, Vol. 2); London (Macmillan); pp. 240–68.
SHARMAN, S. 1951. The Army psychiatrist and military law. *J.R. Army med. Cps.*, **97**: 1–14.

INDEX

N.B.—Authors listed in the General Bibliography (with cross-references to pages on which quoted) are *not* included here, except where otherwise mentioned in the text. In respect of individual names listed, 'Dr.' is, in general, used to denote a *medical* qualification (except in the case of those who are also psychiatric specialists). Psychol. = psychologist; Psychiat. = psychiatrist.

Figures followed by *n* refer to footnotes (commencing) on the pages specified.

Absence without leave (A.W.O.L.). *See* Desertion
Adam, Gen. Sir Ronald F., 24, 37–9, 54, 66, 70, 72, 188n. *See also* Adjutant-General, British Army
Adjutant-General: British Army, 24, 37, 39, 54, 56, 58, 70, 72, 128–9, 131, 188n, 219–20, 223
U.S. Army, 39n
Adjutant-General's Branch, War Office, 14, 37, 39, 196
Advisers in Psychiatry: A.L.F.S.E.A., 22, 210–11
14th Army (S.E.A.C.), 192
B.L.A. (21 Army Group), 21, 118
B.N.A.F., 21, 183, 185
C.M.F., 185, 205, 210, 214
45 and 77 Division, 45
Psychological Warfare Division, S.H.A.E.F., 225n
Aeschylus, 1, 226
Agricultural Companies. *See* Pioneer Corps
Ahrenfeldt, R. H. (Psychiat.), 106n, 139n, 260
Airborne Forces: morale, Malaya 'mutiny', 220–1
and training, 223–4
selection, 43–4, 46–8, 223–4
Air Force, Royal, (R.A.F.): manpower, priority, 32
transfers to Army, 42
Alexander, Gen. Sir Harold (later Field-Marshal Earl), 219, 272

A.L.F.S.E.A., 22, 58, 206, 210–13, 220–1, 235
'Annexure' Scheme, 18–19, 153, 155–9
Anti-aircraft units: morale and training, 223
selection, 36
Apprentices, Army, selection, 48–50
Area Psychiatrists, 17–18, 71, 85, 142–3, 150, 188, 232
Armies: Allied and Dominion, relations with British Army, 223
British, 1st Army. *See* B.N.A.F.
2nd Army. *See* B.L.A.
5th Army (American/British). *See* C.M.F.
8th Army. *See* C.M.F.; M.E.F.
14th Army. *See* S.E.A.C.
Armoured units: intakes, 34, 78
selection, 39–41
Arms Basic Training Units, 45n
Army Act, amendment (and Select Committees), 139n, 221n
Army Council, 36, 39, 272
Army Education Officers. *See* Education Corps, Army
Army Groups, British: 11 Army Group. *See* S.E.A.C.
21 Army Group. *See* B.L.A.
Army Medical Services, 13–14
Artillery, Royal, psychiatric casualties, 164n, 190
Assam. *See* S.E.A.C.
Auchinleck, Gen. Sir Claude (later Field-Marshal), 69n, 271

INDEX

Australian Army Medical Corps, 179
Auxiliary Territorial Service (A.T.S.):
  infestation and mental defect (dullness), 82-3
  morale problems (Training Schools), 213
  officer selection, 68
  personnel selection, 39, 46
  psychiatric disorders, incidence, 276

Bacon, Francis, 97, 196
Baker, A. A. (Psychiat.), 48-50
B.A.O.R., 79-82, 91n, 120-5, 132, 204-5, 213, 266, 268
Barbour, R. F. (Psychiat.), 45, 107, 112, 115, 182-3, 238
Barret, R., 198n
70th Battalions. *See* Young Soldiers' Battalions
'Battle inoculation', 197-9, 201-4
Battle Schools, 197-201, 203
B.E.F.: World War I, 4-8
  World War II, 16-17, 22, 33, 81, 84n, 147, 174-5
Belgium. *See* B.L.A.
Bennet, E. A. (Psychiat.), 21, 58n, 86n
Bhore Committee, 191n
Bion, W. R. (Psychiat.), 40, 60
B.L.A., 21-2, 58, 79n, 118-25, 132, 165, 175-7, 220, 273n. *See also* B.A.O.R.
Blackford, Lord, 272n
B.N.A.F., 21, 58, 183-5, 187
Boards of Control, 20
  England and Wales, 143, 147
  Scotland, 143
Boland, Dr. E. R., 185
Bond, Sir Hubert (Psychiat., Board of Control, England), 143, 147
Borstal Institutions, 116n
Broadcasting, and morale, 221-2
Broadcasting Committee, Army 222
Broadcasting Corporation, British (B.B.C.), 200-201, 222
Browne, E. W., 211-12
B.T.N.I., 79, 87-9
Burma (including Arakan). *See* S.E.A.C.
Butler, Samuel, 123

Cabanès, Dr. A., 2n
Cambridge Psychological Laboratory, 36
Canterbury, Archbishop of, 200n
Cantlie, Gen. Sir Neil (D.G.A.M.S.), 276n
Cherwell, Lord, 73n
Churchill, Sir Winston, 26, 73n, 273n
Civil Defence Officers, selection, 69

Civil Defence Services, man-power, reserved, 32
Civil Liaison Officers. *See* Social workers
Civil resettlement. *See* Ex-servicemen; Prisoners of war, British; Rehabilitation
Civil Resettlement Headquarters, 239, 241n, 245, 247-8
  relations with civil authorities, 237, 241, 247
  with War Office, 245-7
Civil Resettlement Units (C.R.U.s), 238-50
  social adjustment, results, 248-9
  staff, 239-41, 247
  volunteering rate, 240
Civil Service Selection Boards, 69, 73
Clegg, E. A. (Psychiat.), 126
C.M.F., 58, 132-3, 168, 171-3, 185-8, 205-7, 210-11, 214-20
Coates, W. B., 211-12
Collie, Capt. G. F., 229
Columbia University, 4n
'Combatant Tendency', 42
Command Interview Boards, 51
Command Labour Companies, 43, 105, 107, 112-17
Command Psychiatrists, 17, 37, 71, 81, 85, 93, 114-15, 129, 134, 142
  East Africa, 209n
  Eastern Command, India, 207
  Gibraltar, 209n
  Malta, 188
  Northern Command, 33, 37, 78, 82, 94
  Northern Ireland, 79, 87, 102
  overseas, 21
  Scottish Command, 34, 54
  South-Eastern Command, 86n
  West Africa, 209n
Commando units, psychiatric disorders, 43-4
Committees. *See* under specific Committees
Company Commanders' School, 55, 57-8
Conservation of Human Resources Project, 4n
Consultant Psychiatrists:
  to the Army, 16, 19-21, 33, 38, 54, 84, 86n, 88-9, 93, 100, 125, 196, 229-30
  to the Army at home, 20-1
  B.E.F., World War I, 5
  World War II, 16, 33
  India, 21, 58n, 190
  M.E.F., 21, 178-9, 183n
  S.E.A.C. (11 Army Group), 22

INDEX

Convalescent Depots. *See* Depots, base; Psychiatric units, forward
Convalescent Observation Depots, 88, 89n
Copeland, N. (Psychiat.), 97
Corps Psychiatrists, 170-1, 185-8, 191-5
Courts-martial, 12, 14, 95-6, 98-9, 139n, 224, 261-3, 268, 271
Crew, Prof. F. A. E., 55, 92
Crime, military. *See* Disciplinary problems
Crocker Committee, 68n, 71
Curle, A., 241n, 247
Cutler, Dr. E. C., 188n

Dante, 137
Death penalty, and abolition, in British Army, 7, 117, 271-5
Delinquency, military. *See* Disciplinary problems
De Maré, P. B. (Psychiat.), 209n
Depots, base, morale and psychiatric disorders, 185, 214-15, 221
  in Convalescent Depots, 152-3, 168, 179-81, 187, 189, 232
  in Reinforcement Holding Units, 170-1, 181, 187, 204
  in Training Depots, Reinforcement, 185, 187, 214
  in Transit Camps, 187, 204, 211, 214
De Quincey, T., 97
Desertion and absenteeism (A.W.O.L.), 7, 78-9, 101-2, 107, 108n, 109, 115, 117-25, 127-9, 132-3, 171-3, 204-5, 214, 218, 231, 271-5
  incidence, British Army, World Wars I and II, 271-5
Detention Barracks. *See* Penal institutions
Dhotel, Y. (Psychiat.), 2n
Dicks, H. V. (Psychiat.), 224-5
Directorates, War Office: of Army Kinematography, 222
  of Army Psychiatry (A.M.D. 11), 19-20, 23, 209n
  and disciplinary problems, 105
  and 'Hate training' (in Battle Schools), 200
  and officer selection, etc., 69, 71-2
  and personnel selection, 43-4
  and prisoners of war, repatriated, 237
  of Selection of Personnel, 22-3, 39, 41, 50
Director-General, Army Medical Services (D.G.A.M.S.), 20, 24-5, 38, 66, 72, 84-5, 86n, 88, 148, 229-30, 276n. *See also* Hood, Gen. Sir Alexander
Directors, War Office: of Army Psychiatry, 19, 43-4, 71-2, 80, 91n, 104, 113, 127, 183, 222-3, 229-30, 232, 239
  of Labour, 85-6, 89
  of Military Training, 21, 36-7, 39, 109, 202, 221
  of Organization, 239, 246
  of Selection of Personnel, 56, 91, 230, 232, 247
Directors-General, Medical Services, Royal Navy, Army, and R.A.F., 147
Discharge, psychiatric, from Army. *See* Disciplinary problems; Mental defect; Psychiatric disorders
Disciplinary Barracks, U.S. Army, 139-40
Disciplinary problems, military psychiatric, 97-140, 260-70, 271-5. *See also* Desertion; Mental defect; Morale; Penal institutions; Psychiatric disorders; Rehabilitation
  criticism of psychiatrists, 101, 103, 106
  delinquents, military,
    chronic and 'psychopathic', 93, 102-7, 112-17, 119, 123, 125, 127-8, 134, 136-9, 262-70
    classification and segregation, 107, 111, 113-14, 122, 127, 131, 134, 136, 139, 260-1
    disposal, and discharge from Army, 93, 98-106, 110-11, 113-115, 117, 126-9, 132-8, 139n, 260-70
    psychiatric examinations, 12, 95-96, 98-101, 106, 118, 125, 128-9, 135, 137, 264-6, 268-9
    psychiatric reports, 96n, 100-101, 105, 129, 137, 139n, 264, 269
    prisoners of war, repatriated, 227, 231, 243-5
    sexual offenders, 139n
    young soldiers, and immaturity, 107-112, 115-17, 123-4, 134, 273n
Disposal of military psychiatric cases. *See* Disciplinary problems; Forward psychiatry; Mental defect; Psychiatric disorders
45 and 77 Division, 45, 105, 117, 235, 237-8
Divisional Psychiatrists, 170, 188, 191-5
Drever, Prof. J. H. (Psychol.), 38

INDEX

East Africa, 21, 189n, 209–10
Education Corps, Army, 36–7
Eisenhower, Gen. Dwight D., 4n
Emergency Medical Service (E.M.S.), 17–21, 142, 147–8, 150, 154–5, 159, 176
Engineers, Royal, psychiatric casualties, 182
Essex, Earl of, 219n
Exhaustion, Battle (Combat) and Campaign, 4–15, 22, 30, 99, 123–4, 147–9, 151, 153, 158, 164, 166, 171–3, 175–6, 178, 180, 182–5, 192, 198, 204. *See also* Forward psychiatry
Ex-servicemen, problems of civil resettlement, 249–50

Farmer, E. (Psychol.), 36–7
Field Medical units: Advanced Dressing Stations (A.D.S.), [= M.D.S.], 192
 Casualty Clearing Stations (C.C.S.), 169, 186, 191–2
 Field Ambulances, 179–80
 Field Dressing Stations (F.D.S.), 169, 175
 Main Dressing Stations (M.D.S.), 169, 192, 195
 Regimental Aid Posts (R.A.P.), 169, 171, 174
Field Punishment Camps, B.L.A., 118–19, 122
Films, psychological aspects, and morale, 221–2
Fletcher, Dr. R. T., 268n
Forward psychiatry, 163–95
 opposition, and criticism of, 166–7, 183–4, 188, 190
 organization, 167–71
 overseas theatres, 173–95
 psychiatric casualties, incidence, 166, 174–6, 180–2, 183n, 184, 186, 189–90, 194, 207
 precipitating factors, 164–8, 171–174, 176, 180–2, 189–90, 192–4, 205–9, 272n, 273–5
 results of treatment, forward, 166, 169–70, 175–81, 184, 186–7, 193–5
 treatment and disposal, 169–71, 174–95
France. *See* B.E.F.; B.L.A.
Functional disorders. *See* Sickness rate

Gates, Col. P. H. (Inspector of Military Prisons), 136
General Service Corps, intake scheme, 23, 41–2, 45n, 59, 95
General Staff Branch, War Office, 196

German Army. *See* Officer selection; Personnel selection
Germany. *See* B.A.O.R.; Morale, enemy
Gibraltar, 21, 58, 189n, 209–10
Gilbey, Maj. G. H., 109–10
Ginzberg, Prof. E., 4n
Gregg, Dr. Alan, 26n
Grinker, R. R. (Psychiat.), 184

Hackney, A., 35n
Hance, Gen. Sir Bennett (late D.G.I.M.S.), 191n
Hargreaves, G. R. (Psychiat.), 33–4, 37–9, 78, 82, 94
Harris, H. B. (Psychiat.), 75
Hobley, Maj. A. J., 115–16
Hood, Gen. Sir Alexander (D.G.A.M.S.), 24–5, 66, 72, 229
Horder, Lord, M.D., 147
Hospitals, psychiatric, civil:
 civil mental hospitals, 144–6, 280
 India, 191n
 E.M.S., and Neurosis Centres, 17–18, 21, 142, 147–8, 150, 154–5, 159, 176, 280
Hospitals, psychiatric, military:
 B.E.F., World War I, 5–8
 World War II, 16–17, 174
 B.L.A., 175–6
 B.N.A.F., 184
 C.M.F., 186
 India, 190–1
 M.E.F., 18, 21, 178–9, 181
 U.K., 16–19, 143n, 176, 280–1
 psychoneuroses, 147–54, 201–2
 psychoses, 143–6
Howard-Vyse, Gen. Sir Richard (British Red Cross and Order of St. John), 230
Hunter, H. D. (Psychiat.), 185

Illiteracy, 33, 87, 91–2, 137, 178n
India, 21, 58, 68–9, 190–1
Industrial Health Research Board, 31n, 36
Industrial psychology, 31, 50
Industry, British: man-power, reserved, 32
 psychiatric disorders, 31n
 selection, 37
Infantry: battle stress, severe, in, 171–173, 182, 205–6
 desertion in, 124, 204–5
 intakes, 34, 78, 205
 mental defectives (dullards) unsuitable for, 90–1, 189
 psychiatric casualties, 172–3, 182
 training and morale, 204–7

306

INDEX

Infestation, parasitic (pediculosis, scabies), 82–3
Intakes, Army. *See also* General Service Corps
   mental defect (dullness), incidence, 34, 37, 78
   psychiatric disorders, incidence, 34
Isolated areas overseas, psychiatric problems, 209–10
Italy. *See* C.M.F.

James, G. W. B. (Psychiat.), 20–1, 178, 180, 182
Japan. *See* Morale, enemy
Judge Advocate-General's Branch, War Office, 100

Kelnar, J. (Psychiat.), 225
Kenton, C. (Psychiat.), 184
Kipling, R., 6n, 206n

Laignel-Lavastine, Prof. M. (Psychiat.) 2n
Leaderless Group Tests, 60–2
Leader Training Battalions, 59, 68
Le Bon, G., 233n
Lewis, Prof. A. (Psychiat.), 19, 155–6
Lewis, C. Day, 163, 164n
Lewis Committee, 139n, 221n, 261–2
London County Council (L.C.C.), 18, 148
Long-Term Treatment Scheme (military psychotics), 145n, 146

MacKeith, S. A. (Psychiat.), 21, 185, 205–6, 214
Mackenzie, D. L. (Psychiat.), 80, 209n
Main, T. F. (Psychiat.), 21, 78, 117–18, 197–9, 202–4, 215–18, 221–2
Malaya. *See* A.L.F.S.E.A.; S.E.A.C.
'Malingering', 5, 7, 78, 86, 103, 164n
Malta, 21, 164n, 188–90
Man-power, wastage and conservation, 4, 31, 34–5, 37–8, 43, 47–8, 50, 77–8, 87–8, 102–3, 118, 127–8, 155–7, 159, 172, 177, 193, 223–4, 261–4, 266, 268
Matas, J. (Psychiat.), 194
May, P. R. A. (Psychiat.), 106n, 139n, 260–70
Medical categories, low: disposal, 34–5, 46
   morale, 43
Medical (Recruiting) Boards (Centres), civilian: World War I, 30, 273n
   World War II, (Ministry of Labour and National Service), 31–2, 37, 94–5, 107, 141, 174, 277–81
M.E.F., 18, 21, 58, 123n, 124n, 145, 165, 168, 171, 177–83, 183n, 185, 203–4, 221–2, 271–2. *See also* M.E.L.F.
M.E.L.F., 136
Mental defect and dullness, 23, 37, 39–41, 76, 77–96. *See also* Pioneer Corps
   after-care, 95n
   and desertion and absenteeism, 78–9, 101–2, 117–19, 123, 127, 273
   and disciplinary problems, 77n, 78–81, 86, 91n, 95–6, 97–8, 100–102, 104, 106–7, 113, 117–19, 123, 125–8, 137, 189, 270, 273
   disposal and discharge, 82–96, 102, 143, 280–1
   criticism of psychiatrists in relation to, 94–5
   incidence, in intakes and units, 23, 34, 78, 141, 277–81
   and infestation, 82–3
   and military training, difficulties in ordinary units, 77, 81, 84–5, 90–1, 189
   in special units, 84–5, 87–8
   and morale, 77, 83, 86–7, 89
   and psychiatric disorders (instability), 78, 81, 84, 86, 90, 91n
   rejections at intake, 141, 277–81
   and sickness rate, 81–2, 86, 91n, 189
   and stability, emotional, 86, 95
   U.S. Army, 77n, 83, 94–5, 277–81
   and venereal disease, 81–2, 86, 91n, 212–13
Mental Health, Expert Committee on, 3n, 25n
Mental Nursing Orderlies, 145–6, 153–4
Mental Testing, Advisory Committee on, 38–9
Middle East. *See* M.E.F.; M.E.L.F.
Military Corrective Establishments (M.C.E.s). *See* Penal institutions
Military Provost Staff Corps (M.P.S.C.), 130, 135–7, 139
Military Testing Officers, 57–8, 62–3
Milne, A. (Psychiat.), 195
Ministry of Health, 20, 147, 159, 270
Ministry of Home Affairs, N. Ireland, 143
Ministry of Labour and National Service, 20, 22, 31–2, 37, 94, 141, 159, 228, 230, 237, 241, 277, 280. *See also* Medical (Recruiting) Boards
Ministry of Pensions, 15, 20, 146–7, 159, 237
Moderator, Church of Scotland, 200n, 207n

INDEX

Montgomery, Lt.-Gen. B. L. (later Field-Marshal Viscount), 200–201, 219
Morale, enemy, and psycho-social structure (civil, military and political): Germany, 224–5
Japan, 225
Morale, military: in depots, reinforcement units, transit camps, etc., 152–3, 168, 170–1, 179–81, 185, 187, 189, 204, 211, 214–15, 221, 232
and desertion and absenteeism, 117–18, 122–5, 204–5, 214, 218, 271–5
and disciplinary problems, 108–9, 115, 117–18, 122–5, 138, 204–7, 215–21, 271–5
of Forces overseas, 209–10, 221–2
group, lesions of, 130, 183–4, 215–21
and leadership, 13, 51, 108, 124–5, 138, 197, 204, 207–8, 218–20, 273–5
in low medical categories, 43
of mental defectives (dullards), 77, 83, 86–7, 89
of officer cadets (O.C.T.U.s), 52
of prisoners, military, 126, 133n, 135–8
of prison staff, military (M.P.S.C.), 130
and psychiatric casualties, 164, 168, 170–3, 182, 189–90, 206–7, 272n, 273–5
psychological (psychiatric) aspects of, 196–8, 202–25
of psychoneurotics, 150–1, 153, 157, 209
and selection, inadequate, 183–4, 205–6, 208–9, 212–13, 272n, 273–5
and training, 196–225, 272n, 273–5
unit, effect on: of chronic delinquents, 103, 106, 128, 138
of mental defectives (dullards), 85, 91, 189
and venereal disease, 207, 212–13
Morale Committee, British Army, 223
Moran, Lord, *M.D.*, 52n, 73n
'Mutinies': Airborne, Malaya (A.L.F.S.E.A.), 220–1
collective complaints not permitted, 219, 221
in Military Prisons and Detention Barracks, 130
Salerno (C.M.F.), 215–20
Myers, Dr. C. S. (Psychol.), 38

Nass, Dr. L., 2n

Navy, Royal: Detention Quarters, Naval, 132
man-power, priority, 32
psychiatric treatment, 21
transfers to Army, 42
Neal, Dr. J. B., 12n
Netherlands. *See* B.L.A.
Neurosis Centres. *See* Hospitals, psychiatric, civil
Neuroses. *See* Exhaustion; Forward psychiatry; Hospitals, psychiatric; Psychiatric disorders
Non-Commissioned Officers (N.C.O.s), 51–2, 69, 88, 108–9, 130, 165, 182, 263
North Africa. *See* B.N.A.F.; M.E.F.
Northern Ireland. *See* B.T.N.I.
'Northfield Experiment', 152–3
Northfield Military Hospital (Psychiatric), 149–53
North-West Europe. *See* B.E.F.; B.L.A.
Norway (Narvik), 174
Nursing Orderlies. *See* Mental Nursing Orderlies
Nursing Sisters (Q.A.I.M.N.S.), 145n, 153

O'Connor, Gen. Sir Richard N. (Adjutant-Gen.), 72
Officer Cadet Training Units (O.C.T.U.s), 33, 51–4, 59, 68, 73–75, 197
Basic, 59, 68
'Officer Rating', 59
Officer Reception Unit, 232
Officer selection, 23, 51–76
German Army, 53n, 54–5, 64
N.C.O.s, 69
new methods,
A.T.S., 68
emergency commissions (W.O.S.B.s), 20–1, 23, 54n, 57–75, 76n
opposition, and criticism of, 58n, 63–6, 71–3
overseas theatres, 21, 23, 58, 68–9
psychiatrists' role, 54, 58–9, 62–7, 71–2
psychologists' work and advice, 58–9, 67, 71–2, 74–5, 76n
regular commissions, 67, 71
removal of psychiatrists and psychologists, 71
validation, 73–4
old methods, 51–2, 54n, 73–4
criticism of, 53, 65–6
rejection rate, 53

308

INDEX

psychiatric disorders, 52–3, 56, 67–8, 75
   results, new and old methods, 73–4
   U.S. Army, 53n
Oliver Committee, 129–32, 135n
Opinion surveys, A.L.F.S.E.A. and C.M.F., 206, 210–12
Organic disease (infectious, toxic, traumatic):
   in aetiology of psychiatric casualties, 6, 192–4
   of psychiatric disorders, 144, 193–194, 209–10
   and morale, 208–10
Overseas, psychiatric services, 16–17, 21–3, 58, 68–9, 173–95, 209–10. *See also* under specific Forces and theatres overseas

Parachutists (paratroops). *See* Airborne Forces
Patton, Gen. G. S., 5n, 164n, 272n
Pearce, J. D. W. (Pychiat.), 87
Penal institutions, military: Field Punishment Camps, 118–19, 122
   Military Corrective Establishments, 80, 131n, 132–9
   psychiatrists' contribution, potential, 139–40, 260–3, 269
   Military Prisons and Detention Barracks, 79–80, 102, 105, 117–119, 122, 124n, 125–40, 261–3, 269
   disturbances ('mutinies'), 130
   investigations, official, 129–30
   Special Training Barracks, C.M.F., 132–3
   staff (M.P.S.C.), 130, 134–9, 262–3
   U.S. Army, 139–40
Pensions, for psychiatric disability (related to military service), 10, 144, 147, 158
Penton, C. F. (Board of Control, England and Wales), 143
Penton, J. C. (Psychiat.), 79, 108n, 112n, 119–25, 204–5
Personnel selection, 13, 15, 22–3, 29–50, 76. *See also* Mental defect
   German Army, 37n, 38, 39n
   inadequate, effects of, 32, 34–5, 93–94, 98–9, 106–7, 124, 165, 174, 177–8, 184–5, 205, 208–9, 212–13, 272n, 273–5
   opposition and criticism, 31–2, 35–6, 40
   psychiatrists' role, 41
   psychologists' work, 50n
   and training, 31, 40
   U.S. Army, 38, 39n

Personnel Selection Officers, 23, 42, 45, 48, 59, 92, 111, 113–15, 156, 235
Phillips, R. J. (Psychiat.), 119–20, 174–5
Philpott, S. J. F. (Psychol.), 38
Physical Development Centres, 43
Piercy, Lord, 73
Pioneer Corps, 23, 34, 41–2, 46, 79–91, 94–6, 102, 113, 126, 128, 157, 220
   Agricultural Companies, 157–9
   Pioneer Training Pool, N. Ireland, 87–89
   Pioneer Training School, 89
Plato, 251
Prison Commission (England and Wales), 116n, 129
Prisoners of war, British, repatriated:
   disciplinary problems, 227, 231, 243–5
   ex-European (Germany, Italy), 235, 238, 240
   ex-Japanese, 235–6, 240
   experimental rehabilitation schemes, R.A.M.C., Crookham, 230–2, 235
   Special Reception and Training Unit (C.R.U.), 238–9
   morale, low, 231
   officers, psychological reactions, and psychiatric disorders, 227, 242
   rehabilitation, military, 232
   sickness and invaliding rate, 227
   psychological reactions (P.O.W. syndrome), and psychiatric disorders, 210, 226–37, 241–5, 249
   rehabilitation, and civil resettlement, 44–5, 226–50
   military, and selection, 227, 232, 237
   sickness and invaliding rate, 227, 231
   World War I, experience, 226, 229, 232, 234–5
Prisoners of war, German and Italian, 19, 224–5
Prison Medical Service (civil), 128–9
Prisons, military. *See* Penal institutions
Prophylaxis, psychiatric, 3, 25–6, 31, 50, 159, 171, 197–8, 203, 207, 273–5
Psychiatric Centres. *See* Hospitals, psychiatric
Psychiatric disorders, British Army. *See also* Exhaustion; Forward psychiatry; Hospitals, psychiatric; Mental defect
   and desertion and absenteeism, 7, 78–9, 101–2, 117–19, 123, 127, 273
   discharge from Army, 23, 34, 42, 102–6, 143–6, 153, 276–81

INDEX

Psychiatric disorders—*cont.*
and disciplinary problems, 7, 14, 78–9, 97–8, 101–7, 113, 117–19, 123, 125–8, 137, 139n, 144
incidence, World War I, 9–10
World War II, 23, 141, 183n, 210n, 276–81
instability, in mental defectives (dullards), 78, 81, 86, 90, 91n
in officer cadets (O.C.T.U.s), 75
in officers, 52–3, 56, 67–8, 75
overseas, isolated areas, incidence and disposal, 210n
precipitating factors, 209–10
rejections at intake, 141, 277–81
treatment and disposal, 35, 42–3, 141–62, 210n, 276–81
and venereal disease, 212–13
Psychiatric disorders, U.S. Army. *See also* Psychiatry, U.S. Forces
rejections at induction, incidence, disposal and discharge, 276–81
Psychiatric social workers, 160
Psychiatric units (centres), base, 168–170, 186–7. *See also* Hospitals, psychiatric, military
Psychiatric units (centres), forward:
Advanced [= Main Filtration], 168–70, 181, 186–7. *See also* Hospitals, psychiatric, military
Exhaustion, Army, Corps, and Divisional [= Forward Filtration], 168–70, 175–6, 186–7, 191–2
Filtration, 168–9, 181
Forward, 168, 186
Main, 168
Rehabilitation, and Convalescent Depots, 168–70, 179–81
Psychiatrists, British Army. *See also* Advisers in Psychiatry; Area, Command, and Consultant Psychiatrists; Psychologists and Psychiatrists, Expert Committee; and under individual names
opposition, and criticism of, 26–8, 36, 40, 58n, 63–6, 71–3, 76, 94–5, 101, 103, 106, 148, 151, 166–7, 183–4, 188, 190, 251–2
in World War I, 6
in World War II, 15–18, 21, 32–3, 67, 72, 141–2, 154, 183, 185, 188, 190, 197, 209n, 252
Psychiatrists, U.S. Forces, 5n, 171–3, 184–5, 252–3
Psychiatry, British Army: applications to civil life, 3–4
before World War II, 4–13
during World War II, 8n, 13–28
lessons learnt, 252–9
psychiatric disorders, statistics, 276–81
Psychiatry, French Army: World War I, experience, 4
Psychiatry, U.S. Forces: applications to civil life, 4n
World War I, experience, 8, 10–11, 31, 170n
World War II, experience, and post-war developments, 4n, 5n, 8n, 139–40, 171–3, 183n, 252–4
psychiatric disorders, statistics (Army), 276–81
Psychological warfare,
Germany, psychiatric advice on, 225
selection of personnel, 69
Psychologists. *See* Officer selection; Personnel selection; Selection tests; and under individual names
Psychologists and Psychiatrists in the Services, Expert Committee on, 25–6
Psychoneuroses, British Army, 147–62. *See also* Psychiatric disorders
disposal and discharge, 148, 150–61
hospitals, E.M.S., and Neurosis Centres, 147–8, 150, 154–5
hospitals, military, 147–54
criticism of psychiatrists, 151
nursing staff, 153–4
therapy, 149–52, 154, 158
Psychoses, British Army, 143–6. *See also* Psychiatric disorders
disposal and discharge, 144–6
hospitals, civil, 144–6
hospitals, military, 143–6
nursing staff, 145–6
therapy, 145–6
Psychosomatic disorders. *See* Sickness rate
'Pulheems' medical classification, 45n, 268

Q.A.I.M.N.S. *See* Nursing Sisters

Radio. *See* Broadcasting
Raven, J. C. (Psychol.), 33
Reallocation. *See* Personnel selection
Reallocation Centre, C.M.F., 186–7
Reconnaissance Corps, selection, 39–40
Rees, J. R. (Psychiat.), 16, 31, 37, 73, 84–5, 88–9, 94–5, 125, 147–8, 155, 159, 190, 201. *See also* Consultant Psychiatrist to the Army
Regular Commissions Boards, 67, 71
Rehabilitation, military and civil: mental defectives (dullards), (military), 87–8

INDEX

military delinquents, (military and civil), 107, 109–16, 119–22, 125, 131–40, 261, 266–8
military psychoneurotics (military and civil), 147–61
physically disabled servicemen (civil), 161–2
prisoners of war, repatriated (military and civil), 44–5, 226–50
psychiatric casualties (military). *See* Forward psychiatry
Rehabilitation Centres, U.S. Army, for delinquents, 139–40
Reinforcement Holding Units (R.H.U.s). *See* Depots, base
Rejections at intake (induction), psychiatric. *See* Psychiatric disorders, British and U.S. Armies
Research and Training Centre (Unit), 59, 69–70, 74, 241n
Research Section, R.A.M.C., Special (Biological), 210–11
Resettlement, civil. *See* Prisoners of war, British
Rest Centres, Army, 180, 185
Review of Sentences Boards: B.L.A./B.A.O.R., 119–22, 132, 266, 286
M.E.L.F., 136
Ritchie Committee, 71
Rodger, A. (Psychol.), 31, 36
Rodger, T. F. (Psychiat.), 22, 34, 54n, 57
Royal Army Medical College, 20
Rudolf, G. de M. (Psychiat.), 209n

Sandiford, Dr. H. A., 19
School of Infantry, 197
S.E.A.C., 22, 165–6, 191–5, 207–9, 211n, 213, 235. *See also* A.L.F.S.E.A.
Selection. *See* Officer selection; Personnel selection
Selection, vocational (civil life), 31
Selection Boards. *See* Civil Service, and War Office, Selection Boards; Regular Commissions Boards
Selection Centres,
  Army, 42–5, 111, 113–14, 117, 230, 235
  A.T.S., 46
Selection Groups (S.G.), 79n, 80n
S.G. 4 and 5. *See* Mental defect; Pioneer Corps
Selection tests and procedures, 33–4, 36–9, 47, 79n, 80n, 111, 113–14, 120–2, 126–7
N.C.O.s and officers, 33, 54–62, 70, 75
Selection Training Unit, Army, 44

Self-inflicted wounds, 7, 194
Sexual offenders. *See* Disciplinary problems
Sexual promiscuity. *See* Venereal disease
S.H.A.E.F., 69
Shakespeare, 29, 138, 213n
'Shell-shock.' *See* Exhaustion
Sicily. *See* C.M.F.
Sickness rate (functional and psychosomatic disorders): in mental defectives (dullards), 81–2, 86, 91n, 189
and morale, 210n, 272n
peptic ulcer, incidence, 276
in prisoners of war, repatriated, 227, 231, 236
Social crises, psychological effects of, 2
Social workers (Civil Liaison Officers), in C.R.U.s, 241
Southborough Committee, 12–13, 15, 22, 29–30, 40n, 141, 198n, 273n
South-East Asia. *See* A.L.F.S.E.A.; S.E.A.C.
Special Reception and Training Unit, 238–9
Special Training Barracks, C.M.F., 132–3
Special Training Units (S.T.U.s). *See* Young Soldiers' Training Units
Statistics, military psychiatric. *See* Psychiatry, British Army, and U.S. Forces
Sterility and impotence, fear of, 213
Suetonius, 51
Suicide, and 'attempted suicide', 49, 75, 129, 210n
Sutherland, J. D. (Psychol. and Psychiat.), 54n, 58, 70

Tank regiments. *See* Armoured units
Temple, Dr. William (Archbishop of Canterbury), 200n
Thomson, Prof. G. H. (Psychol.), 34
Torrie, A. (Psychiat.), 71–2
Training, military. *See also* Mental defect
of delinquents, 110, 114, 126, 131–5, 138
'Hate training', and criticism, 199–201, 207
and morale, 196–225, 272n, 273–5
'Noise training' (air-raid and battle), 201–4
of prisoners of war, repatriated (re-training), 227
psychological (psychiatric) aspects of, 21, 197–208, 223–4
of psychoneurotics, 148–9, 151–2

INDEX

Training, military—*cont.*
 selection, importance of, 31, 46–50
Training Centres (Units),
 A.T.S., 46
 Infantry, 84–5, 90
 Primary, 46, 59, 86, 95, 205
Training Depots, Reinforcement. *See* Depots, base
Transit Camps. *See* Depots, base
Treatment, military psychiatric cases. *See* Forward psychiatry; Hospitals, psychiatric; Psychiatric disorders
Treatment Centres. *See* Hospitals, psychiatric
Trist, E. L. (Psychol.), 58, 240, 241n
Tunbridge, Dr. R. E., 21, 188, 190

Ungerson, B. (Psychol.), 75

Venereal disease, and sexual promiscuity: and immaturity (instability), emotional, 212–13
 and mental defect (dullness), 81–2, 86, 91n, 212–13
 and morale, low, 207, 212–13
 and selection, inadequate, 212
Vinchon, J. (Psychiat.), 2n
Vinci, Leonardo da, 1–2
Virgil, 158n
Volunteers, British Army, 107–8, 124, 273n

War neuroses. *See* Exhaustion
War Office Medical Boards, 21
War Office Selection Boards (W.O.S.B.s), 20–1, 23, 54n, 57–75, 76n, 152
 overseas theatres, 21, 23, 58, 68–9
War Office Selection Centre, 45, 71, 117n
Wavell, Gen. Viscount (later Earl), 58
Wechsler, D., 270n
Welfare problems, 86–7, 97, 115, 124, 131, 133n, 157, 204, 206, 210, 213, 220–1, 223, 231, 236, 241, 247–9, 269, 272n, 273–5
Wells, A. F., 211–12
West Africa, 21, 189n, 209–10
White, A. A. (Psychiat.), 192, 194, 207–9
Wilde, J. F. (Psychiat.), 175
Wilson, A. T. M. (Psychiat.), 19, 78, 86, 117–18, 197–8, 230–1, 236–7, 239
Wingate, Maj.-Gen. Orde, 208n
Wishart, J. W. (Psychiat.), 157–8, 183–185
Wittkower, E. D. (Psychiat.), 55, 57
World Health Organization, Expert Committee on Mental Health, 3n, 25n

Yellowlees, H. (Psychiat.), 16
Young Soldiers' Battalions (70th Battalions), 85, 107–9
Young Soldiers' (Special) Training Units (Y.S.T.U.s), 43, 105, 107, 110–12, 115–17

Zilboorg, G. (Psychiat.), 26n

For Product Safety Concerns and Information please contact our EU representative GPSR@taylorandfrancis.com
Taylor & Francis Verlag GmbH, Kaufingerstraße 24, 80331 München, Germany

www.ingramcontent.com/pod-product-compliance
Lightning Source LLC
Chambersburg PA
CBHW071154300426
44113CB00009B/1202